NEONATAL THERAPEUTICS

NEONATAL THERAPEUTICS

T. F. Yeh, M.D.

Professor of Pediatrics
College of Medicine
University of Illinois
Deputy Chairman
Division of Neonatology
Cook County Hospital
Chicago, Illinois

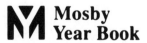

Mosby
Year Book

St. Louis   Baltimore   Boston   Chicago   London   Philadelphia   Sydney   Toronto

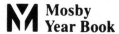

Mosby
Year Book

Dedicated to Publishing Excellence

Assistant Managing Editor, Text and Reference: Jan Gardner
Production Project Coordinator: Carol Reynolds
Proofroom Supervisor: Barbara Kelly

Mosby-Year Book, Inc.
11830 Westline Industrial Drive
St. Louis, MO 63146

1 2 3 4 5 6 7 8 9 0 RV 95 94 93 92 91

Library of Congress Cataloging-in-Publication Data
Neonatal therapeutics / [edited by] T.F. Yeh — 2nd ed.
   p. cm.
Rev. ed. of: Drug therapy in the neonate and small infant. c1985.
Includes bibliographical references.
Includes index.
ISBN (invalid) 0-8151-9758-3
   1. Infants (Newborn)—Diseases—Chemotherapy. 2. Infants—Diseases—
Chemotherapy. I. Yeh, Tsu F. II. Drug therapy in the neonate and small infant.
   [DNLM: 1. Infant, Newborn, Diseases—drug therapy.   WS 420 N4393]
RJ253.7.C45N46   1991
615.5'8'0832—dc20   91-6602
DNLM/DC   CIP
for Library of Congress

This book is dedicated to the patients of _____ *the Neonatal Intensive Care Unit of Cook County Children's Hospital and their families; and to the memory of my parents, C. Z. Huang and S. C. Yeh.*

CONTRIBUTORS

Rama Bhat, M.D.
Associate Professor of Pediatrics
College of Medicine
University of Illinois
Chicago, Illinois

Ian Carr, M.D.
Professor of Pediatrics
Chicago Medical School
Director, Pediatric Cardiology
Chicago Medical School
Chicago, Illinois

Shoichi Chida, M.D.
Attending Physician
Department of Pediatrics
School of Medicine
Iwate Medical University
Morioka, Japan

Cheng T. Cho, M.D., Ph.D.
Professor of Pediatrics
Chief, Section of Pediatric Infectious
* Disease*
Department of Pediatrics
University of Kansas Medical Center
Kansas City, Kansas

Jung-hwan Choi, M.D.
Visiting Research Fellow
Department of Pediatrics
The Pritzker School of Medicine
University of Chicago
Chicago, Illinois

Maria Lourdes Cruz, M.D.
Department of Pediatrics
College of Medicine
University of Cincinnati
Cincinnati, Ohio

David J. Durand, M.D.
Attending Physician
Division of Neonatology
Children's Hospital of Oakland
Oakland, California

Michael E. Evans, Ph.D.
Professor and Chairman
Department of Pharmacology
Indiana University
Indianapolis, Indiana

Howard A. Fox, M.D.
Clinical Professor of Pediatrics
Hahnemann University School of
* Medicine*
Philadelphia, Pennsylvania
Chairman, Department of Pediatrics
Monmouth Medical Center
Long Branch, New Jersey

Tetsuro Fujiwara, M.D.
Professor and Chairman
Department of Pediatrics
Iwate Medical University
Morioka, Japan

Arthur Garson, Jr., M.D.
Professor of Pediatrics and Medicine
Chief of Pediatric Cardiology
Baylor College of Medicine
Texas Children's Hospital
Houston, Texas

Hilda Goldbarg, M.D.
Assistant Professor of Pediatrics
The Chicago Medical School
Director, Pediatric Neurology
Cook County Hospital
Chicago, Illinois

Ronald Grifka, M.D.
Fellow Pediatric Cardiology
Baylor College of Medicine
Texas Children's Hospital
Houston, Texas

Vivian Harris, M.D.
Professor of Radiology
College of Medicine
University of Illinois
Director of Pediatric Radiology
Cook County Hospital
Chicago, Illinois

William C. Heird, M.D.
Professor of Pediatrics
Department of Pediatrics
Columbia University
College of Physicians and Surgeons
New York, New York

Norman M. Jacobs, M.D.
Associate Professor of Clinical Pediatrics .
College of Medicine
University of Illinois
Director, Pediatric Infectious Diseases
Cook County Children's Hospital
Chicago, Illinois

Eunice G. John, M.D.
Professor of Clinical Pediatrics
College of Medicine
University of Illinois
Chicago, Illinois

Lily C. Kao, M.D.
Attending Physician
Division of Neonatology
Children's Hospital of Oakland
Oakland, California

Sudha Kashyap, M.D.
Attending Physician
Babies Hospital (Presbyterian Hospital)
New York, New York

Kwang Sik Kim, M.D.
Associate Professor of Pediatrics
University of Southern California School
of Medicine
Division of Infectious Diseases
Children's Hospital of Los Angeles
Los Angeles, California

Mineo Konishi, M.D.
Attending Physician
Department of Pediatrics
Iwate Medical University School of
Medicine
Morioka, Japan

Kwang-sun Lee, M.D.
Professor of Pediatrics, Obstetrics and
Gynecology
The Pritzker School of Medicine
University of Chicago
Chicago, Illinois

Lawrence D. Lilien, M.D.
Director of Nursery
Fairview General Hospital
Cleveland, Ohio

Julie A. Luken, M.D., F.A.A.P.
Associate Professor of Pediatrics
University of Health Sciences
The Chicago Medical School
Assistant Professor of Pediatrics
College of Medicine
University of Illinois
Chicago, Illinois

Albert D. Moscioni, Ph.D.
Assistant Professor of Surgery
Department of Surgery
Vanderbilt University School of
Medicine
Nashville, Tennessee

William Oh, M.D.
Professor of Pediatrics
Brown University Program in Medicine
Department of Pediatrics
Women and Infant's Hospital of Rhode
Island
Providence, Rhode Island

Hemendra B. Patel, M.D.
Attending Physician
Division of Neonatology
Cook County Hospital
Chicago, Illinois

Rosita S. Pildes, M.D.
Professor of Pediatrics
University of Illinois
Chairman, Division of Neonatology
Cook County Hospital
Chicago, Illinois

Tonse N. K. Raju, M.D.
Associate Professor of Pediatrics
College of Medicine
University of Illinois
Chicago, Illinois

Devyani S. Raval, M.D.
Assistant Professor of Pediatrics
College of Medicine
University of Illinois
Attending Physician
Division of Neonatology
Cook County Hospital
Chicago, Illinois

Shirley Reitz, Pharm.D.
Assistant Professor
Department of Clinical Pharmacy
University of South Dakota
Vermillion, South Dakota

Ruth Andrea Seeler, M.D.
Pediatric Hematologist
Professor of Pediatrics
College of Medicine
University of Illinois
Chicago, Illinois

Maria Serratto, M.D.
Professor of Pediatrics
College of Medicine
University of Illinois
Chief, Cardiac Catheterization and
  Exercise Laboratories
Division of Pediatric Cardiology
Cook County Hospital
Chicago, Illinois

Gopal Srinivasan, M.D.
Professor of Pediatrics
The Chicago Medical School
Senior Attending Physician
Division of Neonatology
Cook County Hospital
Chicago, Illinois

Reginald C. Tsang, M.B.B.S.
Professor of Pediatrics, Obstetrics and
  Gynecology
Director, Division of Neonatology
College of Medicine
University of Cincinnati
Cincinnati, Ohio

Dharmapuri Vidyasagar, M.D.
Professor of Pediatrics
Director of Nursery
Department of Pediatrics
College of Medicine
University of Illinois
Chicago, Illinois

Sambasivarao Voora, M.D.
Chief, Division of Neonatology
St. Vincent Health Center
Erie, Pennsylvania

Angela Wilks, M.D.
Assistant Professor of Pediatrics
College of Medicine
University of Illinois
Attending Physician
Division of Neonatology
Cook County Children's Hospital
Chicago, Illinois

Paul Y. K. Wu, M.D.
Professor of Pediatrics
University of Southern California
Director, Division of Neonatal-Perinatal
  Medicine
Los Angeles County-University of
  Southern California Medical Center
Los Angeles, California

T. F. Yeh, M.D.
Professor of Pediatrics
College of Medicine
University of Illinois
Deputy Chairman
Division of Neonatology
Cook County Hospital
Chicago, Illinois

FOREWORD

Drug therapy in neonates and infants requires a thorough understanding of disease process coupled with continually updated knowledge of new treatment methods and pharmacokinetics. The first edition of this book provided a valuable resource to medical students, pediatricians, and neonatologists who provide care to sick neonates.

The second edition reviews current state-of-the-art use of natural vs. bovine surfactant in respiratory distress syndrome as well as the use of immunoglobulins in sick neonates. Additional new chapters cover therapy or prevention of bronchopulmonary dysplasia, fluid therapy, and intraventricular hemorrhage. New insights are provided for the definition of and controversies in therapy of neonatal seizures. In addition, Dr. Yeh and his colleagues have done an outstanding job in bringing former chapters up to date.

The second edition of this book will again provide a useful and practical guide for the understanding of pathophysiology of commonly observed problems in the neonate and appropriate therapeutic intervention.

R. S. Pildes, M.D.
Professor of Pediatrics
College of Medicine
University of Illinois
Chairman, Division of Neonatology
Cook County Children's Hospital
Chicago, Illinois

PREFACE

Five years have elapsed since the publication of the first edition of this monograph. The favorable reception of the first edition and the progress in the discipline over the past 5 years amply justify revision of the book.

This book is written essentially for pediatricians and neonatologists in practice. I believe that it provides more information on general management and drug therapy than is currently available in general textbooks but does not treat the pharmacology of drugs in unnecessary detail. To reflect the content of the book more accurately the title has been changed to *Neonatal Therapeutics.*

The general format of the first edition has been retained. Each chapter begins with a brief description of pathogenesis and general management followed by a more detailed discussion on drug therapy. We have expanded and revised some chapters extensively. I am particularly indebted to Dr. Fujiwara for his new chapter on surfactant therapy and to Dr. Kao for her chapter on bronchopulmonary dysplasia. Other new chapters included in this edition cover fluid and electrolyte balance, immunotherapy, transfusion of blood products, and prevention of intraventricular hemorrhage. I hope the second edition will provide adequate coverage on most of the current neonatal problems. In addition, the format of the illustrations and tables has been improved and kept consistent throughout the book.

I thank all the contributing authors who have made this new edition possible. I thank Lula B. Johnson for her secretarial work; and Kevin Kelly and Bethany Caldwell of Mosby–Year Book for editorial guidance.

I hope the reader will enjoy this book and find it useful in the management and therapy of the common problems in the neonate.

T. F. Yeh, M.D.

CONTENTS

Pharmacology

Pharm

Substance Abuse

XV

NEONATAL THERAPEUTICS

1

Factors Modulating Drug Therapy and Pharmacokinetics

Michael E. Evans, Ph.D.

Rama Bhat, M.D.

Dharmapuri Vidyasagar

The goal of drug therapy is to produce an appropriate and desired pharmacologic effect in each patient. This requires the administration of an appropriate dosage that accounts for individual variations in genetic makeup, disease processes, and patient history—all of which may influence the disposition and biological effects of the drug. The effects of most therapeutic agents are related to the drug concentration at the site of action, the length of time the concentration is maintained, and the rate at which active levels are achieved. Thus the major factors that modulate individual variability in drug response are drug disposition in the body and sensitivity of the body to the drug. In general, although individual differences to drug response do exist at the molecular level, these are often of lesser magnitude than differences resulting from individual variation in drug disposition. In this respect, therefore, age-related changes in drug disposition are of major concern in drug therapy.

DOSAGE

Until 15 to 20 years ago drug dosing in infants was empirically based on several rules in which weight, height, age, or body surface area were used to calculate the neonatal dose as a fraction of the adult dose. These parameters are important correlates of many physiologic functions in development that change in accordance with body weight (e.g., lean body mass), body length (e.g., long axis of the heart), or body surface area (e.g., oxygen uptake and basal metabolic rate). Although none of these rules are ideal in neonatal dose determination, body surface area appears to be the most applicable, as this parameter has been shown to best correlate with a number of physiologic parameters that have importance for drug kinetics. It should be noted that significant differences in calculated dosage may arise depending on the method selected. For example, the ratio of body surface area to body weight in the full-term neonate is more than twice the adult value. Thus a neonatal medication dosage calculated on the basis of this ratio would be twice as large as that calculated on the basis of body weight. The use of body surface area in dose determination is not optimal either, however, as the relative weight of various tissues and organs changes significantly during development.

Differences in pharmacodynamic aspects of drugs in the neonate also may complicate the use of drugs in pediatrics, as demonstrated by the diminished responsiveness of the cardiovascular system to digitalis, which is associated with a decreased number of receptor sites in the neonate.[2]

PHARMACOKINETICS

It is generally accepted that the newborn cannot be treated therapeutically as a small adult. It should also be appreciated that the qualitative differences between infants and adults in anatomic composition and physiologic functions that contribute to the altered disposition of drugs in the neonate are not always uniform in development. Furthermore, the great variability in kinetic properties (absorption, protein binding, metabolism, distribution, and excretion) according to birth weight and gestational age and the possible existence of abnormalities and pathologic syndromes further complicate the therapeutic approach in the pediatric patient.

The science of pharmacokinetics involves the application of mathematical and biochemical techniques to describe the disposition of chemicals. The physiologic factors that determine the concentration and duration of a chemical at the local site of action are absorption, distribution, and elimination. In general the rate for each of these factors is well described by first-order exponential kinetics in which the absolute rate of the process is proportional to the concentration. The higher the chemical concentration, the higher the absolute rate of the process; as the concentration becomes smaller, the absolute rate of the process decreases proportionally. On a proportional scale (i.e., the absolute amount of the drug that is absorbed, distributed, or eliminated per unit time divided by the total amount of drug available for this process), the rate of the process under first-order kinetics is a fixed value.

This principle is illustrated by the equation $\frac{dx}{x} = Kdt$, where $\frac{dx}{dt}$ is the change in x per unit time (t) and x is the absolute concentration at time (t). A negative sign is used to indicate loss of x. Thus for a first-order process the half-life of the reaction is dependent on a fixed-rate constant *(K)* and independent of concentration *(x)*. Processes that generally follow first-order kinetics include passive diffusion or filtration across membranes and metabolism. These processes underlie the physiologic parameters of absorption, distribution, and renal clearance. In first-order kinetics the rate of decrease is such that the time required for a specified percent loss is a constant and is independent of the starting concentration. However, not all substances follow first-order (fixed-rate constant) kinetics. The elimination-rate constant, for example, can become smaller as dose or serum concentrations become larger, resulting in dose-dependent elimination kinetics. Ethanol, aspirin, and phenytoin are three common examples of chemicals that exhibit a dose-dependent elimination in the therapeutic range. As the dosage is increased for these compounds, the elimination half-life is increased and the plateau steady-state concentration is disproportionally increased.[8] This deviation from first-order kinetics is characteristic of a saturation process in which the rate of the reaction becomes limited owing to a finite biochemical/physiological capacity and approaches a fixed value (zero-order kinetics). Explanations for zero-order kinetics include possible inhibitory effects of metabolites, saturation of a rate-limiting enzyme involved in membrane transport, or metabolism of a compound.

COMPARTMENT MODELS

In a comprehensive treatment of chemical disposition, the structural complexity of the body and the multiplicity of ways in which it deals with foreign compounds can result in exceedingly complicated pharmacokinetic analyses. Fortunately many of the quantitative formulas that are derived can be simplified through the use of compartment models. In these models the body is conceived as a series of compartments that have characteristic input and output rates for each particular chemical. A *compartment* is defined as a kinetically distinguishable "pool" in terms of the chemical concentration-time profile.

A realistic approach for describing the disposition of chemicals is the two-compartment open model shown in Figure 1–1. This system designates an initial, rapid distribution for the chemical throughout a small central compartment and a slower, second distribution to a larger peripheral compartment. The model is described as an open system because the chemical is eventually cleared or eliminated from both compartments. The two compartments do not necessarily correspond to specific anatomic entities but rather are theoretical spaces postulated to account for the rate of distribution of chemicals throughout the various body fluids and tissues.

The rate of uptake of a chemical from the plasma into the various body fluids and tissues is controlled by several forces, including the rate of blood flow through the tissues, the tissue mass, and the partition characteristics of

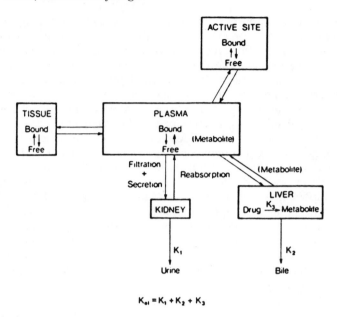

FIG 1-1.
Two-compartment open model for drug disposition. K_{el} is the sum of all methods of irreversible elimination (K_1, K_2, K_3).

the chemical between the plasma and tissue. In the final analysis, chemicals are distributed into the tissues in a highly complex manner and exhibit a concentration gradient even at the subcellular level. Fortunately many of these tissue compartments exhibit sufficiently similar properties to be considered either as large groups or as too small to be detected. Thus in a physiologic sense chemicals are considered to be distributed into the various tissues by a limited, multiple-compartment model that consists of four major compartments based on perfusion and partition characteristics (Table 1–1). Distribution for most chemicals, however, can be considered under a two-compartment model system.

TABLE 1-1.
Major Tissue Groups in Limited Multiple-Compartment Model

1	2	3	4
High perfusion	Low perfusion	Low perfusion	Negligible perfusion
Lean tissue	Lean tissue	Fat tissue	Bone
Heart	Muscle	Adipose tissue	Teeth
Lung	Skin	Bone marrow	Ligament
Hepatoportal			Cartilage
system			Hair
Kidney			
Endocrine glands			
CNS			

Group 4 (bone, teeth, and so on) contributes little to the distribution of most chemicals and, except for select chemicals (i.e., calcium, lead, tetracycline), can be ignored in most pharmacokinetic analyses. Most of the highly perfused lean tissues in group 1, as well as the major portion of the extracellular fluid, are in rapid equilibrium with the plasma and can be considered both mathematically and physiologically as part of the central compartment. A major portion of the adipose tissue in group 3 anatomically has a boundary contiguous with the muscle and skin of group 2 tissues, and distribution of chemicals into the tissues of groups 2 and 3 as a factor of time can be considered as a single compartment. Therefore, a two-compartment model consisting of:

Central compartment
  Plasma
  Group 1 tissues
  Extracellular fluid
Peripheral compartment
  Group 2 tissues
  Adipose tissue (major portion)

is normally sufficient to achieve an accurate assessment in the disposition of most chemicals.[8]

The two-compartment open model for describing chemical disposition has three defining characteristics: (1) chemicals are absorbed and eliminated only through the central compartment (i.e., plasma); (2) the transfer of chemicals between the central and peripheral compartment is reversible; (3) loss of the chemical from the central compartment by either metabolism or end-organ elimination is irreversible.

Further expansion of the two-compartment model to three-, four-, and five-compartment models can be made for select chemicals to provide for a best-fit description of the plasma concentration–time curve. The disposition of lead, for example, is best described by a three-compartment model, which consists of the central compartment (compartment 1), the slowly perfused tissues (compartment 2), and bone (compartment 3).[9]

PRINCIPLES OF PHARMACOKINETICS

Essentially four factors determine the intensity and duration of effect from a chemical: (1) the total amount of chemical absorbed (f); (2) the volume of distribution (Vd); (3) the degree of protein binding; and (4) the rates of absorption, distribution, and elimination. For most drugs, four different first-order rate constants are evident. These constants are associated with absorption (K_a), distribution to (K_{12}) and from (K_{21}) the peripheral compartment, and the elimination rate constant $(K_e$ or $K_{el})$. K_{el} is the sum of all the methods of irreversible elmination of the chemical from the central compartment ($K_{el} = K_m + K_r + K_1 + K_L$) and includes metabolism (K_m), renal (K_r) and fecal excretion (K_1), and pulmonary exhalation (K_L).

Because elimination (K_{el}) is often a first-order rate constant, the relative fraction of drug that is eliminated from the body in any given time period is a constant, irrespective of the absolute amount of drug in the body.

The total amount of drug present in the body (x) at time (T) can be described according to the equation $x = x_0 e^{-KelT}$ where x_0 is the amount of the drug present in the body at time zero. For most drugs elimination is usually considered in terms of biological half-life, the time required for any given drug concentration to decrease by half ($t^1/_2$). The half-life, or $t^1/_2$, for any drug is mathematically defined as the time required for $\dfrac{x}{x_0} = 0.5$. More generally, $t^1/_2 = (t_2 - t_1)$, if $\dfrac{x(t_2)}{x(t_1)} = 0.5$. For $t_2 = t$ and $t_1 = 0$, $(t_2 - t_1) = t$; and $t = t^1/_2$, if $\dfrac{x(t)}{x(0)} = 0.5$ [more simply written as $\dfrac{x}{x_0} = 0.5$]. Rearrangement and integration of the equation provide the mathematical relationship between half-life and elimination rate: $t^1/_2 = 0.693/K_{el}$.

It is important to understand that K_{el} is not the inverse of half-life. For example, because K_{el} may equal 0.5 hour^{-1}, the half-life is not 2.0 hours. The rate constant K_{el} describes the rate of elimination at any time in terms of a proportion of the total amount of drug in the body. As the drug begins to be eliminated, however, the absolute rate decreases as the total amount of drug in the body decreases. Thus biological half-life of a drug with $K_{el} = 0.5$ hour^{-1} is not 0.5 hour but 0.693/0.5 hour^{-1}, or 1.30 hours.

ABSORPTION

Absorption is defined as the movement of the chemical from the site of administration (or exposure) to the circulatory system. This movement is dependent primarily on the passage of the substance across the membrane of the cells of the intervening tissues. The principal routes of absorption for therapeutic agents involve the gastrointestinal tract, the respiratory system, and the skin, but other routes such as subcutaneous or intramuscular injection also may be important in certain instances. The rate of absorption will affect both the time to and duration of peak plasma concentration but not the area under the concentration-time curve. A slow absorption rate will both delay the time to peak plasma concentration and prolong the duration of peak effect. For chemicals administered chronically, the absorption rate generally is unimportant to the final steady-state plasma concentration of the compound. The effects of a single administration, however, may be greatly reduced in intensity and prolonged by a slow absorption process. The completeness of absorption is important in the intensity of effect for both single and chronic administration.

Under multiple dosage either at intervals or as a continuous infusion, the plasma concentration of the chemical, mathematically and physiologically, approaches a steady-state equilibrium, which is approximately 90% of maximum after four half-lives of the drug and more than 98% of maximum after seven half-lives (Fig 1–2). The mean steady-state plasma level (*Cpss*) obtained

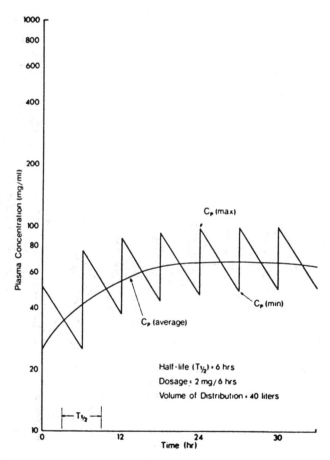

FIG 1–2.
Under multiple dosage, plasma concentration of chemical approaches a steady-state equilibrium that is approximately 90% of maximum after four half-lives of the drug, and more than 98% of maximum after seven half-lives.

is directly proportional to the dosage rate (*D/T*) and inversely proportional to the efficiency of removal of the drug from the plasma, or clearance (c). In equation form:

$$Cpss \ = \ \frac{\text{Dosage rate}}{\text{Plasma clearance}} = \frac{D/T}{c}$$

The *Cpss* can be predicted based on volume of distribution (V_d) and half-life of the drug according to the equation *Cpss* = 1.44 $t^{1}/_{2}$ (dose/V_d) *T*, where *T* equals the dosing interval. The fluctuation between the peak levels (*Cp max*) and the trough levels (*Cp min*) is dependent on the ratio of the half-life to dosage interval. The smaller the dosage interval in relation to the half-life or as a continuous infusion situation is approached, the less difference between *Cp max* and *Cp min*. Conversely, large doses given less frequently can result in greater fluctuations and possible toxic levels at the *Cp max* in spite of the absence of toxicity at mean *Cpss*. When dosage administration by either infusion or individual doses is ended, the concentration of the chemical in the body is decreased 90% from the maximum steady-state value within four half-lives.

ALIMENTARY TRACT

In oral absorption two cellular boundaries separate the gastrointestinal canal from the circulatory system: the epithelial lining of the canal and the endothelial wall of the blood capillary. Because the capillary endothelium has a highly porous structure (40 A) and is readily penetrated by most chemicals, the epithelium of the gastrointestinal tract constitutes the effective membrane barrier in oral absorption. Absorption by the gastrointestinal tract for most chemicals is due to passive diffusion or the un-ionized molecule across the epithelium. Thus it is dependent on the lipid solubility of the chemical, the concentration gradient of the molecules available for diffusion, the time available for absorption, and the available surface area.

Maturational changes in the amount of gastric secretions, motility, and blood flow of the gastrointestinal tract occur throughout life, from birth to old age. Because drug absorption is regulated by both pH-dependent diffusion and gastric emptying, it also varies in an age-related manner. During the first month of life, the gut undergoes maturation until a steady state is reached, then a slow decline in the secretions, motility, and blood flow occurs.[2] The major factors that affect drug absorption in the neonate are described in Table 1–2. The newborn has a gastric pH of 6 to 8, but the pH drops to 1 to 3 within a few hours after birth. A relative state of achlorhydria and a rise in pH then ensue, however, and persist until about the third year of the child's life, when the pH reaches adult levels. Newborns also have a higher pH in the small intestine, which allows bacterial flora, normally restricted to the

TABLE 1–2.
Factors Affecting Oral Absorption of Drugs in the Newborn

Factors	Differences in Newborn	Effect on Oral Drug Absorption	References
Gastric pH	High (6–8)	Affects nonionic diffusion and chemical stability of drugs	Weber and Cohen[10]
Small intestine pH	High		
Microbial flora	Decreased and qualitatively different	Variable; may alter patterns of metabolism	Weber and Cohen[10]
Peristalsis	Irregular and unpredictable	May lower total amount; may cause greater variation in amount and rate	Smith[7]
Gastric emptying time	Slower	Decreases rate of absorption for drug absorbed in duodenum	Smith[7]

colon, to colonize it. The gastric emptying time in newborns is prolonged to about 6 to 8 hours but will decrease to adult values by approximately 6 to 8 months of age. In addition, peristalsis in the newborn is very irregular and only partially dependent on the feeding pattern.

Malabsorption in the neonate can also be associated with an increased deconjugation of bile acids in the small intestine caused by small bowel contamination, and steatorrhea related to inadequate solubilization of fat in the duodenum owing to low bile acid secretion.[5] Thus in most cases, oral absorption of therapeutic agents in the newborn is often delayed, reduced, or both when compared with absorption in adults.

EPIDERMIS

The term *percutaneous absorption* is used to denote the passage of a substance from outside the body through the epidermis and its subsequent diffusion into the dermis and entry into the blood and lymphatic vessels. Based on case reports of drug toxicity, percutaneous absorption in the neonate generally was believed to be more rapid and extensive than in the adult; however, many of these reports involved drug application to broken skin, which greatly increases percutaneous absorption. Studies on transepidermal water loss and carbon dioxide excretion, both measurements of the stratum corneum barrier, have shown no significant differences between adults and neonates. Additionally, histologic studies on the stratum corneum from the epidermis do not indicate a substantial visible increase in thickness of the epidermis of newborns compared with that of older children and adults. Another major factor in percutaneous absorption in the neonate is the relatively large proportion of surface area to body weight.

INTRAMUSCULAR AND SUBCUTANEOUS ADMINISTRATION

Absorption following intramuscular or subcutaneous administration depends mainly on the regional blood flow, which may be very different among specific muscles and tissues. In the neonate the absorption pattern may change considerably during the first 2 weeks of extrauterine life in relation to maturational changes of the relative blood flow of the various muscles and tissues, particularly in association with the presence of hypoxic conditions. Absorption from intramuscular or subcutaneous sites in the neonate is often reduced because of decreased regional blood flow and reduced skeletal muscle mass and subcutaneous fat tissue. A different bioavailability for drugs is therefore not surprising in the neonate. It should be remembered, however, that depending on the physicochemical properties of the compounds, there may be either increased or reduced absorption in the neonate.

DISTRIBUTION

After absorption, chemicals are rapidly distributed by blood flow throughout the body. The initial phase of distribution reflects cardiac output and regional blood flow: highly perfused organs, such as the heart, liver, brain, and kidney, receive most of the available chemical during the first few minutes after absorption. The second phase of distribution involves slower delivery of the chemical to muscle, viscera, skin, and fat and requires from several minutes to several hours. This second phase is distinguished by the reduced blood flow of these tissues and organs and their larger fraction of total body mass. The diffusion of the chemical from the blood into the tissues—the third phase of distribution—is superimposed on the first two phases. For most chemicals diffusion into the interstitial tissues occurs rapidly because of the relatively large capillary pore size (40 A). The final distribution pattern for any chemical is dependent on the lipophilicity of the compound and its affinity for the various tissues in the body. Because pharmacologic activity is dependent on concentration at the site(s) of action, the final site(s) and volume of distribution will greatly influence the degree of activity of the compound.

VOLUME OF DISTRIBUTION

Body composition, in terms of lipid, protein, and water, is an important determinant of drug distribution. For example, the distribution of drugs having low lipid solubility (e.g., digoxin), correlates much better with lean body weight than with total body weight, as very little drug is distributed in fat tissue. Interindividual variability in pharmacokinetic parameters in the adult frequently is intimately connected with the amount of depot body fat.

DRUG-PROTEIN BINDING

The degree of binding to plasma proteins influences the overall disposition of a drug. According to pharmacologic principles, only the unbound fraction of a drug is therapeutically active. Alterations in protein binding can significantly affect the pharmacologic response, tissue distribution, hepatic and renal clearance, and consequently, the half-life of a drug. For the majority of drugs, binding to serum albumin is quantitatively the most important and often accounts for almost the entire drug binding in plasma.[1] Because drug binding is usually reversible, the albumin-drug complex serves as a circulating drug reservoir that releases more drug as free drug is distributed, metabolized, or excreted. Thus albumin binding decreases the maximum intensity but increases the duration of action of many drugs. When binding is subnormal, single doses of drugs may have to be decreased to avoid toxicity.

Such dosage adjustments are necessary for drugs whose albumin-bound phase represents a major fraction of the total drug in the body (i.e., high affinity for albumin and small volume of distribution). Thus under conditions of hypoproteinemia or reduced affinity of the protein for the drug, or both, free-drug concentration is a greater fraction of the plasma drug level, and the result is a greater peak intensity of pharmacologic activity. The quantitative effect of hypoalbuminemia on the extent of albumin binding varies greatly among drugs. Even mild degrees of hypoalbuminemia (30 g/L) can lead to a doubling of the free-serum fraction of phenytoin during chronic therapy. Epidemiologic studies have also shown that adverse reactions to prednisone, phenytoin, and diazepam are more common in hypoalbuminemic patients.[3] Renal failure or necrosis also has been shown to decrease drug binding. No consistent correlation has been demonstrated between the extent of binding impairment and the severity of renal insufficiency as reflected by serum creatinine or blood urea nitrogen concentration. Some studies have suggested, however, that the decreased binding of drugs during renal failure may be due in part to a conformational change in the protein-binding molecule, and to the accumulation of free fatty acids or other organic acids that compete with drugs for binding sites.

In the newborn several factors have been shown to be associated with a decreased plasma protein binding. These factors include a reduced protein concentration as well as (1) a qualitatively different albumin (fetal albumin, which shows a lower avidity for drugs), (2) high concentrations of bilirubin and free fatty acids, (3) other endogenous competing substrates, (4) lower blood pH, and (5) depressed renal functions—all factors that are capable of significantly modifying the plasma-protein binding of various compounds.[2]

Several investigators using placental cord blood have demonstrated a significant reduction in the protein binding of drugs in the neonate.[6] During the first few months of life, however, major changes are observed in the structural profile of blood proteins.[4] Thus although plasma albumin in the neonate is present at concentrations equivalent to those found in adults, it is different qualitatively. For example, a significant qualitative difference in fetal and neonatal albumin has been noted for the binding affinity of bilirubin.

EXCRETION

The relationship between biological age and rate of drug elimination is important for several clinical reasons. First, the actions of most drugs are terminated by metabolism, excretion, or both. Failure to recognize an altered rate of elimination in the neonate may result in excessive or subtherapeutic plasma levels of the drug, the former possibly yielding toxic effects. The rate of elimination for a drug determines the dose and dosage interval required to maintain a specific steady-state concentration in the body. Thus failure to adjust dose and dosage interval to account for age-related decrease in drug elimination can result in accumulated toxic levels of drug, as observed with chloramphenicol therapy in infants with gray syndrome. Conversely a rapid elimination rate (as seen in young children given theophylline) may cause a standard regimen of therapy to be inadequate in producing a clinically effective plasma concentration of drug.

Second, age-related changes in the pathway of drug elimination also contribute to drug toxicity. For example, recent studies have shown that theophylline in the neonate is metabolized to caffeine. Both of these methylxanthines have a similar pharmacologic spectrum of activity and can produce toxicity by additive effects. In the adult, by comparison, theophylline is rapidly metabolized to inactive metabolites.

METABOLISM

The majority of drugs and chemicals are biotransformed by four enzymatic pathways. Three of these pathways—oxidation, reduction, and hydrolysis—constitute the phase I type of metabolism and involve a rearrangement of splitting of the molecule at select functional groups. The fourth pathway, designated as the phase II type of metabolism, involves conjugation of the molecule with endogenous, low-molecular-weight polar substances. Phase I reactions generally precede phase II reactions for most chemicals, and often a substance is subjected to several competing as well as sequential pathways of metabolism. The extent of formation of the various metabolites depends on the relative rate of the individual enzymes. A number of factors, including route of administration, disease, age, diet, temperature, and prior exposure to other chemicals, have been shown significantly to affect enzymatic levels and activity.

Quantitatively the most important organ for drug metabolism is the liver, and the total organ size and activity of its drug-metabolizing enzymes change with development, both relatively and absolutely. Numerous studies have shown that it is not possible to generalize regarding drug-metabolizing capacity in newborns as this varies depending on the specific drug as well as the individual.

Drug disposition in the newborn generally is regarded as being substantially different from that of the adult. Some of the differences in neonatal drug distribution and their potential pharmacologic impacts are summarized in Table 1–3. The neonate has a higher water content and less lipid tissue compared with the adult, and distribution volumes for water-soluble and lipid-soluble drugs are altered accordingly.

The increases in V_d for a water-soluble drug acts to decrease the peak plasma concentration and peak effect (intensity) of the drug. Because of the change in V_d, however, the half-life ($t^1/_2$) is increased; therefore, on chronic administration the interval between doses must be increased to prevent excessive accumulation of the drug.

TABLE 1–3.
Factors Affecting Drug Disposition in Neonates, Relative to Adults

| Disposition Parameter | Pharmacologic Effect | | Half-life | | |
| | Neonate | Intensity | Hepatic Metabolism | Renal | |
				Filtration	Transport
Volume of distribution					
Liquid-soluble drug	−	+	0	−	−
Water-soluble drug	+	−	0	+	+
Metabolism	−	0	−	+	+
Renal excretion	−	0	−	+	+
Protein-binding capacity	−	+	−	−	+

+ = increased; − = decreased; 0 = no difference.

A similar consideration with respect to half-life must be made for drugs that are more slowly metabolized or excreted. In this case, however, peak concentration and intensity of effect remain the same as that observed in the adult. In the infant, a decrease in drug-protein binding increases the intensity of effect by providing more free drug without changing the total serum concentration. The half-life, however, is decreased for drugs that are eliminated by filtration owing to an increased amount of free drug for renal clearance. Conversely, a decrease in protein-binding capacity for drugs that are excreted by transport processes increases half-life because of the redistribution of the increased free drug throughout the extracellular water.

Many other factors undoubtedly may influence drug delivery in the neonate. In this regard, the use of drugs in the neonatal period can be hazardous if the biological peculiarities of this period of life are not taken into account. Adjustment of the dosage to body size is at best an approximation. The well-known sensitivity of the newborn to various pharmacologic agents is dependent on a number of different factors, such as immature absorptive capacity, slow elimination processes, changes in body composition, and altered threshold of pharmacologic receptors. Optimum dosage regimes for the various drugs used in the neonatal period can be derived by the application of pharmacokinetic methods. These methods can also be of great value in determining the influence of various disease states on the disposition of drugs during the neonatal period.

REFERENCES

1. Anton HA, Solomon HM: Drug protein binding. *Ann NY Acad Sci* 1973; 226:221–223.
2. Boerth RC: Decreased sensitivity of newborn myocardium positive inotropic effects of ouabain, in Morselli PL, Garattini S, Sereni F (eds): *Basic and Therapeutic Aspects of Perinatal Pharmacology.* New York, Raven Press, 1975, pp 191–199.
3. Greenblatt DJ, Koch-Weser J: Clinical toxicity of chlordiazepoxide and diazepam in relation to serum albumin concentrations. *Eur J Clin Pharmacol* 1974; 7:267–269.
4. Kapitulnik J, et al: Increase in bilirubin-binding affinity of serum with age of infant. *J Pediatr* 1975; 86:442–445.
5. Lester R: Diarrhea and malabsorption in the newborn. *N Engl J Med* 1977; 297:505–509.
6. Rane A, Lunde PKM, Jalling B, et al: Plasma protein binding of diphenylhydantoin in normal and hyperbilirubinemic infants. *Pediatr Pharmacol Ther* 1971; 78:877–881.
7. Smith CA: *Physiology of the Newborn.* Springfield, Ill: Charles C Thomas, 1959, p 327.
8. Wagner JG: *Fundamentals of Clinical Pharmacokinetics.* Drug Intelligence Publications, vol 13. Hamilton, Ill: Hamilton Press, 1975, p 112.
9. Waldron HA, Stofen D: *Sub-clinical Lead Poisoning.* New York, Academic Press, 1974, p 98.
10. Weber WW, Cohen SN: Aging effects and drugs in man, in *Handbook of experimental pharmacology,* vol 28 of Concepts in Biochemical Pharmacology, edited by JR Gilette and JR Mitchell. Berlin: Springer-Verlag, 1975, pp 213–233.

2

Drugs During Pregnancy and Lactation

Angela Wilks, M.D.

Sambasivarao Voora, M.D.

Tsu F. Yeh, M.D.

PLACENTAL TRANSFER OF DRUGS

The pregnant woman is exposed to an average of four prescription drugs during the 9 months of fetal confinement. If nonprescription drugs are included, the number of drug exposures ranges from 8.7 to 11.[9] Most drugs do find their way to the fetal side of the placenta, with the extent and degree of transfer dependent on (1) physicochemical characteristics of the drug, (2) maternal drug concentration in the plasma, (3) physiologic properties of the placenta, and (4) blood flow changes of the fetal maternal unit.

In general, drugs that cross the placenta with relative ease have molecular weights of less than 500, high lipid solubility, a low affinity for protein binding, and a low degree of ionization. Most local anesthetics have molecular weights less than 500. Heparin has molecular weights greater than 1,000 and is more restricted to crossing the placental barrier. Ampicillin is about 10% protein bound, as compared with dicloxacillin, which is 96% protein bound, with resultant high levels of ampicillin in the amniotic fluid and the fetus. Many physiologic changes that take place in the pregnant woman have the potential to, and do, affect the maternal blood concentration of a drug. This affects the degree of drug available to the placenta and hence the degree of transfer across and to the fetus.

During pregnancy, the total volume of water and plasma in the body increases by as much as 50% by the eighth month of pregnancy. This will effect an increase in the apparent volume of distribution and a decrease in plasma albumin and α-glycoprotein. Most acidic drugs (e.g., phenytoin) are bound to plasma albumin, and most basic drugs (e.g., propranolol) to α-

16

glycoprotein. This may result in a larger fraction of unbound drug and decreased total drug concentration.

The increase in renal blood flow and glomerular filtration rate may lead to subtherapeutic concentration of a drug because of an increase in drug clearance. In addition, during pregnancy there is decreased gastrointestinal motility, with delay in gastric emptying time and transit times. This can alter the amount and degree of absorption of drugs taken orally.

As the placenta matures, the trophoblastic epithelium thins from 26 μm to 2 μm (the latter at term), with increased transplacental diffusion. Different disease states, such as diabetes, can also alter the permeability characteristics of the placenta. Uterine blood flow increases during pregnancy to approximately 10% of resting maternal cardiac output by term. Any condition that alters the uteroplacental blood flow can alter the drug delivery to the fetus, for example, hypotension resulting from sympathetic blockade.

DRUG EFFECTS ON THE FETUS AND NEONATE

Most drugs given to the pregnant woman reach the fetus, with the potential of having adverse effects. Table 2–1 is a list of some of the more common drugs used during pregnancy and their reported effects on the fetus. For details, the reader is referred to a book specific for this purpose.[2]

As with any drug, the risk of giving the drug to a pregnant woman must be weighed against the potential risk to the fetus. It is the physician's responsibility to anticipate effects in both the mother and the fetus.

DRUGS IN BREAST MILK

The incidence of breast-feeding has almost doubled in the last decade, and the trend seems to be continuing. Because of this increase and the increase in frequency of pregnancy in women with chronic disease, the clinician often faces the problems of prescribing drugs to a nursing mother, the presence of drugs in breast milk, and the safety of the infants that are breast-fed. These problems have been compounded by the lack of systematic human pharmacokinetic data for most drugs. In this chapter, we review the current literature on commonly used drugs. For detailed information, the reader is referred to a book specific for this purpose.[2]

TRANSPORT OF DRUGS ACROSS MILK-BLOOD BARRIER

Almost all drugs present in the maternal circulation are detected in breast milk to a certain extent. Drugs entering the perialveolar interstitial space from capillary circulation have to cross the milk-blood barrier prior to entry into

TABLE 2–1.
Effects on Fetus and Neonate of Commonly Prescribed Drugs

Drug	Fetal/Neonatal Effects
Analgesics	
Acetaminophen	Nephrotoxic effects
Indomethacin	Premature closure of patent ductus, oligohydramnios, pulmonary hypertension, reduced fetal urine output
Narcotics	Withdrawal symptoms, respiratory depression, apnea, bradycardia, death, (heroin) decreased incidence of hyaline membrane disease (HMD), thrombocytosis, (methadone) increased T_3 and T_4 levels, small for gestational age (SGA)
Salicylates	Platelet dysfunction, intrauterine death, low birth weight, methemoglobinemia, decreased factor XII
Anesthetics	
General	Depression at birth, apnea
Local	Seizures, hypotension, neurologic depression, myocardial depression, bradycardia, methemoglobinemia, mydriasis, neurobehavioral disturbances
Anticoagulants	
Coumarin derivatives (warfarin sodium)	Contraindicated in pregnancy. Fetal warfarin syndrome, hemorrhage, CNS defects, spontaneous abortion, stillbirth, prematurity
Heparin	Does not cross placenta; calcium deficiency
Magnesium sulfate	Respiratory depression, hypotonia, potentiation of neuromuscular weakness in conjunction with aminoglycosides
Anticonvulsants	
Phenobarbital	Hemorrhage, malformations in combination with phenytoin
Phenytoin	Fetal hydantoin syndrome (craniofacial and limb), hemorrhage, tumors (neuroblastoma, ganglioneuroblastoma)
Valproic acid	Neural tube defects, fetal valproate syndrome
Antidiabetic agents	
Chlorpropamide	Not recommended in pregnancy, severe hypoglycemia
Insulin	Drug of choice for diabetes mellitus in pregnancy; congenital anomalies
Tolbutamide	Thrombocytopenia
Antiemetics and antihistamines	
Cimetidine	Transient liver impairment (one case)
Diphenhydramine	Cleft palate
Promethazine	Impaired platelet aggregation, respiratory depression
Anti–human immunodeficiency virus (azidothymidine; AZT)	No information available
Antihypertensive agents	
Captopril	Contraindicated in pregnancy; fetal abnormalities, stillbirth

Hydralazine	Thrombocytopenia, fetal death, birth defects second or third trimester
Methyldopa	Decreased intracranial volume, mild hypotension, decrease in midtrimester losses
Propranolol	Bradycardia, apnea, hypoglycemia, growth retardation
Reserpine	Nasal stuffiness, inguinal hernia, microcephaly, hydronephrosis, hydroureter
Anti-infective agents	
Ampicillin	Depresses maternal plasma and urinary estriol, interfering in fetal placental unit assessment
Amphotericin	No evidence of adverse fetal effects
Chloroquine	Fetal death, prematurity, abortion
Erythromycin (Estolate)	Contraindicated in pregnancy
Isoniazid	(Combination therapy) psychomotor retardation, convulsions, potential neurotoxicity, meningomyelocele, hypospadias
Rifampin	Limb malformations, CNS anomalies
Sulfonamides	Jaundice, hemolytic anemia, kernicterus
Tetracycline	Yellow staining of teeth, enamel hypoplasia, inhibition of and delay in bone growth, inguinal hernia, hypospadias
Antineoplastic agents	
Laetrile	No studies in pregnancy; possible gestational cyanide poisoning
Methotrexate	Oxycephaly, hypertelorism, large anterior or posterior fontanelle, growth retardation
Vincristine	Low birth weight, kidney malformation
Antithyroid agents	
Propylthiouracil	Fetal goiter
Sodium iodide (^{131}I)	Contraindicated in pregnancy; teratogenic
Potassium iodide	Contraindicated in pregnancy, hypothyroidism, goiter
Bronchodilators	
Aminophylline (theophylline)	Withdrawal, in vitro chromosome breakage of human lymphocytes, apnea
Cardiovascular agents	
Bretylium	No adverse effects reported; potential for fetal hypoxia and bradycardia secondary to reduced uterine blood flow
Digoxin	Treat supraventricular tachycardia in fetus; premature labor
Nitroglycerin	(?)Malformations; experience limited in pregnancy; reduced fetal beat to beat variability
Verapamil	Prolonged arteriovenous conduction in fetal ewe
Tolazoline	(?)Malformations; experience limited in pregnancy
Diagnostic agents	
Methylene blue	Hemolytic anemia, methemoglobinemia, jaundice

(Continued)

TABLE 2-1. *(cont.)*

Metrizamide	Hypothyroidism, jaundice
Radiopaque medium (Renografin)	Intestinal tract opacification, fetal hypothyroidism
Diuretics	
Furosemide	Diuresis, increased urinary sodium and potassium
Thiazide	Thrombocytopenia, hypoelectrolytemia
Environmental agents	
Bromide	Congenital hip dislocation, polydactyly, GI malformations, clubfoot, intrauterine growth retardation, hypotonia
Carbon monoxide	Stillbirth, fetal brain damage
Hexachlorophene	(?)Malformations
Lead	Growth retardation, abortion, congential anomalies
Mercury	Seizures, mental retardation, involuntary movements, defective vision
Naphthalene	Hemolysis, jaundice
Pesticides	Abortion, congenital malformations
Hormones	
Androgens and estrogens	(?)VACTERL syndrome, adenocarcinoma of vagina, penile abnormalities, cleft lip and palate, labioscrotal fusion, tracheoesophageal fistula, limb and renal anomalies, heart defects
Progestins	(?)VACTERL syndrome, hypospadias, masculinization of female
Immunoglobulins	
Hepatitis, rabies, tetanus	No reported risk to fetus
Miscellaneous	
Aspartame	Contraindicated in patients with phenylketonuria
Laminaria (cervical softening)	Fetal death
Penicillamine	Death, cutis laxa, growth retardation, abnormalities
Povidone-iodine (vaginal douche)	Hypothyroidism, increased iodine levels in amniotic fluid
Saccharin or cyclamate	(?)Behavioral problems (e.g., hyperactivity, emotionalism)
Fluoride	Positive effect on growth and development of fetal bones and teeth
Muscle relaxants	
Isoxsuprine	Fetal tachycardia, hypotension, hypocalcemia, ileus, neonatal respiratory depression, heart rate variability, respiratory depression
Narcotic antagonist	
Narloxone	(?)Enhanced fetal asphyxia
Neuropsychotropics	
Diazepam	Withdrawal, hypotonia, cleft lip or palate, inguinal hernia

Imipramine	Withdrawal symptoms, limb reduction, cleft palate, CNS anomalies
Lithium	Cardiovascular abnormalities, cyanosis, hypotonia, bradycardia, nephrogenic diabetis insipidus, neonatal goiter
Phenothiazine	Withdrawal symptoms
Radiation therapy	Contraindicated in pregnancy (all efforts to protect fetus if substantially justified)
	Nondisjunction of chromosomes, microcephaly, mental retardation, predisposition to later malignancies
Recreational drugs	
Cigarettes	Low birth weight, decreased cord RBC zinc level
Cocaine	Impaired fetal growth, abruptio placentae with increased stillbirth rate, malformations, transient EEG abnormalities
Ethanol	Fetal alcohol syndrome, spontaneous abortion, growth retardation, developmental and behavioral dysfunction in infants
Heroin	Lower incidence of hyaline membrane disease after 32 weeks' gestation, low birth weight, SGA, withdrawal at 48 hours, lower incidence of jaundice, long-term effects on growth and behavior
Lysergic acid diethylamide (LSD)	Limb anomalies, chromosome breaks
Marijuana	Impaired fetal growth
Pentazocine and tripelennamine (T's and blue's)	Low birth weight, withdrawal symptoms within 7 days of delivery
Sedatives	
Chloral hydrate	Large doses result in intrauterine death
Thalidomide	Phocomelia, cardiovascular anomalies, ear anomalies
Stimulants	
Amphetamine	Withdrawal symptoms, hypoglycemia, irritability, tremors, limb deformities, biliary atresia, seizures
Caffeine (excess)	Late spontaneous abortion
Ephedrine	Minimum neonatal tachycardia
Oxytocin	Fetal bradycardia, hyponatremia, hyperbilirubinemia, seizures
Tocolytic agents	
Ritodrine	Increased fetal heart rate, hyperglycemia, neonatal hypoglycemia, ketoacidosis, death
Terbutaline	Increases fetal heart rate, fetal hyperglycemia, neonatal hypoglycemia
Vaccines	Live virus vaccines contraindicated in pregnancy. Live oral polio virus vaccine if pregnant patient at substantial risk of exposure to wild virus

(Continued)

TABLE 2–1. *(cont.)*

Vitamins	
Cholecalciferol (vitamin D)	Supravalvular aortic stenosis, elfin facies, mental and
Excess	growth retardation, inguinal hernia, strabismus
Deficiency	Defective tooth enamel, neonatal rickets, hypocal-
	cemia, seizures
Isotretinoin (Accutane)	Contraindicated in pregnancy; teratogenic cranial facial
	abnormalities; cardiac, thymic, CNS anomalies;
	branchial arch–mesenchymal tissue defects
Phytonadione	No fetal risk reported
Pyridoxine (deficiency)	Seizures

milk. The milk-blood barrier, like other biologic membranes, acts as a lipid barrier with water-filled pores. Drug transportation can occur through water-filled pores, plasma cell membranes, and interalveolar spaces (Fig 2–1). The possible mechanisms of transportation include (1) diffusion (passive or facilitated), (2) active transport, (3) pinocytosis, and (4) reverse pinocytosis, or emiocytosis.

The concentration of a drug in milk is influenced by several of its characteristics, including (1) size of the molecule, (2) ability to bind to proteins, (3) solubility, (4) pH, (5) dissociation constant (pK), and (6) degree of ionization. The concentration of the drug in milk is, however, independent of the volume of milk secreted. This has been shown in animal experiments, which supports the hypothesis that mammary excretion is a diffusion process.

Maternal Factors

Four basic parameters—absorption, distribution, biotransformation, and elimination—determine the amount of drug available for transfer across biologic membranes. These pharmacokinetic parameters are in turn influenced by factors (some of which may be related to the altered body composition caused by pregnancy) including concurrent disease state, route and duration of drug administration, individual variation in metabolism, and elimination and drug interaction (e.g., multiple-drug therapy or presence of nicotine in mothers who smoke). The excess fat deposited during pregnancy may persist during lactation and alter the distribution of fat-soluble drugs and chemicals. In addition, absorption and elimination rates during pregnancy may not return to prepregnancy levels, and can influence plasma drug concentration in the lactating period.

Infant Factors

Once the infant is nursed with milk containing drugs, the amount of drug that reaches the pharmacologic receptors again depends on the same four pharmacologic parameters in the infant: absorption, distribution, biotransformation, and elimination.

Certain physiologic variations characteristic of the newborn, especially premature infants, may influence the bioavailability of a drug ingested through milk. These variations include gastric emptying time, gastrointestinal motility, gastric pH, pool size of bile salts, and the diet itself.

Most drugs are metabolized and excreted via liver and kidney, whose functioning may not be mature in the newborn infant, especially a premature infant. Hence drug accumulation may occur despite low levels of drugs in the ingested milk. Premature infants also have less albumin in plasma, which results in increased free-drug concentration.

Safety of Drug to Infant

The clinician facing the problem of prescribing a drug for a nursing mother should address the following questions:

1. Is it absolutely necessary for the mother to take the drug?
2. Do the maternal benefits outweigh the risk to the infant?
3. Is there an alternative drug (e.g., ampicillin vs. sulfonamides in a nursing mother with a urinary tract infection) that poses less risk to the infant?

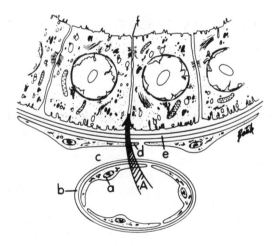

FIG 2–1.
Milk-blood barrier of mammary gland alveolus. *Arrow (A)* shows passive diffusion of material in lumen of blood vessel into lumen of alveolus. All un-ionized molecules must cross the endothelial cell of the blood vessel *(a)*, basement membrane of blood vessel *(b)*, interstitial breast space *(c)*, myoepithelial cell of alveolus *(d)*, basement membrane of alveolus *(e)*, and interalveolar spaces *(f)*. (From George DI Jr, O'Toole TJ: *J Am Dent Assoc* 1983; 106:204–208. Used by permission.)

If the clinician decides that drug therapy in the nursing mother is necessary, the next question is whether that particular drug can be given directly to the infant when necessary.

In general, when a drug can be given directly to the infant, the drug can also be given to the mother; however, risk to the infant always exists, and the infant needs to be observed closely for symptoms of drug toxicity.

Minimizing the Effect of Drugs in Breast Milk

The following adjustments may be made to reduce the effects on the infant:

1. Use a short-acting form of the drug to minimize the chances of accumulation.
2. Avoid feeding during the expected peak plasma levels (e.g., feed the infant prior to dosing the mother).
3. Use preparations that can be given at longer intervals (e.g., once per day vs. three to four times per day).
4. Use single-dose regimens instead of several-day courses whenever applicable.
5. Consider temporarily discontinuing breast-feeding or using previously expressed milk during the course of medication.

PRESENCE OF COMMONLY USED DRUGS IN BREAST MILK

Analgesics

Acetylsalicylic acid (aspirin) is an organic acid and is highly bound to plasma proteins, which renders it less permeable across the milk-blood barrier. The milk-plasma concentration ratio has been reported to vary between 0.6 and 1.0. Occasional aspirin intake by the nursing mother is safe; however, side effects such as easy bruising and metabolic acidosis have been reported.

Narcotic analgesics such as *codeine, meperidine,* and *morphine* are excreted in small amounts and may be used safely in therapeutic doses. Heroin may be excreted in significant amounts in addicts; Cobrinik and colleagues[5] reported successful treatment of infants with withdrawal symptoms through breast-feeding by their mothers.

The milk-plasma ratio of *methadone* varies from 0.3 to 1.89, and no adverse effects have been reported in breast-fed infants. Marijuana is concentrated in breast milk, and the effects on the infant are not known.

Antibiotics and Other Antimicrobial Agents

Penicillins are present in breast milk and are usually safe, but in theory can cause sensitivity in the infant.

Sulfonamides are excreted in breast milk in various concentrations depending on their protein binding and pK. Sulfonamides can produce kernicterus in breast-fed neonates with hyperbilirubinemia, and hemolytic anemia in those with glucose-6-phosphate dehydrogenase deficiency. Contrary to previous reports, a recent study[15] of secretion of sulfisoxazole in human milk revealed a concentration of 1% of the maternal dose, which is of no significant risk to a healthy infant beyond the neonatal period.

Although *tetracycline* is present in breast milk in up to 20% to 90% of maternal serum levels, no significant levels have been detected in the serum of infants, which may be indicative of poor absorption from the gastrointestinal tract. Because of the possibility of tooth discoloration and enamel hypoplasia in infants, it is better that nursing mothers avoid the use of tetracycline.

Erythromycin is a base, and the concentration in breast milk can reach several times that of maternal serum levels; however, no adverse reactions have been reported in the breast-fed infant.

Clindamycin appears in breast milk in concentrations of 0.7 to 3.8 μg/mL, and the case of a breast-fed infant with bloody diarrhea was reported which might represent clindamycin-induced enterocolitis.[17]

Metronidazole appears in breast milk at levels equal to that in serum and may cause vomiting and bloody dyscrasias in the infant. Although previous investigators have contraindicated breast-feeding in mothers receiving metronidazole, following the U.S. Food and Drug Administration's approval of a single-dose (2 g) regimen for treatment of trichomoniasis, Erickson and colleagues[8] reported peak concentrations 2 to 4 hours after the dose, which declined rapidly over the next 24 hours. Hence temporary discontinuation of breast-feeding for 24 hours seems more appropriate.

Chloramphenicol is excreted in breast milk at levels equal to approximately 50% of maternal plasma level, which may depress infant bone marrow production; however, the Committee on Drugs[7] of the American Academy of Pediatrics lists chloramphenicol under drugs that are compatible with breast-feeding.

According to O'Brien,[19] *cephalexin, cephalothin, chloroquine, oxacillin,* and *para-aminosalicylic acid* are safe. *Isoniazid* reaches concentrations that are similar to maternal plasma levels, and it is necessary to watch the infant closely for signs of hepatitis.

Anticoagulants

Oral anticoagulants are either coumarin or indanedione derivatives. *Coumarin* derivatives include dicumarol (*bis*-hydroxy-coumarin), *warfarin,* and *acenocoumarol.* There is evidence that all of the coumarin derivatives are safe to use in nursing mothers. Neither warfarin nor acenocoumarol has been detected in breast milk. The levels of dicumarol have not been measured, but no alterations have been detected in clotting time in breast-fed infants.

Indanedione derivatives include *anisindione, phenindione,* and *diphen-*

adione. Phenindione has been proved to cause hemorrhage in infants of nursing mothers receiving phenindione and is contraindicated.

Anticonvulsants

The milk-plasma concentration ratio of phenytoin is 0.45. An infant's plasma level at steady-state concentration has been found to be 0.5 μg/mL, which is not harmful to the infant when maternal plasma levels are in the therapeutic range.

The milk-plasma concentration ratio for several antiepileptic medications was measured by Kaneko and co-workers.[14] The ratio for *phenobarbital* ranged between 0.4 and 0.6. When maternal plasma levels are between 10 and 30 μg/mL, no significant effect is noted in the infant; decreased responsiveness and excessive sleeping may be seen when maternal plasma levels exceed 30 μg/mL.

Carbamazepine reaches a milk-plasma concentration ratio of 0.4.[14] Carbamazepine is effectively cleared by infants, and no adverse effects have been noted.

Antithyroid Drugs

Iodine has been known to be present in breast milk and is reported to cause goiter in the infant whose nursing mother received iodine for hyperthyroidism or as an antitussive preparation.

Thiouracil is actively transported into breast milk and reaches a level 3 to 12 times higher than that in maternal serum; breast-feeding is contraindicated. *Propylthiouracil,* however, in a daily dose of 200 to 300 mg, has been reported to be safe.[13]

Methimazole has the potential for interfering with thyroid function in the infant and is contraindicated.

Cardiovascular Agents

The milk-plasma concentration ratio of *digoxin* varies from 0.7 to 0.9. Even in cases of maternal toxicity, the amount of drug ingested by the infant is only one-twentieth the recommended maintenance dose; it is therefore safe for nursing mothers to use digoxin.

Propranolol is a weak base and may concentrate in breast milk. In three lactating women, the milk-plasma concentration ratio varied from 0.33 to 1.65. The amount ingested by a neonate is 0.1% of the maternal dose; therefore, propranolol can be freely used by nursing mothers.

The milk-plasma concentration ratio of active *hydralazine,* an antihypertensive drug commonly used during pregnancy, varies from 0.5 to 1.3. Negligible amounts ingested in each feeding (0.013 mg per feeding) do not affect the infant.

Hydrochlorothiazide has been demonstrated in breast milk but has not been detected in the infant's plasma.

Alpha-methyldopa does not pose a risk with the usual therapeutic maternal doses.[25]

Contraceptives

There is considerable controversy regarding the effects of contraceptive agents present in breast milk. Both *estrogen* and *progestin* components are present in breast milk. Gynecomastia was reported in an infant whose mother was receiving large doses of an estrogen-containing oral contraceptive; however, no consistent long-term adverse effects on growth and development have been reported.[6]

Antianxiety Drugs

Diazepam and its active metabolite, *desmethyl diazepam,* are excreted in significant concentrations. The milk-plasma concentration ratio varied markedly. Drowsiness has been reported in an infant whose mother was receiving 30 mg diazepam daily.[21] Discontinuation of breast-feeding is suggested if large doses are required.

Antidepressants

The excretion of trycyclic antidepressants (e.g., *imipramine* and *amitriptyline*) into breast milk is negligible. *Lithium* has been shown to be present in breast milk in significant amounts, and flaccidity, cyanosis, and heart murmur have been noted in infants. One recent report,[24] however, indicated no harm to nursing infants whose mothers were receiving lithium.

Antipsychotic Drugs

Chlorpromazine and other *phenothiazines* appear in breast milk in small amounts, and maternal doses of 100 mg/day do not appear to cause symptoms in the infant.

Radiopharmaceuticals

With the advent of computed tomography and ultrasound, the use of radiopharmaceuticals for diagnostic purposes is decreasing; however, it is not unusual for a nursing mother to take one of these drugs for diagnostic or therapeutic purposes. As there are demonstrable amounts in breast milk and significant effects on the infant, the best approach is to discontinue breast-feeding temporarily until all radioactivity clears from milk. This interval will depend on the maternal dosage, half-life, and metabolism of the given isotope.

The concentration of *radioactive iodine* (^{125}I and ^{131}I) in breast milk can reach 5% of maternal dose and may persist up to 1 to 3 weeks.[12, 19] Also, ^{125}I presents the risk of thyroid cancer. When used for therapeutic purposes, radioactivity can be detected in breast milk up to 2 weeks with Gallium 69 and for 3 days when technetium (^{99m}Tc, ^{99m}Tc-MAA, or [99m]Tc-04) is used.[20, 23] *Radioactive sodium* may persist in breast milk for 96 hours.

Social Drugs

Ethanol is excreted in breast milk and reaches concentrations equal to that in maternal blood. Studies by Kesaniemi[16] revealed that in both moderate social drinking (blood concentration 50 μg/dL) and heavy habitual drinking (blood concentration 100 μg/dL) the maximum blood alcohol concentration in the infant (1.9 μg/dL and 3.7 μg/dL, respectively) did not have any effect on the infant. Maternal blood alcohol levels exceeding 300 μg/dL, however, can cause mild sedation or sleepiness in the infant. Intoxicated mothers should not breast-feed their babies, and mothers with chronic alcoholism who cannot stop drinking should be discouraged from breast-feeding. Excessive alcohol ingestion also can lead to reduction of the milk ejection reflex. Pseudo-Cushing's syndrome was reported in a 4-month-old infant girl breast-fed by a mother who consumed excessive amounts of alcohol.

Although *nicotine* is excreted in breast milk and can be found in the milk of even light smokers (one to four cigarettes per day),[22] no deleterious effects have been noted, even in infants of heavy smokers (one to one and one-half packs per day).[10] A decrease in milk production has been reported in heavy smokers.[22]

Caffeine does not diffuse freely into breast milk, and concentration in milk is lower than in maternal plasma; however, infants excrete caffeine slowly, and irritability and poor sleeping may be seen in the infant.[1]

Cocaine should not be taken during breast-feeding. One infant was found to have symptoms of cocaine intoxication, and there was persistence of cocaine and its primary metabolite, benzoylecgonine, in maternal milk as long as 36 hours after use.[4]

Pollutants in Breast Milk

Pesticides and environmental pollutants have been known to be present in breast milk.[11] *Organochlorine pesticides* include *DDT* (dichlorodiphenyl-trichloroethane), *hexachlorobenzene,* and *chlordane.* Several investigators have shown breast-milk concentrations of DDT higher than the 50 parts per billion maximum set for cow's milk by the World Health Organization. The long-term consequences of these compounds are not known, and unless the milk is heavily contaminated it is safe to continue breast-feeding. Hexachlorobenzene in breast milk has been reported to cause porphyria.[3]

TABLE 2-2
Reported Signs or Symptoms of Drugs in Lactating Infants

Drug	Sign or Symptom
Methotrexate*	Possible immune suppression, unknown effect on growth or association with carcinogenesis
Bromocriptine	Suppresses lactation
Cimetidine†	May suppress gastric acidity in infant, inhibit drug metabolism, and cause CNS stimulation
Clemastine	Drowsiness, irritability, refusal to feed, high-pitched cry, neck stiffness
Cyclophosphamide*	Possible immune suppression, unknown effect on growth or association with carcinogenesis
Ergotamine	Vomiting, diarrhea, convulsions (doses used in migraine medications)
Gold salts	Rash, inflammation of kidney and liver
Methimazole	Potential for interfering with thyroid function
Phenindione	Hemorrhage
Thiouracil	Decreased thyroid function (does not apply to propylthiouracil)

*Data not available for other cytotoxic agents.
†Drug is concentrated in breast milk.

TABLE 2-3.
Drugs That Mandate Temporary Cessation of Breast-feeding*

Drug	Recommended Alteration in Breast-Feeding Pattern
Metronidazole	Discontinue breast-feeding 12–24 hr to allow excretion of dose.
Radiopharmaceuticals	Radioactivity present in milk. Consult nuclear medicine physician before performing diagnostic study so that radionuclide with shortest excretion time in breast milk can be used. Prior to study the mother should pump her breast and store enough milk in freezer for feeding the infant; after study the mother should pump her breast to maintain milk production but discard all milk pumped for the required time that radioactivity is present in milk.
Gallium 69	Radioactivity in milk present for 2 wk.
Iodine 125	Risk of thyroid cancer; radioactivity in milk present for 12 days.
Iodine 131	Radioactivity in milk present 2–14 days, depending on study.
Radioactive sodium	Radioactivity in milk present 96 hr.
Technetium 99m ^{99m}Tc macroaggregates, ^{99m}Tc O$_4$	Radioactivity in milk present 15 hr to 3 days.

*From Committee on Drugs, American Academy of Pediatrics: *Pediatrics* 1983; 72:375. Used by permission.

Environmental pollutants such as *polychlorinated biphenyls* (*PCBs* and *PBBs*) also are present in breast milk. Although toxic effects are reported when contamination with PCBs and PBBs occurs,[18] there is no evidence of either immediate or long-term hazard from low levels of exposure to these chemical pollutants.

The report of the Committee on Drugs of the American Academy of Pediatrics[7] provides ready, helpful information to the clinician in prescribing drugs to a nursing mother. Because most drugs are safe for a nursing mother to use, it is advantageous to remember the few drugs that are contraindicated or the drug therapy during which temporary cessation of breast-feeding is indicated.

The drugs listed in Tables 2–2 and 2–3 are contraindicated during breast-feeding.

REFERENCES

1. Berlin CMJN: Excretion of methyl xanthines in human milk. *Semin Perinatol* 1981; 5:389–394.
2. Briggs GC, Freeman RK, Yaffe SJ: *Drugs in Pregnancy and Lactation,* ed 2. Baltimore, Williams & Wilkins Co, 1986.
3. Cam PC: A new skin epidemic in infants. *Ann Dermatol Venereol* 1960; 87:393–396.
4. Chasnoff IJ, Lewis DE, Squires L: Cocaine intoxication in a breast-fed infant. *Pediatrics* 1987; 80:836–838.
5. Cobrinik RW, Hood RT, Chusid E: The effect of maternal narcotic addiction on the newborn infant. *Pediatrics* 1959; 24:288–304.
6. Committee on Drugs (American Academy of Pediatrics). Breastfeeding and contraception. *Pediatrics* 1981; 68:138–140.
7. Committee on Drugs (American Academy of Pediatrics). The transfer of drugs and other chemicals into human breast milk. *Pediatrics* 1983; 72:375–383.
8. Erickson SH, Oppenheim GI, Smith GH: Metronidazole in breast milk. *Obstet Gynecol* 1981; 57:48–50.
9. Fanaroff AA, Martin RJ: *Neonatal-Perinatal Medicine—Diseases of the Fetus and Infant,* ed 4. St Louis, CV Mosby Co, 1987, 293.
10. Ferguson BB, Wilson DJ, Schaffner W: Determination of nicotine concentrations in human milk. *Am J Dis Child* 1976; 130:837–839.
11. Giacoia GP, Catz CS: Drugs and pollutants in breast milk. *Clin Perinatol* 1979; 6:181–196.
12. Honour AJ, Myant NB, Rowlands EN: Secretion of radioiodine in digestive juices and milk in man. *Clin Sci* 1952; 11:447–462.
13. Kampmann JP, et al: Propylthiouracil in human milk. *Lancet* 1980; 1:736–738.
14. Kaneko S, Sato T, Suziki K: The levels of anticonvulsants in breast milk. *Br J Clin Pharmacol* 1979; 7:624–629.
15. Kauffman RE, O'Brien C, Gilford P: Sulfisoxazole secretion into human milk. *J Pediatr* 1980; 97:839–841.
16. Kesaniemi YA: Ethanol and acetaldehyde in the milk and peripheral blood of lactating women after ethanol administration. *J Obstet Gynaecol Br Commonwealth* 1974; 81:84–86.

17. Mann CF: Clindamycin and breastfeeding (editorial correspondence). *Pediatrics* 1980; 66:1030.
18. Miller RW: Pollutants in breast milk. *J Pediatr* 1977; 90:510–511.
19. O'Brien TE: Excretion of drugs in human milk. *Am J Hosp Pharm* 1974; 31:844–854.
20. Palmer KE: Excretion of ^{125}I in breastmilk following administration of labelled fibrinogen. *Br J Radiol* 1979; 52:672–676.
21. Patrick MJ, Tilstone WJ, Reavey P: Diazepam and breast-feeding. *Lancet* 1972; 1:542–543.
22. Perlman HH, Dannenberg NM, Sokoloff N: The excretion of nicotine in breast milk and urine from cigarette smoking. *JAMA* 1942; 120:1003–1009.
23. Pittard WB III, Mer Katz R, Fletcher BD: Radioactive excretion in human milk following administration of technetium (Tc[99m]) macroaggregated albumin. *Pediatrics* 1982; 70:231–234.
24. Sykes PA, Quarrie J, Alexander FW: Lithium carbonate and breast-feeding. *Br Med J* 1976; 21:1299.
25. White WB, Andreol JW, Cohn RD: Alpha-methyldopa disposition in mothers with hypertension and in their breast-fed infants. *Clin Pharmacol Ther* 1985; 37:387–390.

3

Infants of Drug-dependent Mothers

Gopal Srinivasan, M.D.

Infants of drug-dependent mothers (IDDM) are at risk for a number of problems both perinatally and postnatally. Most drugs potentially can cross the placenta, and their effects on the fetus and neonate depend on (1) dose, (2) duration of addiction, (3) ability of the mother and fetus to metabolize the drug, and (4) response of the fetus to the offending agent. Genetic differences can modulate the severity of impact of a given drug. The effects may be caused by the drug itself or by one of its metabolites. The malformations can be nonspecific or can have a pattern of specificity, such as that of fetal alcohol syndrome.

Higher incidence of abortion, stillbirth, meconium-stained amniotic fluid, maternal anemia, premature rupture of membranes, placenta previa, abruptio placentae, and multiple births can be associated with maternal drug abuse. A higher incidence of neonatal syphilis, gonorrhea, hepatitis, and human immunodeficiency virus infection also has been reported. Increased incidence of intrauterine growth retardation (IUGR) and prematurity increases the risk for poor outcome.

Neonatal withdrawal syndrome is easily recognizable. Seventeen percent to 90% of IDDM show signs of withdrawal. Symptoms are due to autonomic and central nervous system dysfunction. The classic signs of withdrawal are tremors, irritability, hypertonia, high-pitched cry, frantic sucking of hands, vomiting, diarrhea, poor feeding, excessive sweating, nasal congestion, frequent sneezing and yawning, low-grade fever, and tachypnea; convulsions have also been reported. Most infants undergoing withdrawal will have seven or more of these symptoms. The severity and duration of symptoms may vary depending on individual tolerance and the presence of other factors discussed previously.

Mortality is high among IDDM, due to immaturity, aspiration pneumonia, malformation, and sudden infant death syndrome (SIDS). Infants born to opiate-abusing mothers have decreased ventilatory response to carbon diox-

TABLE 3–1.
Differences and Similarities Between Infants of Heroin Addicts and of
Methadone-Dependent Mothers

Effects	Heroin	Methadone
Increased incidence of prematurity	+	−
Intrauterine growth retardation	+	+
Acceleration of lung maturity	+	−
Decreased incidence of jaundice	+	−
Onset of withdrawal symptoms	Early	Late
Head circumference less than 3rd percentile	+	+*
Autonomic nervous system imbalance	+	+
Excessive sweating	+	+
Postnatal transient high blood pressure	−	+
Sudden infant death syndrome	+	+

*Significantly "greater incidence."

ide. Pneumograms in these infants may appear abnormal, with increased total sleep time, duration of apneas, and respiratory rate and may explain the increased incidence of SIDS.[17]

An increased incidence of congenital malformations has been reported by Ostrea and Chavez.[13] The reported malformations were cardiac anomalies (ventricular septal defect, patent ductus arteriosus, interrupted aortic arch), genitourinary tract anomalies (hypospadias, posterior urethral valve, multicystic kidney), hydrocephalus, and malrotation of the intestines.

DRUGS ASSOCIATED WITH NEONATAL WITHDRAWAL SYNDROME

Narcotics

Heroin and methadone abuse in pregnancy has profound effects on the fetus and neonate. The differences and similarities between infants of heroin addicts and infants of methadone-dependent mothers are listed in Table 3–1.

Postnatal depression caused by (1) drug overdose, (2) shift in the oxyhemoglobin curve to the right, (3) respiratory alkalosis secondary to tachypnea from CNS effects, (4) excessive sweating, and (5) sleep disturbances has been reported with heroin and methadone addiction. Although the incidence of premature birth is only slightly higher in methadone addicts than in the general population, it is significantly higher (18% to 25%) among heroin addicts. Infants of heroin addicts have lower levels of serum bilirubin due to induction of glucoronyl transferase. Codeine (in prescription cough syrups) can also result in withdrawal symptoms.

Barbiturates

Seizures have been reported in infants soon after birth from withdrawal from short-acting barbiturates. Because long-acting barbiturates have a prolonged half-life, infants may not show signs of withdrawal at the time of hospital discharge.

Analgesics, Tranquilizers, Sedatives

Neonatal abstinence syndromes have been reported following the maternal use of diazepam (Valium) chlordiazepoxide (Librium), hydroxyzine (Atarax), glutethimide (Doriden), ethchlorvynol (Placidyl), propoxyphene hydrochloride (Darvon), and pentazocine (Talwin). There are very few case reports of withdrawal syndrome, however, compared with the large-scale use of analgesics, tranquilizers, and sedatives in pregnant women. Although no known teratogenic effects have been reported, these drugs should be used with caution during pregnancy.

Sympathomimetics

Amphetamines have been linked to biliary atresia,[11] and teratogenic effects and behavior disturbances were noted in experimental animals exposed to amphetamines in utero. No teratogenecity has been reported in human neonates.

Phencyclidine

Phencyclidine [(1-phenylcyclohexyl)piperidine], an arylcyclohexamine, is popular among teenagers because of its low cost and availability. Phencyclidine crosses the placenta. Rapid oxidative hydroxylation is the major pathway for conversion of the drug to its inactive metabolites, which are excreted in the urine. In addition to abstinence syndrome, dysmorphic features, neurologic abnormalities, and microcephaly have been reported as a result of maternal addiction in pregnancy; these findings are suggestive of teratogenic effects.[9]

Cocaine

Cocaine acts as a CNS stimulant while peripherally causing vasoconstriction, tachycardia, and rapid rise in blood pressure. Cocaine use during pregnancy is associated with increased rate of spontaneous abortion and abruptio placentae, resulting in increased incidence of prematurity and stillbirth.[3, 7] Cocaine users had infants with lower weight, length, and head circumference than nonusers.[18]

Infants exposed to cocaine were noted to have significant depression of interactive behavior and poor organizational response to environmental stimuli by Brazelton neonatal behavioral assessment.[3] The severity of abstinence syndrome of infants exposed to cocaine was not significantly different from a methadone group.[15] Hypertension, tachycardia, and cerebral infarction have been reported after a large dose of intravenous cocaine by the mother prior to delivery.[4] The preliminary reports suggesting 15% incidence of SIDS have not been confirmed in subsequent study.[1] Doberczak et al.[8] reported transient CNS irritability and abnormal neonatal EEG after intrauterine exposure to cocaine.

Increased incidence of genitourinary tract malformation has been noted among infants born to cocaine-dependent women compared with polydrug users and non-drug-dependent women.[6] Other teratogenic effects include skull defects, exencephaly, interparietal encephalocele, and parietal bone defects without herniation of brain tissue or meninges[2]; skull defects are similar to those observed in mice exposed to cocaine, and the exact mechanism of teratogenicity is unknown. On the other hand, no evident symptoms or teratogenicity was noted in one report.[12]

Maternal cocaine use during breast-feeding has been reported to cause clinical manifestations of cocaine intoxication in the infant, including tachycardia, tachypnea, hypertension, irritability, and tremors. Therefore, breast-feeding during cocaine abuse is contraindicated.

TREATMENT

Treatment should be instituted as early in pregnancy as possible to avoid the adverse effects of drugs on the development of the fetus. Intrapartum fetal monitoring during labor and delivery and prevention of maternal withdrawal with methadone or meperidine will prevent morbidity from fetal distress, aspiration, and birth asphyxia. Naloxone is not a recommended treatment for respiratory depression at birth in IDDM because the drug may precipitate acute withdrawal symptoms including seizures.

In the neonatal period therapy is directed not only at treatment of withdrawal syndrome but also at problems secondary to prematurity and IUGR. Supportive care includes correction of hypoglycemia and polycythemia, provision of adequate calories and fluids, and management of problems resulting from prematurity.

Not all infants undergoing withdrawal require therapeutic intervention with drugs. In an effort to standardize observations, several scoring systems have been developed. In a simple scoring system suggested by Kahn et al.,[10] the severity of abstinence syndrome is graded as follows:

Grade I: Mild but recognizable as abnormal
Grade II: Symptoms only when disturbed
Grade III: Symptoms at frequent intervals, even when undisturbed

A quiet, comforting environment with gentle handling, swaddling, and frequent feeding may be sufficient in mildly symptomatic cases (grades I and II). Treatment with drugs is indicated only when symptoms interfere with adequate weight gain and well-being (grade III). These signs and symptoms include marked irritability even when undisturbed, seizures, and vomiting or diarrhea. Various pharmacologic agents used for treatment of withdrawal are listed in Table 3–2.

The dosage of the drug to be used is titrated, beginning with the smallest recommended dose and increased until the desired response is achieved. Once the neonate is asymptomatic for 2 or 3 days, the drug dosage is tapered. The tapering process is started by lowering the dose and decreasing the frequency of administration. This process should be continued every 2 to 3 days as long as symptoms of withdrawal do not reappear. Therapeutic regimens vary considerably among institutions and the choice of the pharmacologic agent is arbitrary, indicating that an optimum regimen has not been established. Phenobarbital or chlorpromazine is preferred in our nursery because of their safety and easy availability. Paregoric is recommended for infants with diarrhea.

Paregoric

Paregoric (camphorated tincture of opium) has been the most popular opiate for treatment of withdrawal symptoms since the nineteenth century. It is simple to administer and appears to restore normal CNS function, as measured by the sucking behavior of infants. Paregoric cannot be used if vomiting is present, and constipation may be a problem during treatment. Twenty-four to 28 hours are needed to reach the proper dose to control symptoms adequately, and a prolonged period is necessary for tapering of the drug. The total duration of the therapy is 20 to 45 days. Paregoric contains camphor, a known CNS stimulant. Camphor is absorbed rapidly and excreted slowly because of its lipid solubility, and requires glucuronide conjugation. Laudanum (tincture of opium) does not contain camphor and is preferable whenever a narcotic is used. However, caution must be exercised in using the correct dilution, as laudanum is a 10% solution equivalent to 1% mor-

TABLE 3–2.
Drugs Used for Treatment of Neonatal Withdrawal Syndrome*

Drug	Dose	Route of Administration	Interval Between Doses (hr)
Paregoric	0.05–0.1 mL/kg	PO	4–6
Phenobarbital	1–2 mg/kg	IM or PO	6
Chlorpromazine	0.5–0.7 mg/kg	IM or PO	4–6
Diazepam	0.3–0.5 mg/kg	IM or PO	8

*From Pildes R, Srinivasan G: Infants of drug dependent mothers. *Curr Pediatr Ther* 1986; 12:713–715. Used by permission.

phine, whereas paregoric contains 0.04% morphine. Laudanum must be diluted 25 times to obtain the same dilution as paregoric; it then can be used similarly to paregoric.

Phenobarbital

Phenobarbital adequately controls the symptoms of withdrawal with the exception of vomiting and diarrhea. This drug can be given intramuscularly or orally. It is an effective anticonvulsant and can be administered intravenously for seizures. Phenobarbital acts as a generalized nonspecific CNS depressant. No standard dose or schedule is available for phenobarbital therapy. In our nursery the drug is given in a dose of 1 to 2 mg/kg every 6 hours and adjusted according to the response. It has been our practice to give a loading dose of 10 to 20 mg/kg IV if seizures are a part of the withdrawal syndrome. The total duration of therapy usually ranges between 10 and 14 days. Excessive sedation is a side effect that may lead to inadequate fluid and caloric intake.

Chlorpromazine

Chlorpromazine has been used in our nursery when vomiting is one of the symptoms of abstinence syndrome. The pharmacokinetics of chlorpromazine have not been well studied in infants. It can be given intramuscularly or orally in a dose of 0.5 to 0.7 mg/kg every 4 to 6 hours. Side effects include occasional hypothermia and cardiovascular effects resulting in hypotension. Extrapyramidal signs may be seen in infants who receive more than 2.8 mg/ kg/day.

Diazepam

Diazepam has been used effectively for treatment of abstinence syndrome. The limited capacity of neonates to excrete diazepam results in rapid achievement of serum concentration and prolonged presence of the drug in circulation. Prolonged half-life accounts for quick tapering of the drug and early discharge. The disadvantages are (1) reappearance of symptoms after discharge, (2) bradycardia, and (3) respiratory depression. The parenteral preparation contains sodium benzoate, which competes with bilirubin for albumin binding sites and increases the risk of toxicity by displacement of albumin-bound bilirubin.

Other Management

Management of the infant also requires sensitivity to the needs of the mother, who may have low self-esteem. Support and encouragement by the hospital staff will improve the mother's self-esteem and promote maternal-infant bonding. Every effort should be made to keep the infant with the mother to promote bonding. Breast-feeding by a drug-dependent mother should be undertaken cautiously. The advantage of promoting maternal-infant bonding must be weighed against the potential risk to the neonate from the drugs excreted in breast milk. Individual variation in drug excretion and tolerance will determine the neurologic status and behavior of the infant. Thus the recommendation of breast-feeding must be individualized and based on the risk-benefit ratio to the neonate.

Social service departments should be involved to assess the family situation prior to discharge and to arrange follow-up visits by a visiting nurse, social worker, and drug counselor to ensure adequate supervision of the child's care. Despite all efforts, 15% to 20% of IDDM require placement in foster homes, either because of child abuse or because the mother is unable to respond to the child's needs.

LONG-TERM PROGNOSIS

Although an increased incidence of SIDS and thrombocytosis has been reported in infants of methadone addicts, only limited information is available on the long-term effects of illicit drug exposure in utero. Irritability, hyperactivity, feeding problems, sleep disturbances, and hypertonicity may persist for several months. The follow-up of children of methadone-maintained mothers has shown these children to have a significantly higher incidence of otitis media, head circumference below the 3rd percentile, neurologic deficits of tone discrepancies, developmental delays, poor fine motor coordination, abnormal eye findings (strabismus, nystagmus), and lower scores on the Bayley mental and motor indices.[14] On the other hand, Chasnoff et al.[5] found the mental and psychomotor development in infants exposed prenatally to drugs, measured by the Bayley Scales of Infant Development, comparable to that in control infants through 2 years of age.

REFERENCES

1. Bauchner H, Zuckerman B, McClain M, et al: Risk of sudden infant death syndrome among infants with in utero exposure to cocaine. *J Pediatr* 1988; 113:831–833.
2. Bingol N, Fuchs M, Diaz V, et al: Teratogenicity of cocaine in humans. *J Pediatr* 1987; 110:93–96.
3. Chasnoff I, Burns W, Schnoll S, et al: Cocaine use in pregnancy. *N Engl J Med* 1985; 313:666–669.
4. Chasnoff I, Bussey M, Savich R, et al: Perinatal cerebral infarction and maternal cocaine use. *J Pediatr* 1986; 108:456–459.

5. Chasnoff I, Burns KA, Burns W, et al: Prenatal drug exposure: Effects on neonatal and infant growth and development. *Neurobehav Toxicol Teratol* 1986; 8:357–362.
6. Chasnoff I, Chisum GM, Kaplan W: Maternal cocaine use and genitourinary tract malformations. *Teratology* 1988; 37:201–204.
7. Cherukuri R, Minkoff H, Feldman J, et al: A cohort study of alkaloidal cocaine in pregnancy. *Obstet Gynecol* 1988; 72:147–151.
8. Doberczak T, Shanzer S, Senie R, et al: Neonatal neurologic and electroencephalographic effects of intrauterine cocaine exposure. *J Pediatr* 1988; 113:354–358.
9. Golden NL, Sokol RJ, Rubin JL: Angel dust: Possible effects on the fetus. *Pediatrics* 1980; 65:18–20.
10. Kahn EJ, Neumann LL, Polk GA: The course of the heroin withdrawal syndrome in newborn infants treated with phenobarbital or chlorpromazine. *J Pediatr* 1969; 75:495–500.
11. Levine JN: Amphetamine ingestion with biliary atresia. *J Pediatr* 1971; 79:130–131.
12. Madden J, Payne T, Miller S: Maternal cocaine abuse and effect on the newborn. *Pediatrics* 1986; 77:209–211.
13. Ostrea EM Jr, Chavez CJ: Perinatal problems (excluding neonatal withdrawal) in maternal drug addiction: A study of 83 cases. *J Pediatr* 1979; 94:292–295.
14. Rosen TS, Johnson HL: Children of methadone maintained mothers: Follow-up to 18 months of age. *J Pediatr* 1982; 101:192–196.
15. Ryan L, Ehrlich S, Finnegan L: Cocaine abuse in pregnancy: Effect on fetus and newborn. *Neonatol Teratol* 1987; 9:295–299.
16. Pildes RS, Srinivasan G: Infants of drug dependent mothers. *Curr Pediatr Ther* 1986; 12:713–715.
17. Ward S, Schuetz S, Krishna V, et al: Abnormal ventilatory patterns in infant of substance-abusing mothers. *Am J Dis Child* 1986; 140:1015–1020.
18. Zuckerman B, Frank D, Hingson R, et al: Effects of maternal marijuana and cocaine use on fetal growth. *N Engl J Med* 1989; 320:762–768.

4

Apnea

Devyani S. Raval, M.D.

Shirley Reitz, Ph.D.

Tsu F. Yeh, M.D.

Apnea is generally defined as cessation of respiration for more than 20 seconds, with or without bradycardia, cyanosis, or both. Incidence of apnea varies from 25% in infants weighing less than 2,500 g[16] to 84% to 90% in infants weighing less than 1,000 g.[1] Half the infants with periodic breathing develop apnea.[16] Apnea occurs most frequently between the fifth and seventh postnatal days and has been considered a contributing factor to significant morbidity and mortality in premature infants.

PATHOPHYSIOLOGY

Two major control systems regulate pulmonary ventilation: the neural and the chemical systems. The neural system primarily encompasses regulation of respiratory rate and rhythmicity; the chemical system primarily involves the maintenance of alveolar ventilation appropriate for the rate of carbon dioxide production. The chemical system is the principal defense against hypoxia. Both control systems have a central and a peripheral component. The central component of the neural control system is governed voluntarily by the cerebral cortex and involuntarily by various groups of neurons within the brain stem. The peripheral component of the neural control system is located on receptors in the upper airway and lung (slowly adapting stretch receptors, rapidly adapting receptors, and J receptors). The central component of the chemical control system is located in the medulla and responds to changes in arterial carbon dioxide pressure (tension) ($Paco_2$), and the peripheral component is located in carotid and aortic bodies and responds to changes in partial pressure of oxygen (Pao_2). The general scheme of ventilatory control is shown in Figure 4–1.[14] Impinging on the brain stem

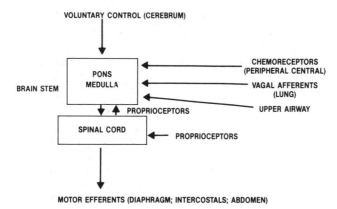

FIG 4–1.
General scheme of ventilatory control.

centers are a variety of chemical and nonchemical stimuli, which are integrated and result in a signal output that has a characteristic amplitude, frequency, and rhythmicity. This output is modulated by ascending and local spinal reflexes in the cord, thus affecting the phrenic, intercostal, and abdominal motoneurons to regulate respiration. The exact mechanisms for the regulation of ventilation in premature infants have not been well established. Various studies suggest that these mechanisms may be imperfect or inadequate, particularly in premature infants.

Physiologic responses to peripheral and central stimuli that are unique to the newborn infant are influenced by the state of oxygenation of the cells, character and intensity of various afferent stimuli, and state of sleep. Unlike adults, whose central and peripheral chemoreceptors are stimulated by hypoxia and hypercapnia, a premature infant subjected to hypoxia responds with an increase and later a decrease in ventilation.[41] Ventilatory response to hypercapnia is less in infants of early gestational age, indicating immaturity of the respiratory center.[42]

Neonates may respond to lung inflation with a gasp and apnea. Moreover the presence of specific laryngeal receptors may cause apnea on instillation of water, milk, or glucose.[18] In a recent study in preterm infants, saline solution and water instillation elicited swallowing, central apnea, and airway obstruction, confirming the presence of upper airway chemoreflex and arousal.[17] Cordero and Hon[15] demonstrated cardiac arrhythmias in newborn infants during nasopharyngeal suctioning, which suggests excessive vagal activity. Autonomic activities such as stooling, feeding, and stretching can induce apnea in the newborn. It has been observed that sudden changes in environmental temperature[37] or exposure to a higher neutral thermal range of environmental temperature can cause apnea.

Various central mechanisms may cause apnea, including hypoxia, depressant drugs, seizures, and state of sleep. During sleep associated with rapid eye movement (REM, active sleep), in addition to increased oxygen consumption,[40] the inhibitory influence on respiratory spinal motor neurons and their afferents not only affect respiratory rate and rhythm but also rib cage stability and synchronization of intercostal muscle and diaphragmatic activity.[13] A recent study has postulated an association between apnea and diaphragmatic workloads with diaphragmatic fatigue.[27]

CAUSES AND CLASSIFICATION OF APNEA

Clinically, various conditions may cause apnea by either producing hypoxia or altering peripheral or central chemoreceptor sensitivity. Conditions associated with apnea are shown in Table 4–1.

Classification of apnea as either central or obstructive is important and helpful for etiologic identification and for initiation of proper management. With the introduction of noninvasive methods that record impedance (pneumograph), heart rate, and air flow (nasal thermistor), improved documentation of frequency, duration, and intensity of neonatal apnea and bradycardia can be achieved.

TABLE 4–1.
Conditions Associated With Apnea

Prematurity (35 weeks)
Environmental factors
  Rapid increase of environmental temperature, vigorous suctioning, feeding, stooling, stretching
Metabolic disorders
  Hypoglycemia, hypocalcemia, hyponatremia
Infection
  Pneumonia, sepsis, meningitis
Respiratory distress
  Progressing hyaline membrane disease, alveolar overdistention with continuous positive airway pressure application, obstruction, postextubation, congenital anomalies of upper airways
Cardiovascular disorders
  Patent ductus arteriosus, congestive heart failure
Gastrointestinal tract disorders
  Feeding, regurgitation, gastroesophageal reflux, necrotizing enterocolitis
CNS disorders
  Depressant drugs, intracranial hemorrhage, seizure, kernicterus, infection, tumors, birth asphyxia
Maldevelopment of upper airway
  Examples include Pierre Robin syndrome, Down syndrome
Other
  Polycythemia, anemia

During normal breathing there are regular fluctuations in impedance and thermistor fluctuations, followed by a decline in heart rate. In obstructive apnea the nasal thermistor signal no longer fluctuates, whereas the impedance tracing continues to exhibit fluctuations that are wider and more erratic. The decrease in heart rate may be mistaken for isolated bradycardias if only an impedance pneumograph is obtained.

In a study[19] of 76 preterm infants with clinical apnea and bradycardia, 433 apneic episodes were demonstrated; 238 (55%) were central, 53 (12.2%) obstructive, and 142 (32.8%) mixed. The majority of the infants, however, had some degree of obstructive apnea.

Several clinical and animal studies have tried to delineate the anatomic site of obstruction. In infants with anatomically normal airways, Mathew et al.[33] suggested that the location of airway obstruction was in the oropharynx, similar to the site of obstruction seen in older children and adults with sleep apnea syndrome. Human and animal experiments have documented that the decrease in genioglossal tone allows the tongue to flop back and come in contact with the posterior pharynx.[39] In addition, neck flexion can raise closing pressure, making the airway more susceptible to collapse.[46] Stark and Bradley[43] have shown that neck flexion in preterm infants markedly diminishes airflow or functionally occludes the upper airway. These infants continue to make ineffectual respiratory efforts without arousing or struggling. The proper neck position reduces the upper airway occlusion and precludes obstructive apnea.

MANAGEMENT

General Principles

Avoidance of Triggering Reflexes
Sudden environmental temperature changes, higher range of neutral thermal environmental temperature, vigorous nasopharyngeal suctioning, feeding, stooling, and stretching have been shown to cause apnea and should be prevented or closely monitored.[16]

Treatment of Underlying Causes
After initiation of normal respiration, attention should be directed to finding the underlying causes of apnea. This includes a thorough history and physical examination; temperature recording; monitoring of blood pressure and blood gases; determination of hematocrit, glucose, electrolyte, and calcium values; complete blood cell count with differential count; and ultrasonography of the head. If clinically indicated, additional tests (e.g., blood culture, spinal tap, abdominal radiography, barium swallow, electrocardiography, electroencephalography, echocardiography, and computed tomography) may be necessary. Once the underlying causes of apnea have been established, appropriate treatment should be started immediately.

Treatment of Hypoxia

A slight (5% to 10%) increase in environmental oxygen can eliminate periodic breathing and decrease the frequency of apnea. This change should be performed with continuous transcutaneous oxygen pressure ($tcPO_2$) monitoring to avoid hyperoxia.

Increasing Afferent Input

Afferent input can be increased by intermittent cutaneous stimulation, which has been shown to decrease apneic episodes.

Proprioceptive Stimulation

Afferent vestibular proprioceptive stimulation by use of a waterbed with an oscillator has led to a significant decrease in apneic episodes. Reduction of frequency of apnea by 25%, 35%, and 29% of central, obstructive, and mixed apneas, respectively, was observed with use of the waterbed[29]; moreover, infants were found to have significantly more quiet sleep, shorter sleep latencies, and less restlessness during sleep.

Treatment With Continuous Positive Airway Pressure

Prolonged apnea occurs during the expiratory phase of the respiratory cycle, when the alveoli tend to collapse. In nonstressed premature infants there are large areas of underventilated but adequately perfused alveoli and progressive decline in thoracic gas volume in the first week of life, when apneic spells become prevalent. Krauss et al.[30] have shown that there is a gradual decline in functional residual capacity (FRC) in apnea associated with "chronic pulmonary insufficiency of prematurity." It therefore seems logical that the low pressure of continuous positive airway pressure (CPAP) may increase the FRC, decrease intrapulmonary shunting, and regularize breathing.

Another mechanism that has been proposed[32] to explain this phenomenon is elimination of the Hering-Breuer deflation reflex with CPAP, which enhances the infant's ability to increase respiratory loads and decrease respiratory rate. Hagan et al.[25] have proposed that rapid distortion of the rib cage triggers an intercostal phrenic inhibitory reflex that terminates inspiration. CPAP probably inhibits this reflex by stabilizing the chest wall. Low pressure (3 to 5 cm HO_2) in CPAP is recommended for transient apnea.

DRUG THERAPY

In the past decade, various respiratory stimulants have been tried for the treatment of "idiopathic apnea." In the neonate the methylxanthines (theophylline, amninophylline, caffeine) and doxapram have been widely studied and used. Because experience with methylxanthines is fairly extensive, they are discussed in detail.

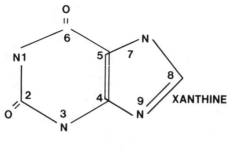

1, 3 dimethyl = theophylline
3, 7 dimethyl = theobromine
1, 3, 7 tri dimethyl = caffeine

FIG 4–2.
Chemical structure of methylxanthine.

Theophylline (Fig 4–2)

Theophylline has been recognized as a respiratory stimulant since the 1920s. Kuzemko and Paala[31] first described the use of rectal theophylline in reducing the frequency of apneic spells in newborn infants. Subsequent studies have confirmed that theophylline decreases both the severity and frequency of apnea in the neonate, although total abolition of apneic spells may not be achieved.

Mechanism of Action.—Several mechanisms have been proposed for the action of theophylline, the most accepted being enhancement of cyclic adenosine monophosphate and catecholamines by inhibition of phosphodiesterase. Studies in preterm apneic infants have shown lower levels of dopamine, norepinephrine, and epinephrine. Other proposed mechanisms of action are alteration of intracellular calcium, which increases skeletal muscle contraction, neuromuscular transmission, and release of catecholamines from the adrenal medulla. Table 4–2 summarizes the pharmacologic effects of methylxanthines. Pharmacokinetic data are shown in Table 4–3.

Absorption.—Theophylline is virtually 100% absorbed when given by mouth in infants, children, and adults. Absorption is hindered by food intake, and in the neonate may be further hindered by relative achlorhydria, prolonged gastric emptying time, or unpredictable peristalsis. Absorption from rectal suppositories is erratic; retention enemas are more reliable.

Aminophylline, an ethylenediamine complex of theophylline (consisting of 70% to 85% theophylline) can be given intravenously or intramuscularly. Intravenous administration causes prompt achievement of therapeutic levels; intramuscular administration causes intense local pain and sloughing and results in somewhat lower levels in the blood.

TABLE 4–2.
Pharmacologic Effects of Methylxanthines

Respiratory
  Increases surfactant production, inspiratory drive, respiratory rate, Pco_2 sensitivity
Cardiovascular
  Increases heart rate and cardiac contractility
  Dilates pulmonary, coronary, and renal vessels
  Reduces peripheral vascular resistance
Alimentary
  Decreases gastrointestinal motility
  Increases gastric secretion
CNS
  Increases CNS stimulation (jitteriness, seizure) and cerebral oxygen consumption
  Decreases cerebral blood flow
Endocrine
  Increases catecholamine and insulin levels
Metabolic
  Increases glucose levels, ketouria, glycosuria
Hematopoietic
  Increases coagulation
Renal
  Increases renal blood flow and diuresis
Musculoskeletal
  Increases muscle contraction
  Decreases fatigue

Distribution.—The apparent volume of distribution (aVD) is significantly larger in the neonate than in older infants and young children, due in part to the lower theophylline protein binding found in neonates. Aranda et al.[3] found that $56 \pm 3.8\%$ of theophylline was bound to protein in adult plasma, whereas only $36.4 \pm 3.8\%$ was bound to protein in the full-term neonate.

Metabolism and Excretion.—Theophylline is metabolized by way of the hepatic cytochrome P-450 monooxygenase system. In children and adults this metabolic pathway results in very little theophylline excreted unchanged in the urine, most undergoing hydroxylation and N-demethylation to form the metabolites 3-methylxanthine (3-MX), 1-methyluric acid (1-MU), and 1,3-dimethyluric acid (1,3-DMU). In the neonate, either the activity or the quantity of enzymes in these metabolic pathways is deficient, resulting in decreased oxidative metabolism of theophylline. The N-methylation pathway is active in the fetal liver as early as 12 weeks of gestation.[5] Several authors have demonstrated the interconversion of theophylline and caffeine.[6, 11, 12] In the neonate the major urinary metabolites include caffeine, 1,3-DMU, 1-MU, and unchanged theophylline.[10] The metabolic pathway of theophylline in newborn infants, children, and adults is shown in Figure 4–3.

TABLE 4–3.
Drugs Used for Treatment of Apnea: Dosage Recommendations and Pharmacokinetic Data

Drug	Loading Dose (mg/kg)	Maintenance Dose (mg/kg)	Recommended Serum Concentration (mg/L)	Apparent Volume of Distribution (L/kg)	Half-life (hr)	Route of Administration
Aminophylline	5.0–6.0	1.1–3.0 q8h	5–15	0.6–0.7	30–33	IV
Theophylline	4.0–5.0	2.0 q12hr 1.0 q8hr	5–15	0.6–1.0	19–30	PO
Caffeine citrate	20	2.5–5.0 q24hr	8–20	0.9	102.9	PO or IV
Doxapram	5.5	1–2.5 qh	1.5–5.0	7.3	8–10	IV

Dosing and Administration.—The therapeutic plasma levels of theophylline range from 5 to 15 μg/mL, although it has been shown that serum concentrations as low as 3 to 4 μg/mL are associated with a decrease in apneic episodes.[35] The recommended loading dose of theophylline is 5.0 to 6.0 mg/kg, which could generate a plasma concentration of 10 μg/mL. Recommended maintenance doses vary widely; most studies recommend 1.1 to 3 mg/kg every 8 hours. Doses recommended by the U.S. Food and Drug Administration for apnea of prematurity (1985) have been criticized for producing subtherapeutic theophylline concentrations.[21, 34] Doses of theophylline during the first 3 weeks of life should also take into account that clearance values in asphyxiated neonates are 20% to 50% lower than in nonasphyxiated babies.[22]

Aminophylline should be given intravenously over 10 to 15 minutes. Peak levels should be obtained 1 hour after intravenous and 1 to 2 hours after oral administration; samples for determination of trough levels should be drawn before the next dose. Toback et al.[44] documented salivary theophylline concentrations in premature neonates that were approximately equal to serum concentrations, suggesting that salivary concentrations may be clinically useful when serum is not readily available.

Percutaneous administration of theophylline can be achieved in the preterm infant with a poorly developed dermis. Evans et al.[20] established the attainment of therapeutic levels of theophylline when a gel containing 17 mg anhydrous theophylline was applied to the upper abdomen of premature infants during the first 3 weeks of life. Absorption of theophylline from a hydrogel disk has also been documented in premature infants.[44] This method of theophylline administration requires further study.

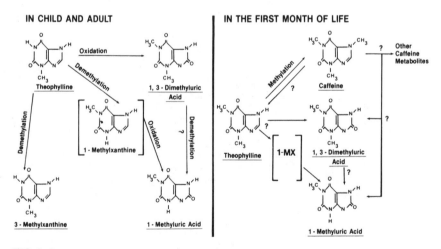

FIG 4–3.
Metabolism of theophylline in the neonate, child, and adult.

Clinical Side Effects.—The adverse effects of theophylline are expressed as an enhancement on the pharmacologic effects, and include (1) tachycardia, arrhythmias; (2) diuresis, glycosuria, ketonuria; (3) hyperglycemia; (4) jitteriness, seizures; (5) vomiting, hemorrhagic gastritis. A heart rate of more than 180 beats per minute and any signs of gastritis require decrease in dosage or cessation of therapy. Drugs such as erythromycin may potentiate the toxic effects of theophylline by competing for metabolizing enzymes. In addition, viral or liver disease, congestive heart failure, and pulmonary edema can increase the half-life of theophylline.

Although it appears that the neonate may tolerate theophylline better than the older population, lack of experience with theophylline overdose in this population limits our ability to draw valid conclusions. Treatment of theophylline overdose in the preterm neonate is symptomatic; more vigorous methods of treatment (e.g., hemoperfusion) have not been studied in the neonate and cannot be advocated at this time.

Caffeine

Caffeine (1,3,7-trimethylxanthine) is structurally related to theophylline (see Fig 4–2), and is prepared synthetically as caffeine sodium benzoate (45% to 52% anhydrous caffeine) and as citrated caffeine (50% anhydrous caffeine). Caffeine sodium benzoate is not recommended in neonates because the benzoate may interact competitively with bilirubin at the albumin binding site. Citrated caffeine may be given orally or intravenously; a parenteral product can be made by the hospital pharmacy department.[36] Caffeine appears to offer several advantages over theophylline, including wider therapeutic index, decreased need for therapeutic monitoring, longer elimination half-life, less frequent dosing, fewer peripheral effects, and potential for effectiveness in some infants not responding to theophylline therapy.

Pharmacokinetics.—Caffeine citrate is absorbed rapidly and completely after oral administration. Caffeine distributes widely in the body, with an average volume of distribution of approximately 0.9 L/kg. Unchanged caffeine accounts for more than 85% of the methylated xanthines and urates found in the urine of infants younger than 1 month of age. By 8 months of age an adultlike pattern of urine caffeine metabolites is reached.[2]

Aranda et al.[4] estimated a half-life of 102.9 hours and clearance of 8.9 mL/kg/hr in premature infants receiving caffeine. Plasma concentrations as low as 3 to 4 μg/mL have been found to abolish apnea and regularize breathing patterns; however, optimal plasma concentrations range from 8 to 20 μg/ml. Concentrations greater than 50 μg/ml have been associated with transient jitteriness.

Dosing Recommendation.—A loading dose of 10 mg/kg caffeine base (20 mg/kg citrated caffeine) yields plasma concentrations between 8 and 14 μg/mL. Because of the long plasma half-life, single daily doses of 2.5 mg/kg caffeine base yield steady-state concentrations between 7 and 19 μg/mL.[4] Pons et al.[38] reported that caffeine elimination half-life varied with gestational and postnatal age; they recommended a maintenance dose of 5.8 (±3.2) mg/kg caffeine base given every 24, 12, 8, or 6 hours in infants younger than 1 month, 1 to 2 months, 2 to 4 months, and older than 4 months of age, respectively.

Long-Term Effects.—There has been some concern about the long-term effect of methylxanthines on growth and development in treated infants; studies in adults given therapeutic doses of theophylline have shown cerebral vasoconstriction and decreased cerebral blood flow. In vitro, methylxanthines have been shown to alter cell division and inhibit cholesterol synthesis. Although a preliminary report from a follow-up study of caffeine-treated neonates at 18 to 36 months has shown no ill effects,[23] further studies are needed in this area.

Doxapram

The use of doxapram as a respiratory stimulant was first described in neonates in 1973 for treatment of depression secondary to the maternal administration of narcotic analgesic drugs.[24] Current trials use doxapram for apnea when the neonate fails to respond to an adequate trial with theophylline.

Mechanism of Action.—It is thought that doxapram acts by stimulating the peripheral (carotid body) chemoreceptors at low doses and by exerting a central stimulating effect at higher doses.

Pharmacokinetics.—There is very little information available regarding the pharmacokinetics of doxapram in neonates. Jamali et al.[28] reported a mean volume of distribution and half-life in premature infants of 7.3 L/kg and 8.2 hours, respectively. Barrington et al.[9] reported an average terminal half-life of 9.9 hours. Doxapram is metabolized by ring hydroxylation to keto-doxapram, an active metabolite.[7]

Dosage Recommendation.—Studies have suggested that the minimum effective concentration of doxapram is 1.5 μg/mL.[9, 28] Concentrations greater than 5.0 μg/mL appear to provide no significant increase in the relief of apnea, but higher incidence of side effects. Based on current pharmacokinetic information, loading doses of 5.5 mg/kg and maintenance doses of 1 mg/kg/hr are recommended[28]; however, doses as high as 2.5 mg/kg/hr may be necessary in some infants unresponsive to lower doses. It is important to remember that the studies defining these recommendations were done in infants already receiving therapeutic doses of theophylline. The doxapram product commercially available in the United States contains benzyl alcohol as a preservative; thus caution is advised when using it in a premature neonate.

Side Effects.—Reported side effects of doxapram appear to be transient and related to its concentration. Abdominal distention, jitteriness, irritability, and vomiting have been associated with serum concentrations greater than 5 μg/mL.[26] Doxapram should be used cautiously, if at all, in infants at risk for seizures or who have had previous seizures.[8] Blood pressure was significantly elevated at doses higher than 1.5 mg/kg/hr.[9]

REFERENCES

1. Alden ER, et al: Morbidity and mortality of infants weighing less than 1000 grams in an intensive care nursery. *Pediatrics* 1972; 50:40–49.
2. Aldridge A, et al: Caffeine metabolism in the newborn. *Clin Pharmacol Ther* 1979; 25:447–453.
3. Aranda JV, et al: Pharmacokinetic aspects of theophylline in premature newborns. *N Engl J Med* 1976; 295:413–416.
4. Aranda JV, et al: Pharmacokinetic profile of caffeine in the premature newborn infant with apnea. *J Pediatr* 1979; 94:663–668.
5. Aranda JV, et al: Metabolism of theophylline to caffeine in human fetal liver. *Science* 1979; 206:1319–1321.
6. Bada SB, et al: Interconversion of theophylline and caffeine in newborn infants. *J Pediatr* 1979; 94:993–995.
7. Bairam A, et al: Kinetics of doxapram and keto-doxapram in newborns. *Pediatr Res* 1989; 25(4 pt 2):64A.
8. Barrington KJ, et al: Physiologic effects of doxapram in idiopathic apnea of prematurity. *J Pediatr* 1986; 108:125–129.
9. Barrington KJ, et al: Dose-response relationship of doxapram in the therapy for refractory idiopathic apnea of prematurity. *Pediatrics* 1987; 80:22–27.
10. Bonati M, et al: Theophylline metabolism during the first month of life and development. *Pediatr Res* 1981; 15:304–308.
11. Bory C, et al: Metabolism of theophylline to caffeine in premature newborn infants. *J Pediatr* 1979; 94:988–995.
12. Boutroy MJ, et al: Caffeine, a metabolite of theophylline during the treatment of apnea in the premature infant. *J Pediatr* 1979; 94:996–998.
13. Bryan AC, Bryan HM: Control of respiration in the newborn. *Clin Perinatol* 1978; 5:269–281.
14. Chernick V: Control of breathing: General principles, in *Breathing in the Fetus and Newborn.* Mead Johnson Symposium on Perinatal and Developmental Medicine, no. 12. Marco Island, Fla, Dec 4–8, 1977, pp 3–6.
15. Cordero L, Hon EH: Neonatal bradycardia following nasopharyngeal stimulation. *J Pediatr* 1971; 78:441–447.
16. Daily WJR, Klaus M, Meyer HBP: Apnea in premature infants monitoring incidence, heart rate changes and an effect of environmental temperature. *Pediatrics* 1978; 43:510–517.
17. Davies AM, Koenig JS, Thach BT: Upper airway chemoreflex responses to saline and water in preterm infants. *J Appl Physiol* 1988; 64:1412–1420.

18. Downing SE, Lee JC: Laryngeal chemosensitivity: A possible mechanism for sudden infant death. *Pediatrics* 1975; 55:640–649.
19. Dransfield DA, Spitzer AR, Fox WW: Episodic airway obstruction in premature infants. *Am J Dis Child* 1983; 137:441–443.
20. Evans NJ, et al: Percutaneous administration of theophylline in the preterm infant. *J Pediatr* 1985; 107:307–311.
21. Gal P, Gilman JT: Concerns about the Food and Drug Administration guidelines for neonatal theophylline dosing. *Ther Drug Monit* 1986; 8:1–3.
22. Gilman JT, et al: Factors influencing theophylline disposition in 179 newborns. *Ther Drug Monit* 1986; 8:4–10.
23. Gunn TR, et al: Sequelae of caffeine treatment in preterm infants with apnea. *J Pediatr* 1979; 94:106–109.
24. Gupta PK, Moore J: The use of doxapram in the newborn. *J Obstet Gynaecol Br Comm* 1973; 80:1002.
25. Hagan R, et al: The effect of stabilization of the rib cage on respiration in preterm infants. *Pediatr Res* 1976; 10:461.
26. Hayakawa F, et al: Doxapram in the treatment of idiopathic apnea of prematurity: Desirable dosage and serum concentrations. *J Pediatr* 1986; 109:138–140.
27. Heldt GP: Development of stability of the respiratory system in preterm infants. *J Appl Physiol* 1988; 65:441–444.
28. Jamali F, et al: Doxapram dosage regimen in apnea of prematurity based on pharmacokinetic data. *Dev Pharmacol Ther* 1988; 11:253–257.
29. Korner AF, et al: Reduction of sleep apnea and bradycardia in preterm infants on oscillating water beds: A controlled polygraphic study. *Pediatrics* 1978; 61:528–533.
30. Krauss AN, Klain DB, Auld PAM: Chronic pulmonary insufficiency of prematurity. *Pediatrics* 1975; 55:55–58.
31. Kuzemko JA, Paala J: Apneic attacks in newborns treated with aminophylline. *Arch Dis Child* 1973; 48:404–406.
32. Martin RJ, et al: The effect of a low continuous positive airway pressure on the reflex control of respiration in the preterm infant. *J Pediatr* 1977; 90:976–981.
33. Mathew OP, Roberts JL, Thach BT: Pharyngeal airway obstruction in preterm infants. *J Pediatr* 1982; 100:964–968.
34. Murphy JE, et al: New FDA guidelines for theophylline dosing in infants. *Clin Pharm* 1986; 5:16.
35. Myers TF, et al: Low-dose theophylline therapy in idiopathic apnea of prematurity. *J Pediatr* 1980; 96:99–103.
36. Nahata MC, et al: Formulation of caffeine injection for I.V. administration. *Am J Hosp Pharm* 1987; 44:1308, 1312.
37. Perlstein PH, Edwards NK, Sutherland JM: Apnea in premature infants and incubator-air-temperature changes. *N Engl J Med* 1070; 282:461–466.
38. Pons G, et al: Developmental changes of caffeine elimination in infancy. *Dev Pharmacol Ther* 1988; 11:258–264.
39. Remmers TE, et al: Pathogenesis of upper airway occlusion during sleep. *J Appl Physiol* 1978; 44:931–938.
40. Rigatto H: Apnea. *Pediatr Clin North Am* 1982; 29:1105–1116.
41. Rigatto H, Brady J, Verduzco RT: Chemoreceptor reflexes in preterm infants: I. The effect of gestational and postnatal age on the ventilatory response to inhalation of 100% and 15% oxygen. *Pediatrics* 1975; 55:604–613.

42. Rigatto H, Brady J, Verduzco RT: Chemoreceptor reflexes in preterm infants: II. The effect of gestational and postnatal age on ventilatory response to inhaled carbon dioxide. *Pediatrics* 1975; 55:614–620.
43. Stark AR, Bradley TT: Mechanisms of airway obstruction leading to apnea in newborn infants. *J Pediatr* 1976; 89:982–985.
44. Toback JW, et al: Usefulness of theophylline saliva levels in neonates. *Ther Drug Monit* 1983; 5:185–189.
45. West DP, et al: Pharmacokinetics and bioavailability of transdermal theophylline in premature and full-term infants. *Clin Res* 1988; 36:908A.
46. Wilson SL, et al: Upper airway patency in the human infant: Influence on airway pressure and posture. *J Appl Physiol* 1980; 48:500–504.

5

Bronchopulmonary Dysplasia

Lily C. Kao, M.D.

David J. Durand, M.D.

Bronchopulmonary dysplasia (BPD) is a complication of mechanical ventilation in newborn infants. Criteria for diagnosis usually include abnormal
chest radiograph, oxygen dependence, and clinical respiratory distress for
more than 28 days in an infant who required mechanical ventilation during
the first week of life.[7] Approximately 15% to 38% of newborns who weigh
less than 1,500 g at birth and who require mechanical ventilation because of
hyaline membrane disease will develop BPD.[50] There is no cure for BPD;
thus our efforts must be directed toward optimizing the infant's pulmonary
function and minimizing iatrogenic complications. In this chapter we review
some of the agents most frequently used to treat BPD, their mechanisms of
action, appropriate dosages, and side effects.

Infants with BPD have abnormal pulmonary function that includes increased respiratory rate, increased airway resistance, increased thoracic gas
volume, decreased dynamic pulmonary compliance, decreased maximal expiratory flow at functional residual capacity, abnormal gas exchange, elevated
oxygen consumption, and increased work of breathing.[23, 49, 53]

A prominent feature of BPD is pulmonary edema, both interstitial and
intra-alveolar.[35] Factors implicated in the cause of this edema include increased capillary permeability and pulmonary vascular pressure, low oncotic
pressure, left ventricular dysfunction, impaired lymphatic drainage, and increased antidiuretic hormone levels.[35, 39] Pulmonary edema causes the decreased dynamic compliance, increased airway resistance, and impaired gas
exchange typical of BPD.

Bronchospasm also plays an important part in BPD symptoms. In contrast
to the small amount of smooth muscle in the airways of healthy infants, who
do not respond to inhaled bronchodilators, infants with BPD have bronchiolar
smooth muscle hypertrophy[41] and clinical and radiographic evidence of airway obstruction.[15] There is often a family history suggestive of an increased
incidence of reactive airway disease.[34] Airway reactivity has been demon-

strated in infants as early as 12 postnatal days and as premature as 26 weeks postconception.[32] In addition, there is evidence that an early increase in pulmonary resistance may precede BPD.[20] These data suggest that infants with BPD are good candidates for bronchodilator therapy and that treatment of this airway obstruction may reduce the severity and incidence of BPD.

DIURETICS

Because of the prominent role of edema in BPD and because diuretics are effective in decreasing pulmonary edema, diuretics were the first agents used to treat BPD. They remain the cornerstone of the pharmacologic treatment of BPD.

Furosemide (Lasix)

Pharmacokinetics.—In neonates, the onset of action of intravenous furosemide occurs within 5 minutes, with peak activity at 20 to 60 minutes and a duration of action of approximately 2 hours. The bioavailability of oral furosemide is less than 20%.[38] At least 94% of plasma furosemide is protein bound.[38]

In infants who weigh less than 1,250 g, furosemide elimination occurs primarily by glomerular filtration. However, by the time infants reach 40 weeks postconception the predominant pathway of elimination may be by the proximal convoluted tubule.[31] The half-life of plasma furosemide in the first 6 weeks of life ranges from 8 to 20 hours.[3, 38]

Mechanism of Action.—The primary diuretic effect of furosemide is to inhibit reabsorption of chloride in the ascending limb of the loop of Henle. Furosemide also decreases reabsorption of sodium and chloride and increases potassium excretion in the distal renal tubule. The magnitude of diuresis is determined by the concentration of intact furosemide present within the renal tubule.[9] Furosemide causes a decrease in renal vascular resistance and increase in renal blood flow that are independent of its diuretic action.

In addition to its renal effects, furosemide has a direct pulmonary vasoactive effect, causing increased venous capacitance, increased oncotic pressure, decreased pulmonary microvascular fluid filtration rate, and increased lymphatic flow. The net result of these actions is a decrease in fluid filtration into the pulmonary interstitium. Furosemide has been shown to decrease vasopressin, an antidiuretic hormone, which is often elevated in infants with BPD.[39] The effects of furosemide may be mediated by prostaglandins and by the renin-angiotensin-aldosterone system.[48] The relative importance of the diuretic and nondiuretic actions of these agents in infants with BPD remains uncertain.

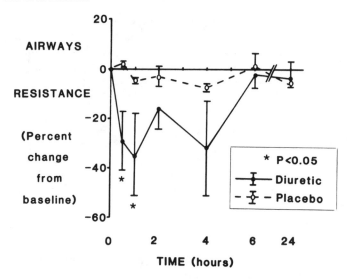

FIG 5–1.
Effect of diuretics and placebo on airways resistance over 24 hours. Resistance
decreased significantly 1 hour after administration of diuretic. Values are mean ± SEM.
(From Kao LC, Warburton D, Sargent CW, et al: *J Pediatr* 1983; 103:624–629. Used by
permission.)

Therapeutic Use in Bronchopulmonary Dysplasia.—We have shown that
there is a rapid, short-term improvement in pulmonary function in infants
recovering from BPD following a single intravenous dose of furosemide (1
mg/kg body weight).[23] Within 1 hour of treatment, airway resistance decreased
36% and dynamic compliance increased 54% (Figs 5–1 and 5–2). By 6 hours,
both compliance and resistance had returned to their baseline values. The
improvement in pulmonary function coincided with an increase in mean
urine output of 226%.

Two studies[17, 30] have shown that a 1-week course of furosemide therapy
causes significant improvement in the pulmonary function of infants with
BPD. The benefits of furosemide therapy for periods longer than 1 week still
remain to be demonstrated in clinical trials, although we believe that long-
term diuretic therapy is helpful for these infants.

Side Effects.—Furosemide causes enhanced excretion of water, calcium,
phosphate, magnesium, sodium, potassium, chloride, and bicarbonate. Hypokalemia, hyponatremia, and hypochloremia can occur within 48 hours of
starting furosemide in infants.[36] One recent study of infants who were hospitalized with severe BPD found that those who died were more likely to
have moderate or severe hypochloremia (less than 80 mEq/L) than those
who survived.[37] Whether this was coincidence or whether the hypochloremia
contributed to their death is unclear.

Urinary calcium excretion in neonates treated with furosemide is 10 to 20 times normal. Although most infants treated with furosemide will maintain a normal serum calcium level, they may develop osteopenia and secondary hyperparathyroidism. The hypercalciuria associated with prolonged furosemide therapy can cause nephrocalcinosis and nephrolithiasis. The incidence of renal calcification diagnosed by serial ultrasound examinations varies from 48% to 64% in infants weighing less than 1,500 g. Most infants with renal calculi are asymptomatic because calculi may pass spontaneously or remain without causing problems. However, nephrolithiasis may cause hematuria, infection, or hypertension. Although age at diagnosis of these calcifications has been reported to vary from 11 days to 5.5 months, we usually detect them in infants who have received at least 1 month of furosemide.

Once renal calcifications are detected, furosemide should probably be discontinued or a combination of furosemide and chlorothiazide should be started. In contrast to furosemide, chlorothiazide decreases renal calcium excretion and leads to dissolution of established renal calcifications. One study suggested that all patients with nephrocalcinosis have either improvement or complete radiographic resolution of the nephrolcalcinosis at the end of 2 years of follow-up.[19] However, renal function may remain compromised.[19] Therefore in infants receiving long-term furosemide therapy renal

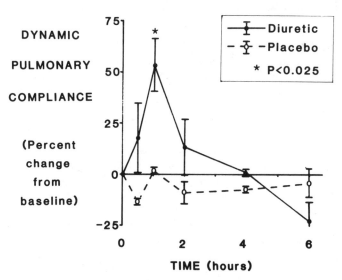

FIG 5–2.
Effect of diuretics and placebo on dynamic pulmonary compliance over 6 hours. Compliance increased significantly 1 hour after administration of diuretic. Values are mean ± SEM. (From Kao LC, Warburton D, Sargent CW, et al: *J Pediatr* 1983; 103:624–629. Used by permission.)

function should be closely monitored and baseline and serial ultrasound examinations performed.

Cholelithiasis has been described in infants receiving both parenteral nutrition and furosemide, possibly because of furosemide-induced reduction in bile flow or increased excretion of biliary calcium.[11]

Adults treated with furosemide for obstructive lung disease develop metabolic alkalosis and compensatory hypoventilation with hypercarbia. Proposed mechanisms for this alkalosis include potassium depletion, renal loss of hydrogen ion, and extracellular fluid space contraction without accompanying bicarbonate loss. Although the same process has been demonstrated in young animals,[22] we have not been convinced that this is a significant cause of hypercarbia in infants with BPD.

Furosemide is potentially ototoxic. In adults the threshold plasma furosemide concentration associated with reversible ototoxicity is 25 µg/mL. Since furosemide has a prolonged half-life in premature infants, parenteral furosemide 1 mg/kg, given more than twice daily, or in excess of 2 mg/kg, may lead to plasma levels associated with ototoxicity.[38] Infants who receive prolonged furosemide therapy, particularly when it is given simultaneously with other potentially toxic drugs, such as aminoglycosides, require periodic and long-term follow-up testing to evaluate hearing.

Furosemide is capable of displacing unconjugated bilirubin from albumin binding sites in vitro. However, it appears that a single dose of furosemide (1 to 1.5 mg/kg) does not change bilirubin binding capacity.[3]

Thiazide Diuretics

Pharmacokinetics.—Chlorothiazide (Diuril) and hydrochlorothiazide (Hydrodiuril) are two thiazides commonly used in neonates. Oral chlorothiazide caused diuresis that peaks between 2 and 6 hours after administration and lasts approximately 8 hours. In a dose of 20 mg/kg, chlorothiazide produces a diuretic response equivalent to that of 1 mg/kg furosemide.[21]

Mechanisms of Action.—Thiazides inhibit sodium reabsorption in both the proximal and distal tubules. The resulting increase of sodium in the lumen of the distal nephron causes enhanced exchange of sodium for potassium and increased excretion of potassium. Chloride is lost in association with the inhibition of sodium reabsorption.

Thiazides also directly cause renal vasoconstriction, resulting in reduced glomerular filtration rate. In contrast to furosemide, thiazides decrease renal excretion of calcium.[24] Thiazides have also been shown to increase thoracic duct lymph flow in animals by an extrarenal effect on water metabolism.

Therapeutic Use in Bronchopulmonary Dysplasia.—We have shown that pulmonary function in infants with BPD improves following combined oral chlorothiazide (20 mg/kg/dose) and spironolactone (1.5 mg/kg/dose) given twice daily.[24, 26] Following 1 week of therapy, airway resistance decreased 41%

and dynamic compliance increased 53% from baseline.[24] There was weight loss during the first 3 days of diuretic treatment, followed by steady weight gain.[24]

The response of infants with BPD to hydrochlorothiazide is less clear. One recent study showed that oral hydrochlorothiazide (2 mg/kg/dose) and spironolactone (1.5 mg/kg/dose) given twice daily for 8 weeks causes increased respiratory system compliance and improved survival of infants with severe BPD.[1] However, another study showed no pulmonary function improvement with this combination of diuretics.[18] One explanation for the difference in response to chlorothiazide plus hydrochlorothiazide may be a difference in their pharmacokinetics and bioavailability.

Side Effects.—Chlorothiazide and hydrochlorothiazide therapy have been associated with abnormal renal losses of sodium, chloride, and potassium. Chlorothiazide causes less calcium excretion than does hydrochlorothiazide.[4, 24]

Potassium-Sparing Diuretics

Spironolactone (Aldactone) inhibits aldosterone-mediated sodium-potassium exchange in the distal tubule. Spironolactone produces only slight diuresis, compared with furosemide, because less than 2% of sodium excretion is aldosterone dependent. Because most sodium is reabsorbed in the proximal renal tubules, spironolactone is relatively ineffective when administered alone. However, it provides significant synergy when combined with a thiazide or loop diuretic that blocks reabsorption of sodium in the proximal tubule. In addition, the potassium-sparing effect of spironolactone partially offsets the potassium losses associated with thiazide administration.[4, 24] Therefore we use a combination of chlorothiazide and spironolactone for treatment of BPD. The diuretic effect of spironolactone is often delayed for 2 to 3 days.

BRONCHODILATORS

Methylxanthines

Pharmacokinetics.—Infants younger than 1 year of age eliminate methylxanthines at a lower rate than do older children and therefore require a much lower dose than older children.[33] Nickerson[34a] proposed the following formula for calculating the daily dosage of theophylline in infants in the first year of life: Daily dose (mg/kg/day) = 8 + Postnatal age (mo). Theophylline dosage should be adjusted according to the serum theophylline levels in each patient. In general, assuming a mean volume of distribution for theophylline of 0.5 L/kg, every 1 mg/kg increase in dose will give a 2 µg/mL increase in serum theophylline concentration.[33]

Intravenous aminophylline contains 79% as much theophylline as does oral theophylline. An oral liquid preparation without alcohol or dyes is ideal for infants and children with BPD. If the patient is taking a rapid-release product, the trough theophylline level should be maintained between 5 and 10 µg/mL. If the patient is taking a sustained-release theophylline preparation, a peak theophylline level should be monitored, because it is a better estimate of the steady-state plasma level.

Mechanisms of Action.—The effect of the methylxanthines as a bronchial smooth muscle relaxant may be due to their ability to enhance intracellular levels of cyclic 3′,5′-adenosine monophosphate (cAMP) by inhibiting phosphodiesterase. There appears to be a relationship between cAMP levels and the degree of smooth muscle relaxation in rabbits.[2] Recent data also show that methylxanthines improve the function of ventilatory muscles and central ventilatory drive, in addition to stimulating ciliary motility and causing a mild diuresis.

Therapeutic Use in Bronchopulmonary Dysplasia.—Rooklin et al.[40] reported a trend toward improvement in pulmonary function after administration of a single intravenous dose of theophylline to infants within the first month of life. We have shown that oral theophylline causes a significant decrease in airway resistance, increase in maximal expiratory flow at functional residual capacity (a measure of small airway function), and increase in dynamic pulmonary compliance in older infants with established BPD.[26] We have also shown that theophylline and diuretics have a synergistic effect on dynamic pulmonary compliance.[26]

A recent study has shown that 1 hour after administration of caffeine, compliance increased and resistance decreased in ventilator-dependent infants with BPD.[14] Because of its wide therapeutic index, long half-life, and minimal side effects, caffeine may have significant advantages over theophylline. However, until further studies have substantiated its efficacy, and it has been compared with theophylline, caffeine should probably not be used routinely for treatment of BPD in infants.

Side Effects.—Sleep disturbances, tachycardia, agitation, and vomiting have all been associated with toxic levels of theophylline, usually greater than 20 µg/mL. Even with theophylline levels in the therapeutic range, behavioral changes may be detected in some infants. Until recently there has been some concern that theophylline increases the metabolic rate in patients with BPD, thereby causing an increase in their already high oxygen consumption.[35] We have recently shown that infants with BPD do not have increased oxygen consumption when they are given theophylline.[27]

β-Adrenergic Agents

Mechanisms of Action.—The β₂-agonists cause bronchodilation, enhance mucociliary transport, increase surfactant production, and may attenuate pulmonary edema mediated by cAMP. The net result of these actions is to de-

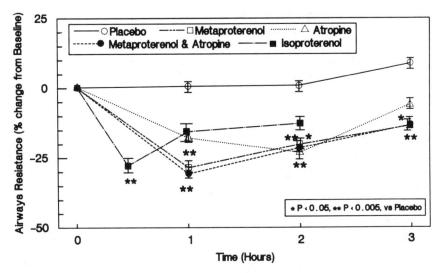

FIG 5–3.
Effects of placebo, isoproterenol, metaproterenol, atropine, and combined metaproterenol and atropine aerosols on airway resistance. Airway resistance decreased significantly 30 minutes after administration of isoproterenol, and 1, 2, and 3 hours after metaproterenol, atropine, and metaproterenol-atropine, respectively. Values are mean ± SEM. (Data from Kao LC, Warburton D, Platzker ACG, et al: *Pediatrics* 1984; 73:509–514, and Kao LC, Durand DJ, Nickerson BG: *Pediatr Pulmonol* 1989; 6:74–80. Used by permission.)

crease pulmonary resistance. Some studies have suggested that these agents also cause an improvement in dynamic lung compliance.[10, 25] However, this increase in compliance may be secondary to the decrease in pulmonary resistance, since compliance is partially dependent on airway resistance at high respiratory frequencies.

Therapeutic Use in Bronchopulmonary Dysplasia.—Clinical trials have shown improvement in pulmonary function in infants with BPD following the administration of the following β-adrenergic bronchodilators: isoetharine (Bronkosol), terbutaline (Brethine), metaproterenol (Alupent), albuterol (also known as salbutamol; Proventil) and isoproterenol (Isuprel).[10, 25, 28, 52]

Beta agonists, when administered as aerosols, are effective bronchodilators with rapid onset of action but short duration of action. We have demonstrated rapid, short-term improvement in airway resistance 30 minutes following isoproterenol inhalation in infants with resolving BPD[25] (Fig 5–3). We have also shown that infants with BPD respond to metaproterenol aerosol with improvement of airway resistance and maximal expiratory flow at functional residual capacity[28] (see Fig 5–3). The onset of action of both isoproterenol and metaproterenol is within 15 to 30 minutes of inhalation. In contrast to isoproterenol, metaproterenol treatment has a longer duration of action and less associated tachycardia.[25, 28]

Side Effects.—The most common adverse effect of treatment with beta agonists in infants is tachycardia.[25] Tremor, palpitation, and hyperexcitability may be more common with oral administration of β_2-agonists, but are rarely noted with inhalation.[45]

Anticholinergic Agents

Mechanisms of Action.—Studies in animals have shown that stimulation of the vagal branches leading to the lung results in bronchial constriction.[12] This parasympathetic bronchial constriction can be prevented by atropine.[51]

Clinical Use.—Inhaled atropine has its predominant effect on the central airways. Since the predominant effect of the β_2-aerosols is on the peripheral airways, one might expect synergy between anticholinergic and β_2-agonists on airway resistance. However, studies in adults have failed to show this anticipated synergy.

We recently compared the effects of inhaled metaproterenol, inhaled atropine, and combined metaproterenol and atropine in infants with BPD.[28] We found that atropine and metaproterenol are equally effective in improving airway resistance and maximal expiratory flow at functional residual capacity. Both agents have a rapid onset of action (15 to 30 minutes), cause maximal improvement within 1 to 2 hours following treatment, and have a duration of action of 3 hours. We were unable to show any consistent synergistic effect of the two agents (see Fig 5–3).

OTHER TREATMENTS

In addition to diuretics and bronchodilators, a number of other pharmacologic agents have been used in an attempt to decrease the incidence or lessen the severity of BPD. The efficacy of these agents should probably still be considered unproved.

Cromolyn Sodium

Mechanisms of Action.—Cromolyn has a number of actions that may be of benefit to the infant with BPD. It stabilizes mast cell membranes, decreases the release of antigen-induced leukotrienes from the lung, inhibits the inflammatory effects of platelet activating factor, and inhibits bronchoconstriction. It has been used to reduce bronchial hyperreactivity in both adults and children.

Clinical Use in Bronchopulmonary Dysplasia.—Because cromolyn blocks bronchoconstriction, in theory it should be of use in managing BPD in some infants. One study showed that treatment of BPD with cromolyn aerosol led to both clinical improvement and a decrease in total white blood cell, polymorphonuclear leukocyte (PMN), and alveolar macrophage counts in specimens obtained from lung lavage.[47] Another study showed improvement in compliance, resistance, and work of breathing after 7 to 10 days of treatment with cromolyn (20 mg q6hr) in infants with BPD.[46]

Steroids

Mechanisms of Action.—The possible mechanisms[5, 29] of action of steroids in the treatment of BPD include increased surfactant synthesis, stabilized cell and lysosomal membranes, inhibition of prostaglandin and leukotriene synthesis, decreased PMN influx into lungs, breakdown of PMN aggregates in the pulmonary microcirculation, reduced bronchoalveolar lavage elastase, enhanced β-adrenergic activity, reduced pulmonary edema, relaxed bronchospasm, and decreased bronchial edema.

Therapeutic Use in Bronchopulmonary Dysplasia.—It appears that dexamethasone therapy (0.5 mg/kg/day for 3 days, then tapered over 1 to 4 weeks) in the early stages of BPD leads to significant short-term improvement in pulmonary function and facilitates weaning the patient from ventilatory support and supplemental oxygen.[5, 29] However, there may be a significant incidence of respiratory deterioration, including need for reintubation and ventilation, following discontinuation of dexamethasone therapy.[8] One study has suggested that dexamethasone improves the status of infants with mild BPD but not of those with established cystic changes.[8]

Cummings et al.[13] noted a significant decrease in mortality or in ventilator dependency at 2 months of age when infants with BPD were given a course of dexamethasone tapering over 6 weeks compared with tapering over 2 weeks.

Side Effects.—Significant morbidity may occur with the use of steroids for the treatment of BPD. Reported complications include sepsis, systemic hypertension, hyperglycemia, gastrointestinal hemorrhage, necrotizing enterocolitis, pneumothorax, periventricular echodensity, periventricular leukomalacia, decreased somatic growth, and adrenal suppression.

Antioxidants

Antioxidants, such as superoxide dismutase (SOD), vitamin E, and vitamin A, have been used in an attempt to prevent or to reduce the severity of BPD. Subcutaneous SOD decreased clinical and radiographic manifestations in 45 infants with BPD, but it did not alter the duration of either mechanical ventilation or supplemental oxygen.[42] At this time SOD therapy should be considered experimental.

Studies have shown conflicting effects of vitamin E on the incidence or severity of BPD.[16, 43] Although infants with vitamin E deficiency might be at increased risk for oxygen-induced pulmonary injury, the use of pharmacologic doses of vitamin E should be considered experimental.

One published controlled trial showed that vitamin A administration decreased both the incidence and severity of BPD[44]; however, this finding has yet to be substantiated by other studies.

CLINICAL APPROACH TO BRONCHOPULMONARY DYSPLASIA

The doses of medications we use to treat BPD are shown in Table 5–1. Because of the prominent role that pulmonary edema plays in BPD, we consider diuretics the most important pharmacologic agents for the treatment of BPD.

For the infant who is not taking enteral nutrition and who is ventilator or oxygen dependent at 3 to 4 weeks of age, we begin a 1-week trial of

TABLE 5–1.
Recommended Medications and Dosage for Treatment of Bronchopulmonary Dysplasia

Medication	Dose	Route of Administration
Diuretics		
Furosemide (Lasix)	1 mg/kg/dose q6–24hr	IV, IM
	2–3 mg/kg/dose q6–24hr	PO
Chlorothiazide (Diuril)	10–25 mg/kg/dose q12hr	PO
Spironolactone (Aldactone)	1–2.5 mg/kg/dose q12hr	PO
Systemic bronchodilators		
Theophylline	5–7 mg/kg loading dose	IV or PO
	2–4 mg/kg/dose q6hr (adjust according to serum level)	
Inhaled bronchodilators		
Albuterol (Proventil)	5 mg/mL solution; 0.05–0.2 mg/kg/dose q2–6hr	Nebulization
Metaproterenol (Alupent)	50 mg/mL solution; 0.2–1.0 mg/kg/dose q2–6 hr	Nebulization
Isoproterenol (Isuprel)	1 mg/mL solution; 0.2–0.5 mL q2–6hr	Nebulization
Atropine*	0.08 mg/kg/dose q2–6hr	Nebulization
Cromolyn sodium (Intal)*	20 mg/dose q6hr	Nebulization
Steroid		
Dexamethasone (Decadron)*	0.5 mg/kg/day for 3 days, then taper over 1–4 weeks	IV

*Probably not indicated for routine use.

intravenous furosemide 2 mg/kg/day divided in two doses. For the infant with severe BPD, we may briefly increase the furosemide dose to 3–4 mg/kg/day, divided into three or four doses. If the infant clinically improves we continue the diuretics; if the infant has no clinical improvement we discontinue the diuretics. The infant who does not improve with the first trial usually receives a second trial 1 to 2 weeks later. Therapeutic effect is reflected by a significant diuresis in the first 24 hours, decrease in respiratory distress, or decrease in respiratory support.

To minimize the complications associated with furosemide, we begin combined oral chlorothiazide (20 to 50 mg/kg/day) and spironolactone (2 to 5 mg/kg/day) as soon as the infant can tolerate enteral medications, usually after feeding has been established. This combination seems to cause less calcium and electrolyte imbalance and to lead to less osteopenia than does furosemide. Infants who are treated with furosemide or with chlorothiazide and spironolactone often require supplemental sodium and potassium chloride to maintain serum chloride levels above 90 mEq/L and sodium levels 128 to 135 mEq/L.

The indications for stopping diuretics are controversial. Our approach is to treat infants with BPD with diuretics as long as they require mechanical ventilation, and usually as long as they require significant supplemental oxygen. Whether the infant who no longer requires supplemental oxygen benefits from continued diuretics has not yet been determined.

We treat the infant with severe BPD, particularly if ventilator dependent, with combined bronchodilators and diuretics. Although we have demonstrated synergy between diuretics and theophylline in the infant with BPD,[26] no studies have shown synergy between diuretics and inhaled bronchodilators; however, it is our subjective impression that the inhaled beta agonists provide significant bronchodilation with less toxicity than theophylline. Although little data are available about the relative efficacy of the various beta agonists in infants, we usually use those agents shown in studies of adults to have the fewest cardiovascular side effects and the greatest duration of action (i.e., albuterol and metaproterenol).

Because of their short duration of action, the inhaled beta agonists should be given every 2 to 6 hours, not every 8 to 12 hours or "as needed." Treatments should be given to ventilated infants by "bagging" rather than "in line" with the ventilator, because most of the medication delivered by the "in line" method is lost in the continuous flow rather than being delivered to the infant. Infants without endotracheal tubes in place should receive treatments via blow-by or CPAP rather than as bagged breaths. There is no evidence that the delivery of aerosols by positive pressure is more effective than is delivery by spontaneous ventilation.

We usually discontinue bronchodilators before we discontinue diuretics in the infant in whom BPD is improving.

We use theophylline only in the infant with severe BPD who is ventilator dependent, and after trying a combination of maximal diuretic doses and inhaled bronchodilator. While there are no studies showing a synergistic effect of theophylline and inhaled β_2-agonist in infants with BPD, we usually continue to use an inhaled β_2-agonist in the patient for whom we have started theophylline. Although theophylline levels of 10 to 20 μg/mL are usually thought to provide maximal bronchodilation, some infants have signs of theophylline toxicity with levels of 10 to 15 μg/mL.[26] Many infants seem to have a bronchodilatory response to lower levels of theophylline.

For infants in whom there is a severe component of bronchospasm that does not respond to either the β_2-agonists or theophylline, a trial of an anticholinergic bronchodilator may be worthwhile.

We consider cromolyn to be an unproved agent in the treatment of BPD and use it only in older patients with severe BPD who are not responding to maximal diuretic and bronchodilator therapy.

We also consider steroids to be unproved in the treatment of most infants with BPD. Although short-term improvement can be accomplished in many of these patients, in our experience the long-term effects are equivocal, and often at the cost of significant side effects.

UNANSWERED QUESTIONS

Although most infants with BPD show progressive improvement of respiratory status, many long-term survivors of BPD have evidence of airway obstruction, hyperinflation, and airway hyperreactivity.[6] A number of questions about the pharmacologic management of both the newborn infant and the older child with BPD remain unanswered. Some of the questions we hope to see answered in the next several years include:

1. How early in the course of BPD are diuretics and bronchodilators effective?
2. Does early treatment decrease the incidence or severity of BPD?
3. Which combinations of diuretics, systemic bronchodilators, and inhaled bronchodilators are most effective?
4. How long should diuretics or bronchodilators be continued?
5. For which infants are steroids indicated?
6. Is there a clinical role for antioxidants, vitamin A supplementation, vitamin E supplementation, or cromolyn?
7. What are the long-term side effects of administering these agents to infants?

REFERENCES

1. Albersheim S, Solimano A, Sharma A, et al: A randomized double-blind controlled trial of long-term diuretic therapy in bronchopulmonary dysplasia. *J Pediatr* 1989; 115:615–620.

2. Andersson RGG: Cyclic AMP and calcium ions in mechanical and metabolic responses of smooth muscles: Influence of some hormones and drugs. *Acta Physiol Scand* 1972; 382(suppl):1–59.
3. Aranda JV, Perez J, Sitar DS, et al: Pharmacokinetics disposition and protein binding of furosemide in newborn infants. *J Pediatr* 1978; 93:507–511.
4. Atkinson SA, Shah JK, McGee C, et al: Mineral excretion in premature infants receiving various diuretic therapies. *J Pediatr* 1988; 113:540–545.
5. Avery GB, Fletcher AB, Kaplan M, et al: Controlled trial of dexamethasone in respirator-dependent infants with bronchopulmonary dysplasia. *Pediatrics* 1985; 75:106–111.
6. Bader D, Ramos A, Lew CD, et al: Childhood sequelae of infant lung disease: Exercise and pulmonary function abnormalities after bronchopulmonary dysplasia. *J Pediatr* 1987; 110:693–699.
7. Bancalari E, Abdenour GE, Feller R, et al: Bronchopulmonary dysplasia: Clinical presentation. *J Pediatr* 1979; 95:819–823.
8. Barrington K, Finer NN: Evaluation of the efficacy of dexamethasone in prevention of severe bronchopulmonary dysplasia. *J Perinatol* 1985; 5:26–32.
9. Brater DC: Determinants of the overall response to furosemide: Pharmacokinetic and pharmacodynamics. *Fed Proc* 1983; 42:1711–1713.
10. Cabal LA, Larrazabal C, Ramanathan R, et al: Effects of metaproterenol on pulmonary mechanics, oxygenation, and ventilation in infants with chronic lung disease. *J Pediatr* 1987; 110:116–119.
11. Callahan J, Haller JO, Cacciarelli A, et al: Cholelithiasis in infants: Association with total parenteral nutrition and furosemide. *Radiology* 1982; 143:437–439.
12. Colebach HJH, Halmagyi DFJ: Effect of vagotomy and vagal stimulation on lung mechanics and circulation. *J Appl Physiol* 1963; 18:881–887.
13. Cummings J, D'Eugenio D, Gross S: A controlled trial of dexamethasone in preterm infants at high risk for bronchopulmonary dysplasia. *N Engl J Med* 1989; 320:1505–1510.
14. Davis JM, Bhutani VK, Stefano JL, et al: Changes in pulmonary mechanics following caffeine administration in infants with bronchopulmonary dysplasia. *Pediatr Pulmonol* 1989; 6:49–52.
15. Edwards DK, Dyer WM, Northway WH: Twelve years experience with bronchopulmonary dysplasia. *Pediatrics* 1977; 59:839–846.
16. Ehrenkranz RA, Bonta BW, Ablow RC, et al: Amelioration of bronchopulmonary dysplasia after vitamin E administration: A preliminary report. *N Engl J Med* 1978; 299:564–569.
17. Engelhardt B, Elliott S, Hazinski TA: Short- and long-term effects of furosemide on lung function in infants with bronchopulmonary dysplasia. *J Pediatr* 1986; 109:1034–1039.
18. Engelhardt B, Blalock WA, DonLevy S, et al: Effect of spironolactone-hydrochlorothiazide on lung function in infants with chronic bronchopulmonary dysplasia. *J Pediatr* 1989; 114:619–624.
19. Ezzedeen F, Adelman RD, Ahlfors CE: Renal calcification in preterm infants: Pathophysiology and long-term sequelae. *J Pediatr* 1988; 113:532–539.
20. Goldman SL, Gerhardt T, Sonni R, et al: Early prediction of chronic lung disease by pulmonary function testing. *J Pediatr* 1983; 102:613–617.
21. Green TP, Thompson TR, Johnson DE, et al: Furosemide promotes patent ductus arteriosus in premature infants with the respiratory-distress syndrome. *N Engl J Med* 1983; 308:743–748.

22. Hazinski TA: Furosemide decreases ventilation in young rabbits. *J Pediatr* 1985; 106:81–85.

23. Kao LC, Warburton D, Sargent CW, et al: Furosemide acutely decreases airways resistance in chronic bronchopulmonary dysplasia. *J Pediatr* 1983; 103:624–629.

24. Kao LC, Warburton D, Cheng M, et al: Effect of oral diuretics on pulmonary mechanics in infants with chronic bronchopulmonary dysplasia: Results of a double-blind crossover sequential trial. *Pediatrics* 1984; 74:37–44.

25. Kao LC, Warburton D, Platzker ACG, et al: Isoproterenol inhalation on airway resistance in chronic bronchopulmonary dysplasia. *Pediatrics* 1984; 73:509–514.

26. Kao LC, Durand DJ, Phillips BL, et al: Oral theophylline and diuretics improve pulmonary mechanics in infants with bronchopulmonary dysplasia. *J Pediatr* 1987; 111:439–444.

27. Kao LC, Durand DJ, Nickerson BG: Improving pulmonary function does not decrease oxygen consumption in infants with bronchopulmonary dysplasia. *J Pediatr* 1988; 112:616–621.

28. Kao LC, Durand DJ, Nickerson BG: Metaproterenol and atropine aerosols improve pulmonary mechanics in infants with bronchopulmonary dysplasia (BPD). *Pediatr Pulmonol* 1989; 6:74–80.

29. Mammel MC, Green TP, Johnson DE, et al: Controlled trial of dexamethasone therapy in infants with bronchopulmonary dysplasia. *Lancet* 1983; 1:1356–1358.

30. McCann EM, Lewis K, Deming DD, et al: Controlled trial of furosemide therapy in infants with chronic lung disease. *J Pediatr* 1985; 106:957–962.

31. Mirochnick MH, Miceli JJ, Kramer PA, et al: Furosemide pharmacokinetics in very low birth weight infants. *J Pediatr* 1988; 112:653–657.

32. Motoyama EK, Fort MD, Klesh KW, et al: Early onset of airway reactivity in premature infants with bronchopulmonary dysplasia. *Am Rev Respir Dis* 1987; 136:50–57.

33. Nassif EG, Weinberger MM, Shannon D, et al: Theophylline disposition in infancy. *J Pediatr* 1981; 98:158–161.

34. Nickerson BG, Taussig LM: Family history of asthma in infants with bronchopulmonary dysplasia. *Pediatrics* 1980; 65:1140–1144.

34a. Nickerson BG: Bronchopulmonary disease following neonatal respiratory failure. *Chest* 1985; 87:528–535.

35. O'Brodovich HM, Mellins RB: Bronchopulmonary dysplasia. Unresolved neonatal acute lung injury. *Am Rev Respir Dis* 1985; 132:694–709.

36. Patel H, Yeh TF, Jain R, et al: Pulmonary and renal responses to furosemide in infants with stage III-IV bronchopulmonary dysplasia. *Am J Dis Child* 1985; 139:917–919.

37. Perlman JM, Moore V, Siegel MJ, et al: Is chloride depletion an important contributing cause of death in infants with bronchopulmonary dysplasia? *Pediatrics* 1986; 77:212–216.

38. Peterson RG, Simmons MA, Rumack BH, et al: Pharmacology of furosemide in the premature newborn infants. *J Pediatr* 1980; 97:139–143.

39. Rao M, Eid N, Herrod L, et al: Antidiuretic hormone response in children with bronchopulmonary dysplasia during episodes of acute respiratory distress. *Am J Dis Child* 1986; 140:825–828.

40. Rooklin AR, Moomjian AS, Shutack JG, et al: Theophylline therapy in bronchopulmonary dysplasia. *J Pediatr* 1979; 95:882–885.
41. Rosan RC: Hyaline membrane disease and a related spectrum of neonatal pneumopathies. *Perspect Pediatr Pathol* 1975; 2:15–60.
42. Rosenfeld W, Evans H, Concepcion L, et al: Prevention of bronchopulmonary dysplasia by administration of bovine superoxide dismutase in preterm infants with respiratory distress syndrome. *J Pediatr* 1984; 105:781–785.
43. Saldanha RL, Cepeda EE, Poland RL: The effect of vitamin E prophylaxis on the incidence and severity of bronchopulmonary dysplasia. *J Pediatr* 1982; 101:89–93.
44. Shenai JP, Kennedy KA, Chytil F, et al: Clinical trial of vitamin A supplementation in infants susceptible to bronchopulmonary dysplasia. *J Pediatr* 1987; 111:269–277.
45. Shim C, Williams MH: Bronchial response to oral versus aerosol metaproterenol in asthma. *Ann Intern Med* 1980; 93:428–431.
46. Shook LA, Pauly TH, Desai NS, et al: Improved lung resistance and compliance during cromolyn therapy in infants with bronchopulmonary dysplasia. *Pediatr Res* 1988; 23:524A.
47. Stenmark KR, Eyzaguirre M, Remigio L, et al: Recovery of platelet activating factor and leukotrienes from infants with severe bronchopulmonary dysplasia: Clinical improvement with cromolyn treatment. *Am Rev Respir Dis* 1985; 131:A236.
48. Sulyok E, Varga F, Nemeth M, et al: Furosemide-induced alterations in the electrolyte status, the function of renin-angiotensin-aldosterone system, and the urinary excretion of prostaglandins in newborn infants. *Pediatr Res* 1980; 14:765–768.
49. Tepper RS, Morgan WJ, Cota K, et al: Expiratory flow limitation in infants with bronchopulmonary dysplasia. *J Pediatr* 1986; 109:1040–1046.
50. Tooley WH: Epidemiology of bronchopulmonary dysplasia. *J Pediatr* 1979; 95:851–855.
51. Vincent NJ, Knudson R, Leith DE, et al: Factors influencing pulmonary resistance. *J Appl Physiol* 1970; 29:236–243.
52. Wilkie RA, Bryan MH: Effect of bronchodilators on airway resistance in ventilator-dependent neonates with chronic lung disease. *J Pediatr* 1987; 111:278–282.
53. Yeh TF, McClenan D, Ajayi OA, et al: Metabolic rate and energy balance in infants with bronchopulmonary dysplasia. *J Pediatr* 1989; 114:448–451.

6

Surfactant Therapy in Neonatal Respiratory Distress Syndrome

Tetsuro Fujiwara, M.D.

Mineo Konishi, M.D.

Shoichi Chida, M.D.

Surfactant therapy in the premature infants with respiratory distress syndrome (RDS) constitutes a major historical milestone in neonatal medicine. Exogenous surfactant preparations of various types have now been evaluated in the treatment of established RDS and prevention of RDS. Although the promise of this therapy seems firmly established, we are at present at one point on a continuum of progress.

The purpose of this chapter is to familiarize pediatricians with the new strategy, surfactant therapy, and to provide an overview of the available surfactant preparations for clinical use, the currently reported results, and the clinical implications of such therapy on the course of RDS.

BRIEF HISTORICAL REVIEW

Soon after the identification of dipalmitoylphosphatidylcholine (DPPC) as the principal surface-active component of pulmonary surfactant and the discovery that deficiency of pulmonary surfactant is the fundamental cause of RDS,[2] aerosols of DPPC were used to treat RDS with little success.[6] However, during the 1970s Enhorning and Robertson[10] demonstrated that the instillation of a crude surfactant fraction, obtained from lung lavage, into the trachea at birth improved the compliance characteristics and prevented the development of lung disease characteristic of RDS in premature rabbit and primate. Adams and co-workers,[1] in fetal lambs, first established that surfactant instillation could prevent the development of RDS in animal models. A reconstituted bovine-based surfactant lipid that could be used in humans was first developed in Japan and successfully tested in infants with established RDS.[13, 15] Subsequently, experimental and clinical investigations have increased exponentially. Attempts to develop an effective exogenous surfactant that could be used in human neonates were begun in a number of laboratories. Since 1985, 15 randomized trials of surfactant therapy for premature infants have been published, in which six surfactant preparations were used. Ten randomized trials have shown the efficacy of surfactant for the treatment of RDS, and other trials are ongoing around the world. The prospect of surfactant therapy in premature infants is now reaching an exciting stage. A number of excellent reviews[21, 28, 30, 37, 39] and a book[34] are currently available.

SURFACTANT PREPARATIONS FOR CLINICAL USE

It is useful to group the available surfactant preparations into three categories: an organic solvent extract of animal lung lavage or of minced lung-saline solution extract with or without additives; natural surfactant isolated from human amniotic fluid; and artificial or synthetic surfactants.

Animal Lung-Based Surfactants

Three bovine-based and one porcine-based surfactant have been made by different techniques.

Surfactant TA.—Surfactant TA (Tokyo Tanabe, Japan) uses as its starting material a crude surfactant isolated from saline extract of minced cow lung. It is extracted with ethyl acetate to remove cholesterol, followed by extraction with chloroform-methanol. To achieve optimum surface activity with less batch-to-batch variability, small amounts of synthetic DPPC, palmitic acid, and triglyceride are added so that the final product contains 84% phospholipids, 7% triglycerides, 8% palmitic acid, and 1% proteolipid-apoprotein (SP-B, SP-C). It is a freeze-dried, white powder. One hundred twenty milligrams (100 mg as phospholipid) is dispersed in a 3 to 4 mL sterile sodium chloride injection (USP) by either sonication or gently shaking, and passed through a 26-gauge needle before it is administered.

Survanta.—Survanta (Abbott Laboratories, North Chicago, Ill.) is a modification of Surfactant TA. It is dispersed in saline solution, autoclaved for sterilization, and frozen for storage. It is thawed to a liquid state before use.

Calf Lung Surfactant.—Calf Lung Surfactant Lipid Extract (CLSE; Rochester; Infasurf, ONY Inc, Buffalo, N.Y.) is an organic solvent extract of a crude surfactant isolated from calf lung lavage by differential centrifugation. It contains 90% to 97% phospholipid, 5% cholesterol-cholesterol esters, and 1% protein (SP-B, SP-C). It is sterilized by flash autoclave. Before use, 90 mg lipid is vortexed with 3 mL physiologic saline solution.

Porcine Surfactant.—Porcine Surfactant (Curosurf; Chiesi Farmaceutici, Parma, Italy) is prepared from a saline extract of minced pig lung, extracted with chloroform-methanol, followed by liquid-gel chromatography. It contains 99% phospholipids and 1% protein, similarly to Surfactant TA or CLSE. It is used as a suspension of 80 mg/mL at 200 mg/kg.

Human Amniotic Fluid Surfactant

This product is produced by collecting amniotic fluid at elective cesarean section for term delivery. The surfactant is then isolated and purified by differential and density gradient centrifugation. It is used as a 60 mg suspension by vortexing with 3.5 mL 0.6% saline solution.

Artificial Surfactants

Three artificial surfactants have been used in premature infants.

1. DPPC-human high-density lipoprotein (HDL) is made from DPPC (1 g) and human HDL (4 mL) mixed with 150 mL 0.9% saline solution, sterilized by irradiation, and given in a dose of 3 to 5 mL into the endotracheal tube at birth.
2. DPPC-phosphatidylglycerol (PG; ALEC, Cambridge, England) is made from two pure DPPC and egg PG in a ratio of 3:1. It has been used in clinical trials both as a powder and as a suspension of 50 to 100 mg in 1 mL cold saline solution.
3. Exosurf (Burroughs-Wellcome, Research Triangle Park, N.C.) consists of DPPC (13.5 mg/mL), tyloxapol (1.0 mg/mL), and hexadecanol (1.5 mg/mL), and is used in a dose of 7 mL/kg.

CLINICAL RESPONSES TO SURFACTANTS

It is useful to group the reported trials of surfactant therapy into two categories: rescue trials and prophylactic trials. The rescue trials have used surfactants to treat infants with established RDS, whereas the prophylactic trials have used surfactants before the infant's first breath or within minutes of delivery to modify the course of RDS in infants at high risk for RDS. Many of the therapeutic benefits of various naturally derived surfactant preparations in RDS have been described in a series of recent randomized prophylactic

TABLE 6–1.
Published Randomized Clinical Trials in Infants With RDS and Surfactants

Strategy	Study	Surfactant	Dose* (mg)	Response	Duration
Prevention					
	Halliday et al.[17]	DPPC/HDL	30	Negligible	
	Enhorning et al.[11]	Infasurf	75–100	Striking	Sustained
	Kwong et al.[25]	CLSE	90	Striking	Sustained
	Shapiro et al.[36]	CLSE	90	Striking	Unsustained
	Merritt et al.[29]	Human AFS	Multiple	Striking	Sustained
	Ten Center[31]	ALEC	Multiple	Not studied	
	Kendig et al.[23]	CLSE	90	Striking	Unsustained
Rescue					
	Wilkinson et al.[40]	ALEC	25	Negligible	
	Hallman et al.[18]	Human AFS	Multiple	Striking	Sustained
	Gitlin et al.[16]	Surfactant TA	120	Striking	Sustained
	Raju et al.[33]	Surfactant TA	120	Striking	Sustained
	Fujiwara et al.[14]	Surfactant TA	120	Striking	Sustained
	CEMSG[7]	Curosurf	200	Striking	Sustained
	Horbar et al.[19]	Survanta	120	Striking	Sustained

DPPC = dipalmitoylphosphatidylcholine; HDL = high-density lipoprotein; AFS = amniotic fluid surfactant; CEMSG = Collaborative European Multicenter Study Group; sustained = effect lasts for at least 72 hours after administration of surfactant.
*Total lipid/kg body weight.

trials, all of which showed statistically significant improvement in respiratory function after surfactant therapy. However, immediate physiologic responses achieved with naturally derived surfactants have not been reproduced with the currently reported synthetic surfactants (Table 6–1).

There is clear experimental evidence to indicate that early surfactant therapy at birth produces a greater and more sustained effect on gas exchange and compliance characteristics than later treatment.[27] However, study groups in different clinical trials reported to date have not been comparable, and the question as to optimal timing of surfactant therapy remains unanswered. Clinical trials comparing the prophylactic or very early vs. rescue strategies are in progress.

Studies with human amniotic fluid surfactant have noted unsustained response in 41% of treated infants with established RDS and 71% of infants treated prophylactically. In both of these studies,[18, 29] infants needed multiple doses of surfactant to sustain therapeutic response. Such relapse is rarely seen in our recent multicenter randomized trials with a single dose of Surfactant TA.[14, 24]

In contrast to the prophylactic trial by Enhorning et al.[11] a recent similar trial using a single dose of CLSE showed that the effects diminished between 24 and 48 hours after surfactant administration.[23] The reason for the variation in response and the identity of the nonresponsive nature in some infants have not been clarified. In addition to demographic variation, a multitude of routine practices, approach to the patent ductus arteriosus, severity of RDS, and dosage of surfactant, or the difference in conventional ventilatory techniques, or the difference and variability in the biophysical and physiologic activity among the different surfactant preparations may account for such variation in response. A major concern about naturally derived surfactants (amniotic fluid surfactant, CLSE) has been quality control. Our recent studies[35] demonstrated that the biophysical properties of Surfactant TA were superior in several respects to those of other naturally derived surfactants (human amniotic fluid surfactant, lung lavage lipid, or phospholipid fraction of a porcine surfactant). Another important variable recently recognized is the variability in sensitivity of surfactants to alveolar protein inhibitors. Surfactant TA is more resistant to alveolar protein inhibitors than other surfactants are.[20] It is unclear whether infants having a more favorable response to surfactant released less inhibitor, had lower effluent protein concentrations, or both. In vitro studies suggest that a higher dose of surfactant can overcome the inhibitory effects of plasma components on surfactant.[12]

EFFECT OF SURFACTANT THERAPY ON COMPLICATIONS OF RESPIRATORY DISTRESS SYNDROME

Surfactant therapy eliminates the surfactant deficiency component of the complex pathophysiology of RDS. Because surfactant therapy reduces the severity of RDS and restores sufficient lung function to permit a reduction in ventilatory support (lower fraction of inspired oxygen [FiO_2] and mean airway pressures), it might be predicted that surfactant therapy would reduce the major morbidity factors of RDS, such as air leaks, bronchopulmonary dysplasia (BPD), and intracranial hemorrhage (ICH). The controlled clinical trials of both prophylactic and rescue types reported the substantial reduction in frequency of the major complications of RDS.

Prophylactic Trials

To date, 104 infants have been treated prophylactically in three controlled trials with naturally derived surfactants, demonstrating a significant impact on the complications of RDS and prematurity (Table 6–2). The 95% confidence interval estimates that pneumothorax (PNTX) decreases between 7% and 28% ($P = 0.003$), and pulmonary interstitial emphysema (PIE) between 18% and 40% ($P < 0.001$). There was no statistically significant reduction in the frequency of ICH and BPD. The 95% confidence interval for the overall increase in survival in the group treated prophylactically is 2% to 31% ($P = 0.009$). Of the prophylactic trials, those of Enhorning et al.[11] and Merritt et al.[29] demonstrated the substantial reduction in mortality. In recent prophylactic trials[30] in which a saline suspension of the DPPC-PG mixture was used, the beneficial effect on gas exchange was found to begin 18 hours after multiple-dose treatments, associated with the substantial reduction in ICH and morbidity.

TABLE 6–2.
Effects of Surfactant Therapy on Complications of RDS

	Prophylactic Trials				Rescue Trials			
	Surfactant (n = 104)	Control (n = 93)	% Difference (95% CI)	P	Surfactant (n = 262)	Control (n = 250)	% Difference (95% CI)	P
%PNTX	10	27	17 (7–28)	0.003	13	27	14 (8–21)	<0.001
%PIE	9	38	29 (18–40)	<0.001	14	37	23 (14–32)	<0.001
%PDA	48	52	4 (−10–18)	NS	53	46	7 (−4–18)	NS
%ICH	37	48	11 (−2–26)	NS	37	47	10 (1–18)	0.043
%ROP	13	8	6 (−2–14)	NS	11	17	6 (−4–15)	NS
%NEC	6	6		NS	4	5		NS
%BPD	38	45	8 (−6–22)	NS	26	34	8 (0.3–16)	0.056
%Death	16	33	17 (2–31)	0.009	19	30	11 (3–22)	0.008

Complications across the studies reported by Enhorning et al.,[11] Kendig et al.,[23] and Merritt el al.[29] (prophylactic trials) were summed with those reported by Hallman et al.[18] Gitlin et al.,[16] Fujiwara et al.,[14] collaborative European multicenter study group,[7] and Horbar et al.[19] (rescue trials). Percent incidences are calculated as percentages of total infants who were evaluated for the complications.

PNTX = pneumothorax; PIE = pulmonary interstitial emphysema; PDA = patent ductus arteriosus; ICH = intracranial hemorrhage; ROP = retinopathy of prematurity; NEC = necrotizing enterocolitis; BPD = bronchopulmonary dysplasia; CI = confidence intervals; P = probability (two-tailed); NS = not significant.

Rescue Trials

In the rescue trials, 262 infants have been treated (see Table 6–2). The incidence of PNTX or PIE is also significantly reduced. The frequency of ICH decreased significantly, from 47% to 37% (95% CI between 1% and 18%; P = .043). The reduction in the frequency of BPD is a marginally significant (P = .056). The 95% confidence interval estimates that between 3% and 22% (P = .008) more infants survive. The trial of Raju et al.,[33] in which a single 120 mg/kg dose of Surfactant TA was used, showed a reduction in mortality from 54% for the control group to 18% for the treated infants. The collaborative European multicenter study group,[7] using a single 200 mg/kg dose of Curosurf, also observed a reduction in mortality from 51% to 31% when treated infants were compared with controls. In both of these studies the rate of death in control infants was much higher than the 17% to 26% observed in other studies. Different patient selection criteria may have contributed to the differences in outcome among the studies.

SURFACTANT THERAPY

Protocol for Rescue Surfactant Therapy

Current techniques for administration of surfactant are somewhat variable. We suggest the following protocol for surfactant therapy.

Preinstillation Ventilation

Mechanical ventilation is provided with a time-cycled, pressure-limited respirator. The ventilator is initially set at a peak inspiratory pressure of 20 to 30 cm H_2O, a positive end-expiratory pressure of 4 cm H_2O, and a respiratory rate of 20 to 30 cpm, with inspiratory time of 1.0 second; no muscle relaxants are used. Subsequent alterations in the ventilator settings are based on blood gas analysis (Pao_2 60 to 80 mm Hg, $PaCo_2$ <50 mm Hg). Following blood gas stabilization, infants who still require more than 7 cm H_2O mean airway pressure and 40% oxygen are treated with surfactant.

Instillation Technique

Surfactant TA (120 mg of lyophilized surfactant lipid in a vial) is suspended in 4 mL saline solution by gentle shaking to give a lipid concentration of 30 mg/mL. The suspension is warmed to 37°C and passed through a 26-gauge needle immediately prior to administration. The infant is briefly detached from the ventilator, and the feeding tube is inserted into the endotracheal tube. In five divided doses, 4 mL/kg of this suspension is instilled into the lungs through an endotracheal tube by way of a catheter that is passed to the tip of the endotracheal tube. To promote uniform distribution and to avoid hypoxia, repeated instillations of surfactant, 0.5 to 1.0 mL each, are followed by manual bagging with 100% oxygen while changing the infant's

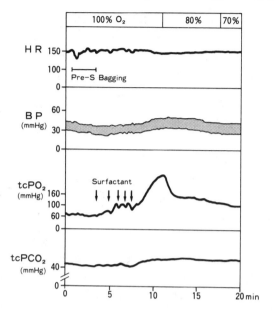

FIG 6–1.
Simultaneous recordings of heart rate *(HR)*, blood pressure *(BP)*, transcutaneous Po_2 *(TcPo$_2$)* and Pco_2 *(TcPco$_2$)* during and after administration of surfactant in a 6-hour old infant boy (26-weeks gestation, birth weight 900 g). He had severe RDS, requiring mechanical ventilation with 90% oxygen. Ventilator settings used were PIP 20 cm H_2O, PEEP 4 cm H_2O, rate 60 cpm (MAP 12.3 cm H_2O). Note that there are immediate effects of surfactant on tcPo$_2$, but no influence on the other parameters. *Arrows* indicate instillation of surfactant. Fio$_2$ decreased to 0.4 by 20 minutes, and to 0.3 by 3 hours after administration of surfactant (data not shown).

position. The ventilator pressures are maintained at 4 cm H_2O higher than the previous settings; the respirator rate is kept at 60 cpm with a 1:1 inspiratory-expiratory ratio to ensure that (tcPo$_2$) is not less than 60 mm Hg. On completion of the instillation, which takes about 5 minutes, the patient is promptly returned to the respirator with the settings used prior to treatment. During the instillation of surfactant, the infant's heart rate, blood pressure, tcPo$_2$, and tcPco$_2$ are recorded (Fig 6–1).

Postinstillation Ventilation
Fifteen minutes after treatment, subsequent adjustments are made, first for Fio$_2$ and then for peak inspiratory pressure and rate, to maintain the normal blood gas values.

Evaluation of Response
All patients are evaluated at set intervals, using treatment age as "time zero" during the first 120 hours after treatment, to determine the initial

response and its duration. Assessment consists of physical examination, including vital signs, arterial blood gases, arterial blood pressures, ventilator settings, mean airway pressure (MAP), FiO_2, and chest radiographs. Each patient is also evaluated for the presence of a patent ductus arteriosus by clinical, radiographic, and echocardiographic criteria. Doppler and contrast echocardiograms are also used for evaluating the left ventricular output, the magnitude of ductal shunting, the presence of tricuspid regurgitation, and right-to-left shunting through fetal pathways.

Responses to Surfactant

The magnitude of initial response is evaluated by the composite changes in arterial-alveolar PO_2 ratio (a/APO_2) and MAP values. The a/APO_2 is an index of oxygenation or physiologic intrapulmonary and extrapulmonary shunt, and MAP is an index of noncompliant lung disease.

According to the protocol described earlier (Protocol for Rescue Surfactant Therapy) we have treated 96 patients with severe RDS within 10 hours of birth with a single dose (120 mg/kg) of surfactant TA. Birth weights ranged from 520 to 2,400 g (25 patients <1,000 g; 44 at 1,000 to 1,499 g; 19 at 1,500 to 1,999 g; 8 at 2,000 to 2,400 g). Sixty-three were boys, 33 girls; 47 were outborn and 49 inborn. Gastric aspirates were collected at birth from all infants, and the stable microbubble rating[32] was measured as an indication of surfactant maturity. Surfactant deficiency was documented in all patients. Based on the magnitude of initial response to a single dose of surfactant TA and its duration, the response patterns are classified into four categories: (1) immediate and sustained response; (2) immediate response, relapse, and recovery; (3) poor or no response; (4) transient response. The response patterns are illustrated in Fig 6–2.

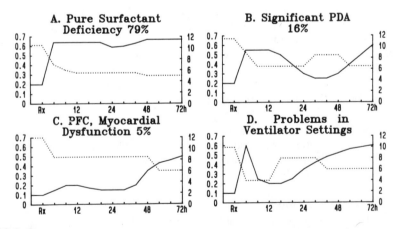

FIG 6–2.
Response patterns in terms of changes in arterial-alveolar oxygen tension ratio (a/APO_2; *continuous line*) and MAP (*dotted line*) after surfactant treatment in infants with RDS. *Left axis,* a/APO_2 ratio; *right axis,* MAP (cm H_2O). For details see text.

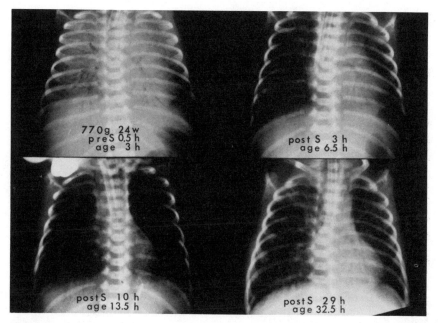

FIG 6–3.
Serial chest radiographs in a 24-week, 770 g infant with severe RDS and hemodynamically significant PDA. Radiograph on the *upper right* was taken 3 hours after surfactant administration; that on the *lower left*, 10 hours after surfactant, corresponds to clinical improvement; that on the *lower right*, taken at age 32.5 hours, is consistent with PDA. Serial echocardiograms showed the presence of a left-to-right ductal shunt at age 6 to 12 hours. Left systolic time interval decreased from 0.33–0.38 to 0.26–0.28 between 24 and 48 hours of age, suggesting a large ductal shunt; concurrently, a/APo$_2$ ratio decreased from the baseline value of 0.45 to 0.25 (44% reduction). Because of the reopening of the PDA after six doses of mefenamic acid, the patient underwent surgical ductal ligation at age 5 days, and had an uncomplicated recovery.

Immediate and Sustained Response (Response A)

This category of response included an increase in a/APO$_2$ greater than 0.2 combined with a decrease in MAP less than 2 cm H$_2$O from the presurfactant values, and these improvements were maintained during the subsequent 120 hours after treatment. Chest x-ray films showed rapid clearing in most cases. From the radiologic standpoint, aeration was nearly complete when evaluated 6 hours after surfactant administration, because the small focal areas of nonaerated lung are too small to be seen on the radiograph.

This response was seen in 79% (76/96) of the surfactant recipients, and may represent "pure RDS," in which surfactant deficiency is the primary factor underlying the disease. This group included 16 infants weighing less than 1,000 g. A slight but not significant decrease in a/APO$_2$ from baseline during remission occurred between 24 and 48 hours after surfactant treatment, but this may be attributed to mild to moderate lung edema due to PDA.

Changes present in serial echocardiographs and radiographs often preceded the appearance of physical signs of PDA (Fig 6–3). Many of these infants were given prophylactically mefenamic acid, a potent prostaglandin synthetase inhibitor to close the PDA; consequently, none of the infants developed a significant PDA during the first week of life. However, nine infants weighing less than 1,000 g underwent surgical ductal ligation afterward (at 10 to 13 days of life) because of PDA reopening. None of the infants weighing more than 1,000 g required surgical PDA ligation.

The sustained response seen in these infants may represent the maintenance of an intra-alveolar surfactant pool size[5] sufficient to counteract inhibitors present in the airways and to prevent the progression of lung disease, thereby decreasing the protein leak into the airways.[21]

Immediate Initial Response, Relapse and Recovery (Response B)

The magnitude of initial response and duration are similar to those seen in category A until about 24 hours after surfactant administration, when there was a gradual decline of a/APO$_2$ accompanied by an increase in MAP by approximately 50% from each of the baseline determinations during remission. These infants comprised 16% (15/96) of the surfactant recipients and may represent hemodynamically significant PDA. This group of infants did not significantly differ from the category A infants in birth weight or gestational age, but had significantly more asphyxia at birth. Asphyxia is known to be an important determinant of decompensation due to a left-to-right shunt through a PDA. Many of these infants recovered after intervention with mefenamic acid. Of these, one infant weighing less than 1,000 g underwent surgical ligation of the duct at age 5 days. Three of the five infants weighing less than 1,000 g had either contraindications to pharmacologic intervention of PDA or were too ill to undergo surgical ligation.

When infants in category B were combined with those in category A, surfactant treatment was successful in 95% of the infants, with 93% suvival rate in this series. Similar results have been obtained in our recent three series of multicenter nonrandomized and randomized trials in a total of 336 infants.

Poor or No Response (Response C)

A poor response was defined as an increase in a/APO$_2$ of less than 0.2, and no response was defined as an increase in a/APO$_2$ of less than 0.1 when evaluated at 6 hours after surfactant therapy, combined with little change in respiratory requirements. This response was seen in 5% (5/96) of the surfactant recipients. All of these infants had severe perinatal asphyxia.

RDS is not simply characterized by surfactant deficiency, and therefore it is not surprising that there are always some unresponsive infants.

Cardiogenic shock or myocardial dysfunction or persistent fetal circulation are the other cardiopulmonary conditions presenting early in the neonatal period as signs and symptoms of respiratory distress, which develop resembling RDS. Five infants had myocardial dysfunction, one of whom had Doppler-detectable tricuspid regurgitaiton, and two larger infants had PFC. These infants were treated with cardiotonic agents. Three of the five recovered.

Transient Response due to Inadequate Ventilator Settings (Response D)

While this response was not seen in this series, in our multicenter uncontrolled trial we encountered a small number of infants who had a transient response that appeared to be related to inadequate ventilator settings.

Low Ventilator Settings Prior to Surfactant Installation.—Because of the fear of acute barotrauma, some attendant physicians in the study did not follow the study protocol, but used higher rates and lower peak inflating pressures. In some extreme cases the presurfactant settings used were PIP 12 to 15 cm H_2O, frequency 80 to 100 cpm, inspiratory time 0.1 to 0.3 seconds, PEEP 2 to 10 cm H_2O, Fio_2 1.0; blood gas levels were Pao_2 40 to 50 torr, $Paco_2$ 50 to 80 torr; and pH was 7.1 to 7.2. Surfactant instillation produced a rapid increase in Pao_2, but this was not sustained (as shown in Fig 6–2,D). The initial settings used in these patients do not seem to be adequate for opening the closed lung units and displacing the fluid from the airways.

Rapid Lowering Ventilator Settings After Surfactant.—In other cases in which the initial settings were adequate, there was a surfactant-induced dramatic increase in Pao_2. At this point both the peak inflating pressure and Fio_2 were reduced too rapidly, resulting in a gradual decline in a/APo_2 (see Fig 6–2,D). Adjustment of the settings led to consistent improvement in oxygenation with decreasing ventilatory requirements.

Certain points about the adjustment of respiratory settings during and after surfactant instillation deserve emphasis. It must be noted that the manner in which surfactant is administered is simply to deliver liquid to the baby's lungs. To provide adequate aeration of the liquid-filled lung at birth, the inflating pressure must be high enough to overcome capillarity in the finer conducting airways. Furthermore, this opening pressure must be applied for a period of time long enough to overcome the viscosity of the fluid that has to be displaced from the airways as the air-liquid interface moves toward the alveoli. All this suggests that initially a higher inflating pressure and a longer inspiratory time should be the preferred settings.

It is important to note that during instillation of surfactant the inflating pressure should be maintained at a few cm H_2O higher than the previous settings to promote uniform distribution of surfactant in the lung and to prevent fluid from plugging the airways. In addition, the settings used prior to treatment should be maintained to produce good air entry into the lung, adequate oxygenation, and ventilation. Lachmann et al.[26] demonstrated that when surfactant-treated preterm animal lungs ventilated with a fixed peak inflating pressure of 25 cm H_2O and a frequency of 40 cpm, a longer inspiratory time (0.9 seconds) resulted in better alveolar recruitment and compliance characteristics than a shorter inspiratory time (0.3 seconds).

Once a clear improvement in the gas exchange has occurred, Fio_2 should be first lowered and then the inflating pressure carefully reduced.

Dosage of Surfactant

In addition to the timing of treatment, either at birth or early vs. late, the dosage of surfactant is also important. There has been no consistency in the dose used in reported clinical trials. Surfactant TA has been used in both low and high doses. Our randomized trial showed that both low-dose (60 mg/kg) and high-dose (120 mg/kg) treatments improved oxygenation with decreased ventilatory requirements, the high-dose surfactant having a more beneficial effect in prolonging the response. The striking and acute improvement in oxygenation and ventilation achieved with the low-dose treatment suggest that initially this dose of surfactant was at least sufficient to neutralize the inhibitors that were already present in the airways before treatment. However, this initial beneficial effect was not sustained in a significant proportion of infants who received the low dose. Our study showed further that infants in the high-dose group had significantly less incidence of both IVH and BPD.[24] Thus the use of an inadequate dose of surfactant may account not only for the variability in response but also for the lack of a substantial reduction in the incidence of IVH in the series reported by others.

Single vs. Multiple Doses of Surfactant

To date, in all clinical trials with Surfactant TA, Survanta, Curosurf, and CLSE, a single dose was used. In the trials using human surfactant a number of cases had to be re-treated. The initial dose used in human surfactant studies is lower than that used in other surfactant studies. When Vidyasager et al.[39] applied the retreatment criteria of Merritt et al.[29] to their patients treated with a single dose of Surfactant TA, only two of the 17 surfactant-treated patients would have required retreatment.

Our recent experience shows that treatment with the single dose of Surfactant TA within 6 hours of age even in very small premature infants (24 to 26 weeks gestation) seldom required re-treatment.

Maldistribution of Surfactant in the Lungs

Maldistribution of the surfactant in the lungs of treated infants may occur especially when surfactant is instilled in a bolus as opposed to divided doses. Eagan et al.[9] observed that improper administration of surfactant occurred in 18% of the infants who received a bolus of Infasurf at birth (i.e., the deposition of surfactant instilled was in the right mainstem bronchus or in the oropharynx). Eagan speculates that the substantial variations in the effectiveness of a single dose of intratracheal instillation of surfactant at birth are likely due to suboptimal administration of surfactant in some clinical trials. Using instillation technique similar to that described earlier here, Charon et al.[3] found that there was homogeneous distribution of technetium-labeled Surfactant TA in the lungs in both the infants who had sustained improvement in a/APO_2 and those who did not. They concluded that gross maldistribution of surfactant is not a major factor associated with suboptimal response to surfactant therapy. Homogeneous surfactant distribution with no improvement in a/APo$_2$ may suggest either surfactant inactivation due to PDA or an increased extrapulmonary right-to-left shunt (clear lung with hypoperfusion).

Potential Toxicity

Remarkably little toxicity has become apparent in the animal and clinical studies of surfactant. One concern about using bovine surfactant is the presence of a small amount of proteolipid apoproteins (SP-B,C) in the preparation; however, attempts to immunize goats with Surfactant TA by a vigorous hyperimmunization technique that was repeated for 6 months were unsuccessful.[4] Also, we have been unable to detect any antibodies against surfactant TA in more than 600 serum samples from the 204 patients treated with surfactant TA.[22]

Follow-up of Surfactant-Treated Infants

Several studies on follow-up of surfactant-treated infants are in progress around the world. Dunn et al.[8] found no differences between the surfactant-treated and control infants with respect to allergic symptoms, respiratory problems, or neurodevelopmental outcome. Vaucher et al.[38] demonstrated improved neurodevelopmental performance among surfactant-treated infants, and speculated that decrease in the frequency of BPD should ultimately lead to improved long-term outcome.

SUMMARY AND PERSPECTIVE

This overview analysis of the current clinical trials of various naturally derived surfactant extracts suggests that use of these preparations to both prevent and treat RDS should be effective in decreasing major morbidity factors of RDS and mortality. The benefits of such therapy greatly exceed the putative hazards. The beneficial effects of surfactant therapy last for at least 72 hours in several studies, but these effects are not consistently seen in other studies. Our clinical experience with Surfactant TA, and a little future projection, suggest that the impact on BPD, ICH, and mortality should eventually be greater. Using our therapeutic regimen with a single dose Surfactant TA, we have had few cases of severe BPD (grade III or higher; i.e., infants who require more than 40% oxygen and are ventilator dependent for a period of months). Although we still see some infants who have mild BPD requiring little or less than 30% supplemental oxygen, the prevalence of such chronic lung disease in tiny infants treated with surfactant does not differ from that in infants without lung disease of comparable gestational age and birth weight who received mechanical ventilation.

Our observations on the 96 RDS patients treated with Surfactant TA suggest that surfactant therapy unmasks the relative contributions of other mechanisms to the whole spectrum of RDS, which includes hemodynamically significant PDA, persistent fetal circulation (clear lung with hypoperfusion), cardiogenic shock, transient myocardial dysfunction with or without tricuspid regurgitation associated with severe perinatal asphyxia, among other problems.

In assessing the effectiveness of surfactant treatment we should consider possible effects of these underlying abnormalities that may complicate the interpretation of the response. Serial echocardiographic and color Doppler examinations are useful in identifying these underlying abnormalities. With early recognition, management, and possible prevention of these circulatory disturbances (PDA, hypotension), it may be possible to increase the significance of surfactant treatment further and to facilitate uncomplicated recovery.

To optimize the effects of surfactant therapy, future refinement will also be needed to better our understanding of surfactant preparations, instillation techniques including pre- and post-surfactant ventilation, as well as weaning guidelines, dose, dose schedule, and patient selection.

The isolation and characterization of three surfactant proteins (SP-A, -B, and -C) have considerably changed our understanding of the nature and properties of pulmonary surfactant and its metabolism. In the 1990s we will have a second- or third-generation surfactant consisting of synthetic lipids and proteolipid apoproteins (SP-B, -C) that are produced by recombinant DNA technology or direct chemical synthesis.

REFERENCES

1. Adams FH, Towers B, Osher AB, et al: Effect of tracheal instillation of natural surfactant in premature lambs: Clinical and autopsy findings. *Pediatr Res* 1978; 12:841–848.
2. Avery ME, Mead J: Surface properties in relation to atelectasis and hyaline membrane disease. *Am J Dis Child* 1959; 97:517–523.
3. Charon A, Taeusch HW Jr, Fitzgibbon C, et al: Factors associated with surfactant treatment response in infants with severe respiratory distress syndrome. *Pediatrics* 1989; 83:348–354.
4. Chida S: Unpublished data, 1985.
5. Chida S, Phelps D, Cordle C, et al: Surfactant associated proteins in tracheal aspirates of infants with respiratory distress syndrome after exogenous surfactant therapy. *Am Rev Respir Dis* 1988; 137:943–947.
6. Chu J, Clements JA, Cotton EK, et al: Neonatal pulmonary ischemia. *Pediatrics* 1967; 40:708–782.
7. Collaborative European Multicenter Study Group: Surfactant replacement therapy for severe neonatal respiratory distress syndrome: An international randomized clinical trial. *Pediatrics* 1988; 82:683–691.
8. Dunn MS, Shennan AT, Hoskins EM, et al: Two year-follow-up of infants in a randomized trial with surfactant replacement for the prevention of neonatal respiratory distress syndrome. *Pediatrics* 1988; 82:543–547.

9. Eagan EA, Kwong MS: Clinical results of multicenter open trial of infasurf. Presented at Ross Laboratories Special Conference: Hot topics '88 in neonatology; Washington, D.C., December 11–13, 1988.

10. Enhorning G, Robertson B: Lung expansion in the premature rabbit fetus after tracheal deposition of surfactant. *Pediatrics* 1972; 50:58–66.

11. Enhorning G, Shennan A, Possmayer F, et al: Prevention of neonatal respiratory distress syndrome by tracheal instillation of surfactant: A randomized clinical trial. *Pediatrics* 1985; 76:145–153.

12. Fuchimukai T, Fujiwara T, Takahasi A, et al: Artificial pulmonary surfactant inhibited by proteins. *J Appl Physiol* 1987; 62:429–439.

13. Fujiwara T: Surfactant replacement in neonatal RDS, in Robertson B, Van Golde LMG, Batenburg JJ (eds): *Pulmonary Surfactant.* Amsterdam, Elsevier, 1984, pp 479–503.

14. Fujiwara T, Konishi M, Nanbu H, et al: Surfactant therapy in RDS: Results of a multicenter randomized trial. *Jpn J Pediatr* 1987; 40:549–568.

15. Fujiwara T, Maeta H, Chida S, et al: Artificial surfactant therapy in hyaline membrane disease. *Lancet* 1980; 1:55–596.

16. Gitlin JD, Soll RF, Parad RB, et al: Randomized controlled trial of exogenous surfactant for the treatment of hyaline membrane disease. *Pediatrics* 1987; 79:31–37.

17. Halliday HL, McClure G, Reid MMc, et al: Controlled trial of artificial surfactant to prevent respiratory distress syndrome. *Lancet* 1984; 1:476–478.

18. Hallman M, Merritt A, Jarvenpaa A-L, et al: Exogenous human surfactant for treatment of severe respiratory distress syndrome: A randomized prospective clinical trial. *J Pediatr* 1985; 106:963–969.

19. Horbar JD, Soll RF, Sutherland JM, et al: A multicenter randomized, placebo-controlled trial of surfactant therapy for respiratory distress syndrome. *N Engl J Med* 1988; 320:959–965.

20. Ikegami M, Ogata Y, Elkady T, et al: Comparison of four surfactants: In vitro surface properties and responses of preterm lambs to treatment at birth. *Pediatrics* 1987; 79:38–46.

21. Jobe A, Ikegami M: Surfactant for the treatment of respiratory distress syndrome. *Am Rev Respir Dis* 1987; 136:1256–1275.

22. Kawashima T, Chida S, Fujiwara T: Measurements of anti-surfactant proteolipid-5-kDa apoprotein antibodies in sera from HMD-patients treated with surfactant TA using an ELISA. *Perinat Med (Jpn)* 1987; 17:473–476.

23. Kendig JW, Notter RB, Cox C, et al: Surfactant replacement therapy at birth: Final analysis of a clinical trial and comparisons with similar trials. *Pediatrics* 1988; 82:756–762.

24. Konishi M, Fujiwara T, Naito N, et al: Surfactant replacement therapy in neonatal respiratory distress syndrome: A multicenter, randomized clinical trial: Comparison of high- vs low-dose of surfactant TA. *Eur J Pediatr* 1988; 147:20–25.

25. Kwong MS, Eagan EA, Notter RH, et al: Double-blind clinical trial of calf lung surfactant extract for the prevention of hyaline membrane disease in extremely premature infants. *Pediatrics* 1985; 76:585–592.

26. Lachmann B, Berggren P, Curstedt T, et al: Combined effects of surfactant substitution and prolongation of inspiration phase in artificially ventilated premature newborn rabbits. *Pediatr Res* 1982; 16:921–927.

27. Maeta H, Vidyasagar D, Raju TNK, et al: Early and late surfactant treatments in baboon model of hyaline membrane disease. *Pediatrics* 1988; 81:277–283.

28. Merritt TA, Hallman M: Surfactant replacement. *Am J Dis Child* 1988; 142:1333–1339.
29. Merritt TA, Hallman M, Bloom BT, et al: Prophylactic treatment of very premature infants with human surfactant. *N Engl J Med* 1986; 315:785–790.
30. Morley CJ: Surfactant therapy for very premature babies. *Br Med Bull* 1988; 44:919–934.
31. Morley CJ, Lloyd D, Duffy P, et al: Ten centre trial of artificial surfactant (artificial lung expanding compound) in very premature babies. *Br Med J* 1987; 294:991–996.
32. Pattle RE, Kratzing CC, Parkinson CE, et al: Maturity of fetal lungs tested by production of stable microbubbles in amniotic fluid. *Br J Obstet Gynaecol* 1979; 86:615–622.
33. Raju TNK, Vidyasagar D, Bhat R, et al: Double-blind controlled trial of single-dose treatment with bovine surfactant in severe hyaline membrane disease. *Lancet* 1987; 1:651–655.
34. Robertson B, Van Golde LMG, Batenburg JJ: *Pulmonary Surfactant.* Amsterdam, Elsevier, 1984.
35. Sasaki M: *Iwate Med J,* in press.
36. Shapiro DL, Notter RH, Morin FC III, et al: Double-blind randomized trial of a calf lung surfactant extract administered at birth to very premature infants for prevention of respiratory distress syndrome. *Pediatrics* 1985; 76:593–599.
37. Shapiro DL, Notter RH, Taeusch W, et al: Surfactant replacement therapy. *Semin Perinatol* 1988; 12:173–260.
38. Vaucher YE, Merritt TA, Hallman M, et al: Neurodevelopmental and respiratory outcome in early childhood after human surfactant treatment. *Am J Dis Child* 1988; 142:927–930.
39. Vidyasagar D, Raju TNK, Shimada S, et al: Surfactant replacement therapy: Clinical and experimental studies. *Clin Perinatol* 1987; 14:713–736.
40. Wilkinson A, Jenkins PA, Jeffrey JA: Two controlled trials of dry artificial surfactant: Early effects and later outcome in babies with surfactant deficiency. *Lancet* 1985; 2:287–291.

7

Resuscitation

Hemendra B. Patel, M.D.

Angela Wilks, M.D.

Devyani Raval, M.D.

Tsu F. Yeh, M.D.

Resuscitation is required at any time for cardiopulmonary arrest. In the birth room it is required for any newborn infant who fails to establish effective ventilation in a reasonable time. In the neonatal intensive care unit it is required any time there is cessation of effective ventilation or circulation. Resuscitation is most often required in the birth room, in the first few minutes of life.

Primary cardiac problems leading to cardiopulmonary arrest are rare in neonates. Primary respiratory arrest causing hypoxia, acidosis, and secondary circulatory failure is common in neonates. Birth asphyxia is the most common cause of cardiopulmonary arrest requiring resuscitation, and is seen in 13% of all deliveries.[10] It can begin at any time before labor, during labor, and in the immediate postpartum period. Immediate intervention is necessary to prevent asphyxial damage to organs. The following factors are associated with birth asphyxia:

1. Maternal conditions
   Age (<16 or >35 years)
   Anemia
   Toxemia of pregnancy
   Medical problems
   Drug abuse
   Antepartum hemorrhage
   Falling estriol level
   Previous neonatal death
   Previous perinatal morbidity

Previous baby with birth defect
Prolonged rupture of membranes
Blood group or type isoimmunization
Poor antenatal care
Malnutrition
2. Intrapartum conditions
Abnormal fetal presentation
Cephalopelvic disproportion
Cesarean section
Precipitate delivery
Prolapsed cord
Narcotic analgesics to mother 2 hours before delivery
Forceps delivery
Prolonged labor
3. Fetal conditions
Multiple pregnancy
Polyhydramnios
Oligohydramnios
Meconium staining
Abnormal fetal growth (large or small for gestational age)
Prematurity
Postmaturity
Abnormal fetal heart rate
Fetal acidosis

PATHOPHYSIOLOGY OF ASPHYXIA

Knowledge of the pathophysiology of acute asphyxia is based on experiments in which asphyxia was induced in newborn animals delivered by cesarean section by sealing their heads in a bag of saline solution before breathing started. Changes occurring in the breathing pattern, heart rate, and arterial blood pressure during acute asphyxia and resuscitation of fetal monkeys are summarized in Figure 7–1.

After a few shallow breaths, the animal stops breathing. This cessation of breathing is called *primary apnea.* After 1 to 2 minutes of primary apnea, gasping starts, with increasing depth and frequency, diminishes slowly to the final gasp, and breathing stops again. This phase is called *secondary apnea or terminal apnea.* The changes in heart rate and arterial blood pressure are parallel. Heart rate falls rapidly or may rise initially and then fall during primary apnea. It stops completely 10 minutes after the last gasp, during secondary apnea. Arterial blood pressure similarly rises initially, then gradually falls through secondary apnea.

If asphyxia is terminated, the response seen depends on the stage of asphyxia. During primary apnea the animal will gasp and develop sponta-

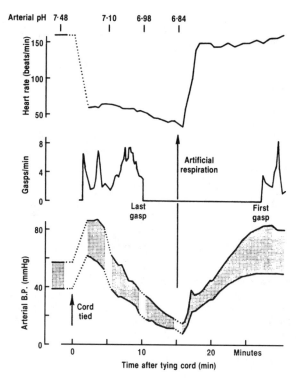

FIG 7–1.
Changes in breathing pattern, heart rate, and arterial blood pressure *(B.P.)* during acute asphyxia and resuscitation in fetal monkey. (From Dawes GS, Hibbard E, Windle W: *J Pediatr* 1964; 65:801–806. Used by permission.)

neous regular breathing. During secondary apnea, gasping and spontaneous breathing will not occur and the animal will die. Assisted ventilation may establish breathing during secondary apnea (Fig 7–2). If given during resuscitation, alkali and glucose[1] cause an increase in cardiac output, help early onset of spontaneous regular breathing, and may decrease subsequent brain damage.[6]

The knowledge obtained from animal experiments helps in management of asphyxia in the human newborn. Clinically, human neonatal asphyxia is never total and continuous; rather, it is partial and intermittent. The human fetus and newborn may be less mature and may be able to tolerate asphyxia of greater magnitude. During primary apnea the infant will start gasping and spontaneous breathing by appropriate sensory stimuli; during secondary apnea assisted ventilation is necessary. In the delivery room it is difficult to determine whether the newborn has primary or secondary apnea.

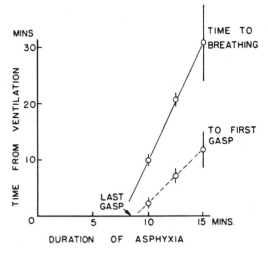

FIG 7–2.
Time from beginning positive pressure ventilation with oxygen until first gasp *(broken line)* to establishment of rhythmic breathing *(solid line)* in newly delivered rhesus monkeys with asphyxia induced for 10, 12½, or 15 minutes at 30° C. *Vertical bars* indicate standard error of the mean in each group. (From Adamsons K, et al: *J Pediatr* 1964; 65:807–818. Used by permission.)

Effects of Asphyxia on Organ Systems

Acute or chronic asphyxia can cause permanent or temporary changes in various tissues (Fig 7–3). These effects depend on the duration and severity of asphyxia.

Biochemical changes during asphyxia are caused by tissue hypoxia, leading to anaerobic metabolism and to formation of lactic acid and other organic acids. Failure of circulation causes accumulation of organic acids in tissues, which leads to metabolic acidosis. Failure of ventilation leads to accumulation of carbon dioxide and respiratory acidosis. The combined effects of these changes are profound mixed acidosis and very low tissue pH. Low tissue pH damages enzymes and cellular metabolism, ultimately causing cell death and tissue necrosis.

Birth asphyxia causes cerebral edema, hemorrhage, and necrosis. It causes respiratory depression at birth, and permanent brain damage as a sequela. It can cause heart failure by decreasing myocardial contractility, and causes hypotensive myocardial ischemia and necrosis.[3]

In the lungs asphyxia initially decreases pulmonary blood flow. It later increases blood flow and pulmonary edema. In preterm infants pulmonary edema leads to desquamation of type II alveolar cells and persistent acidosis, which inhibits surfactant synthesis.[9]

In term infants massive pulmonary hemorrhage is a possible sequela of asphyxia or a result of acute left ventricular failure secondary to myocardial necrosis and fluid overload caused by inappropriate regulation of vaso-pressin.[4] Transient proteinuria and acute tubular necrosis are seen after an episode of asphyxia.[5] Asphyxia is an important predisposing factor in the development of necrotizing enterocolitis.

Asphyxia can cause other biochemical disturbances, such as hypoglyce-mia, hypocalcemia, excessive vasopressin production, hyponatremia, defi-ciency of clotting factors, and hepatic dysfunction.

PRINCIPLES OF NEONATAL RESUSCITATION

Initial Assessment

Resuscitation is more often required in the first few minutes of life than at any other time. Initial assessment in the delivery room will aid the initiation of resuscitation and in following the response to it.

The Apgar score is universally used in the initial assessment of any new-born.[2] The score at 1 minute is a useful guide to the degree of asphyxia and the need for resuscitation; the score at 5 minutes correlates well with long-term survival and brain damage. Although the scoring system is useful for the initial evaluation, 1 minute is too long to wait to make the decision to start resuscitation.

As in any other situation of cardiopulmonary arrest, the signs of circu-

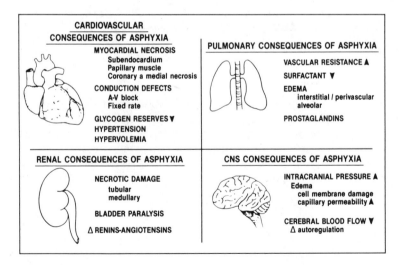

FIG 7–3.
Effects of birth asphyxia on various organs. (From *Cardiovascular Sequelae of Asphyxia in the Newborn.* Report of the Eighty-third Ross Conference on Pediatric Research. Columbus, Ohio, Ross Laboratories. Used by permission).

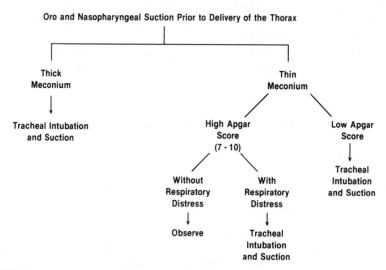

Meconium-Stained Amniotic Fluid

Oro and Nasopharyngeal Suction Prior to Delivery of the Thorax

Thick Meconium → Tracheal Intubation and Suction

Thin Meconium
- High Apgar Score (7 - 10)
  - Without Respiratory Distress → Observe
  - With Respiratory Distress → Tracheal Intubation and Suction
- Low Apgar Score → Tracheal Intubation and Suction

FIG 7–4.
Management of infants with meconium staining. Endotracheal intubation is recommended in infants with low Apgar scores, respiratory distress, or thick meconium staining.

latory and respiratory arrest should be checked. Circulatory arrest is diagnosed by absent or weak pulses, absent heart rate, hypotension (arterial), and poor perfusion. Respiratory arrest is seen as absent breathing or gasping, and cyanosis.

Initial Management

To clear the airway of secretions, the obstetrician should suction the infant's mouth and nose with a bulb syringe on delivery of the head. The newborn is then placed under a preheated radiant warmer with head tilted downward 20° toward the resuscitator. Head and trunk are dried, and a quick examination is done to determine the need for resuscitation. Respiratory efforts, heart rate (by palpation of umbilical cord or auscultation of heart), and color are noted.

Airway

After initial assessment of the newborn, if necessary the airway can be resuctioned with the bulb syringe or suction catheter. Repeated blind suctioning with the catheter may cause bradycardia and apnea secondary to vagal stimulation. In infants with possible meconium aspiration syndrome, endotracheal intubation is recommended if the infant is depressed or in respiratory distress or if the meconium is thick (Fig 7–4).

Breathing

Once spontaneous respiration is absent in neonates, assisted ventilation must be started. It is started by bagging with a face mask. The resuscitation bag should be self-inflating with a pop-off valve and a gas reservoir to deliver 100% oxygen. The face mask should fit nose and mouth without any leakage. Bagging is done for 15 to 20 seconds; then the neonate is checked for spontaneous breathing. If spontaneous breathing is not established, endotracheal intubation should be performed. This provides the best control of the airway.

Circulation

If there is no heartbeat, of if severe bradycardia is unresponsive to effective ventilation with 100% oxygen, external cardiac compression is necessary. Cardiac compression will maintain circulation and blood pressure. The rate of compression (between 100 and 120 per minute) should be synchronized with artificial ventilation. In infants, cardiac compression is done by placing two fingers over the midsternum and compressing the sternum by 1/2 to 1 inch. Encircling of the infant's chest with two hands, with both thumbs on the lower sternum, is an equally effective method for cardiac compression.

The response to all these measures is judged by improvement in heart rate, tone, and color. If there is no improvement, drug therapy is instituted.

DRUG THERAPY DURING RESUSCITATION

Drug therapy forms an essential part of successful resuscitation. It can correct both biochemical changes caused by asphyxia and hemodynamic changes associated with circulatory arrest. In neonates the dosage is based on body weight or body surface area. This calculation requires the actual weight of the infant or knowing how to approximate birth weight with reasonable accuracy.

Routes of Administration

A central arterial line is the best route for drug administration. The arterial line is preferred to a venous line, because it gives access to blood pressure monitoring and arterial blood sampling. The central venous line is an equally good route, because it leads to measurement of central venous pressure. An umbilical venous line in the newborn carries the potential risk for portal vein thrombosis and infection. If used, the catheter should be removed when resuscitation is achieved. The peripheral venous line can be used for administration of drugs. Intracardiac injection can be lifesaving in a given situation, but can cause problems such as hemopericardium, laceration of coronary vessels, pneumothorax, myocardial injury, and arrhythmias. Intramuscular and subcutaneous injections offer slow and unpredictable absorption of drugs and have little if any value during resuscitation. Direct needle puncture of umbilical vessels has the risk for hematoma formation and is difficult to do repeatedly.

Correction of Hypoxia

Hypoxia means lack of oxygen regardless of cause or site involved. Cardiorespiratory arrest leads to severe hypoxia. Tissue oxygenation depends on cardiac output and oxygen carried by blood. The oxygen-carrying capacity of blood depends on partial pressure of oxygen (Po_2), which in turn depends on the fractional concentration of oxygen in inspired gas (Fio_2). Improving the oxygenation of myocardium improves contractility and increases cardiac output. Cerebral function and ultimate recovery depend on adequate oxygen supply to brain; 100% oxygen is used during resuscitation. Oxygen toxicity, from excessively high concentrations of oxygen, can cause rentrolental fibroplasia, a major concern in preterm infants. As soon as possible arterial Po_2 should be determined and Fio_2 decreased.

Correction of Acidosis

To correct respiratory acidosis, it is necessary to establish effective ventilation, reducing the partial pressure of carbon dioxide (PCo_2) to normal or below normal. Metabolic acidosis can be corrected rapidly and transiently by infusion of alkali, but permanent correction is achieved by effective ventilation and circulation.

Sodium Bicarbonate

Sodium bicarbonate ($NaHCO_3$) is used for the correction of metabolic acidosis, especially the lactic acidosis caused by cardiopulmonary arrest. It reduces the hydrogen ion concentration by a simple acid-base reaction, releasing carbon dioxide: $NaHCO_3 + H^+ \rightarrow Na^+ + H_2O + CO_2$. The released carbon dioxide will accumulate in the blood if effective ventilation is not established.

Sodium bicarbonate is available as 4.2%, 7.5%, and 8.4% solutions for parenteral use. In neonates a 4.2% solution is used; any other strength is diluted with distilled water to reduce osmolality. The initial dose of sodium bicarbonate is 1 mEq/kg, infused slowly over 1 to 2 minutes. If blood pH and base deficit are determined, the subsequent dose of bicarbonate is calculated as follows: Sodium bicarbonate (mEq) = 0.3 × Weight (kg) × Base deficit (mEq). If blood gases are not measured, sodium bicarbonate doses of 1 mEq/kg every 10 minutes can be repeated if the infant does not improve. Ventilation is maintained to keep the PCo_2 normal or below normal, since released carbon dioxide from the sodium bicarbonate can cause respiratory acidosis. Accumulation of carbon dioxide will prevent the chemical reaction from proceeding to the right and the pH will remain low. Rapid correction of acidosis by alkali therapy can lead to metabolic alkalosis, intraventricular hemorrhage, hyperosmolality, hypokalemia, and hypernatremia. A paradoxical drop in intracerebral pH can aggravate CNS depression.

Tromethamine

Tromethamine (THAM) is a sodium-free buffer used in the correction of metabolic acidosis in a manner similar to sodium bicarbonate. The base combines with H^+ to raise the pH and Hco_3 without the release of carbon dioxide. It is available as a 0.3 mol/L solution, used in the same dose as bicarbonate. It can cause respiratory depression and hypoglycemia. The use of THAM in neonates is limited.

Correction For Cardiogenic Shock

Hypoxia and acidosis can lead to cardiac dysfunction and cardiogenic shock. Clinically this is manifested as bradycardia, hypotension, poor peripheral perfusion, absent or weak pulses, and shock. Sympathomimetic amines, both synthetic and natural, are useful in reversing cardiogenic shock. They normally regulate the heart rate, force of contraction, vascular tone, and blood pressure.

Epinephrine

Epinephrine is an endogenous sympathomimetic amine that stimulates beta receptors. It improves myocardial contractility and increases heart rate. Epinephrine also increases myocardial oxygen consumption, decreases myocardial efficiency, and produces rhythm disturbances such as fibrillation. Peripherally it acts on alpha receptors, causing an increase in systolic blood pressure and pulse pressure. Diastolic pressure also may be increased slightly. It is rapidly inactivated by the liver and other tissues.

Epinephrine is indicated for cardiac asystole and ineffective slow contractions. Adequate ventilation, external cardiac compression, and at least partial correction of acidosis are desirable before epinephrine is administered.

For neonatal use epinephrine is available as a 1:10,000 solution, given in a dose of 0.1 mL/kg. It is given intravenously through a central or peripheral line or by arterial catheter, although endotracheal instillation has been proved to be equally useful.[7] It is rapidly absorbed from trachea and acts on the heart. Epinephrine administration may be repeated if necessary in the same dose. When all other efforts fail and no other routes are available, intracardiac injections can be given.

Low-dose infusion of epinephrine is useful in maintaining blood pressure and increasing cardiac output. Intravascular volume is restored prior to epinephrine use. This method increases cardiac output, decreases peripheral resistance, and increases systolic blood pressure. Infusion is started at 0.02 to 0.05 μg/kg/min and increased up to 0.5 μg/kg/min depending on response obtained. Higher doses can lead to tachycardia, arrhythmia, vasoconstriction, and poor tissue perfusion.

TABLE 7-1.
Sympathomimetic Amines

Drug	Dose range (μg/kg/min)	Comments
Epinephrine	0.1-0.5	Supports blood pressure in shock; increases cardiac output; low dose decreases peripheral resistance; β_2-adrenergic blocking agent effect
Norepinephrine	0.1-0.5	Mainly acts on receptors, increasing peripheral resistance; mildly inotropic agent; may cause renal ischemia
Dopamine	2-20	Lower dose causes increased renal blood flow and decreases peripheral resistance; mildly inotropic agent; higher dose causes vasoconstriction
Dobutamine	2-20	Useful for cardiogenic shock; minimum peripheral vasoconstriction; no renal effect
Isoproterenol	0.1-0.5	Strong β_1- and β_2-receptor stimulation; decreases peripheral resistance by vasodilation; reduces central venous pressure

Dopamine

Dopamine is the immediate metabolic precursor of epinephrine. It is an agonist, causing an increase in heart rate and increased force of contraction. Peripherally it increases systolic pressure and pulse pressure; diastolic pressure remains same or increases. With low doses it increases renal blood flow, glomerular filtration rate, and fractional sodium excretion. Tachycardia is less marked with dopamine than with epinephrine.

Dopamine is used for cardiogenic and hypovolemic shock. Correction of hypovolemia is essential before beginning dopamine therapy. It is given as a continuous infusion at a rate of 2 to 5 μg/kg/min to a maximum of 20 μg/kg/min, titrated with response obtained. Heart rate, blood pressure, and urine output should be monitored and the infusion rate should be decreased or stopped if tachycardia, arrhythmia, or hypertension develops. Dopamine has a very short half-life in plasma, and its adverse effects will disappear quickly once it is discontinued.

Dobutamine

Dobutamine chemically resembles dopamine. It is a synthetic catecholamine, acting as beta receptor agonist. It increases myocardial contraction, does not produce tachycardia, and does not affect renal blood vessels. It increases peripheral resistance minimally. Dobutamine is administered as a continuous infusion at a rate of 0.5 to 10 μg/kg/min. Higher doses (>20 μg/kg/min) may be required. Heart rate, blood pressure, and cardiac rhythm should be monitored for adverse effects. It has a very short half-life in plasma, similar to that of dopamine. It is mainly useful for treatment of cardiogenic shock.

Norepinephrine and isoproterenol are other sympathomimetic amines used for cardiovascular actions. Their doses and indications are summarized in Table 7-1.

Correction For Hypovolemia

Hypovolemia occurring in an asphyxiated neonate is difficult to differentiate from circulating arrest. It is suspected if after adequate ventilation there is pallor, weak peripheral pulses, poor pulse pressure, arterial hypotension, low central venous pressure, poor capillary filling time (>3 seconds), and persistent metabolic acidosis. Hypovolemia needs to be corrected by volume expansion.

Fluids available for immediate volume expansion are blood, plasma, albumin, and normal saline solution. Blood obtained from the fetal side of placenta, collected aseptically in a heparinized syringe, can be used within 1 hour of delivery. An equally good choice is O-negative, low-titer blood, cross-matched against the mother's blood before delivery. Non-cross-matched O-negative blood is not desirable, because it can cause fatal transfusion reaction as a result of minor group incompatibility. Fresh-frozen plasma and salt-poor albumin are the next best choices. They can cause transient expansion of plasma volume, but on leaving the circulation, can produce edema. Crystalloids are easily available and can rapidly correct plasma volume, restoring tissue perfusion. The agents used are normal saline solution and lactated Ringer's solution. Ten to 20 mL/kg should be given slowly intravenously; and may be repeated if necessary. Decrease in capillary filling time after blanching, normal arterial blood pressure, increase in central venous pressure, correction of metabolic acidosis, and good pulse pressure are signs of correction of hypovolemia. Overcorrection of blood volume can lead to an increase in arterial pressure and can precipitate intraventricular hemorrhage in a small infant.

Miscellaneous Agents

Dextrose

Supplying glucose as a metabolic substrate is important after cardiopulmonary arrest. Blood glucose levels should be determined (using Dextrostix or other available methods). If blood glucose levels are normal, intravenously administered dextrose in water or saline solution at maintenance levels should be administered.

If blood glucose is low, an intravenous push of 200 mg/kg glucose is indicated, followed by 8 mg/kg/min as a maintenance dose.[8] This amount is equal to 2 mL/kg 10% dextrose as push and approximately 5 mL/kg/hr as maintenance fluids. Rapid infusion of 25% or 50% dextrose is not necessary, and may cause vascular injury. Documentation of hypoglycemia is desirable, but not a must, and should not delay administration of glucose.

Calcium

Calcium ion is a potent positive inotropic agent that increases the force of contraction of myocardium. It is indicated during resuscitation for ineffective myocardial contraction and hypotension. Calcium is given slowly as an intravenous push. It can cause severe bradycardia, sustained myocardial contraction, and ventricular (asystolic) standstill. It should be given cautiously in the digitalized neonate, because it can precipitate digitalis toxicity. Calcium is available as calcium gluconate 10% and calcium chloride 10%. The dose is 0.3 mL/kg calcium chloride or 1 mL/kg calcium gluconate (i.e., 5 to 10 mg Ca^{++}/kg). It should be given slowly, accompanied by ECG and heart rate monitoring.

Atropine
Atropine is a vagolytic agent and abolishes the effects of high vagal tone. In adequate doses it reduces vagal tone, increases heart rate, and increases atrioventricular conduction. It is indicated for persistent bradycardia after adequate ventilation and circulation. Atropine is given intravenously in a dose of 0.02 mg/kg, and may be repeated twice if necessary. Adverse effects of atropine are tachycardia and arrhythmia.

Naloxone
Narcotic antagonists are used for reversal of respiratory depression caused by narcotic analgesics. Narcotic analgesics given to the mother during labor can cross the placenta and cause respiratory depression in the newborn infant.

Naloxone, levallorphan, and nalorphine are the available narcotic antagonists. Because levallorphan and nalorphine have substantial agonist actions, naloxone is the drug of choice. It does not cause respiratory depression.

Naloxone is administered intravenously at 0.01 mg/kg, or may be given intramuscularly or subcutaneously at a dose of 0.07 mg/kg.[11] It acts fairly rapidly by any route, with a duration of action that lasts 1 to 4 hours. The infant must be observed for recurrence of respiratory depression and need for repeated medication.

Lidocaine
Lidocaine, a local anesthetic, decreases the automaticity of myocardium. It is indicated to treat ventricular premature beats, ventricular tachycardia, and ventricular fibrillation. It is given as an intravenous bolus followed by continuous infusion, and is metabolized rapidly in liver. Adverse effects are CNS and cardiac actions. Lidocaine causes nausea, vomiting, disorientation, seizures, coma, decrease in cardiac output, heart block, and asystole.

Hypoxia, persistent metabolic acidosis, and electrolyte disturbances can cause ventricular premature beats, ventricular tachycardia, and fibrillation. These metabolic disturbances need to be corrected before using lidocaine. The dose is 1 mg/kg, as a bolus, followed by continuous low-dose infusion if continuous action is required (see Chapter 13).

Bretylium Tosylate
Bretylium tosylate is used for refractory ventricular tachycardia or ventricular fibrillation. It is a sympatholytic drug causing hypotension and stabilizing cardiac rhythm. The dose used is 5 mg/kg IV, which can be increased by 5 mg/kg if necessary, up to 30 mg/kg (see Chapter 13).

REFERENCES

1. Adamsons K, et al: Resuscitation by positive pressure ventilation and trishydroxymethylaminomethane of rhesus monkeys at birth. *J Pediatr* 1964; 65:807–818.
2. Apgar VA: Proposal for a new method of evaluation of the newborn infant. *Anesth Analg* 1953; 32:260–267.
3. Cabal LA, et al: Cardiogenic shock associated with perinatal asphyxia in term infants. *J Pediatr* 1980; 96:705–710.
4. Cole VA, et al: Pathogenesis of hemorrhagic pulmonary edema and massive pulmonary hemorrhage in the newborn. *Pediatrics* 1973; 57:175–187.
5. Dauber IM, et al: Renal failure following perinatal asphyxia. *J Pediatr* 1976; 88:851–855.
6. Dawes GS, Hibbard E, Windle W: The effect of alkali and glucose infusion on permanent brain damage in rhesus monkeys asphyxiated at birth. *J Pediatr* 1964; 65:801–806.
7. Greenberg MI, Roberts JR, Baskin SI: Use of endotracheally administered epinephrine in a pediatric patient. *Am J Dis Child* 1981; 135:767.
8. Lilien L, et al: Treatment of neonatal hypoglycemia with intravenous glucose infusion. *J Pediatr* 1980; 97:295–298.
9. Merritt TA, Farrell PM: Diminished pulmonary lecithin synthesis in acidosis. Experimental findings as related to the respiratory distress syndrome. *Pediatrics* 1976; 57:32–40.
10. Russell G, Lydon Y, Tunstall M: Antenatal prediction of neonatal asphyxia (abstract). *Anaesthesia* 1975; 30:118.
11. Wiener P, Hogg M, Rosen M: Effects of naloxone on pethidine-induced neonatal depression, part I and II. *Br Med J* 1977; 2:228–231.

8

Persistent Pulmonary Hypertension of the Newborn

Tsu F. Yeh, M.D.

Julie A. Luken, M.D.

Persistent pulmonary hypertension of the newborn (PPHN) occurs in a number of circumstances and as a result of a number of underlying mechanisms.[9] It is not a single disease but a situation of fetal circulation that has not made adequate transition to a normal postnatal circulation. In this chapter we summarize the pathophysiology, diagnosis, and management of these disorders; attempt to classify the syndrome into several groups; and discuss appropriate treatment.

FETAL AND NEONATAL PULMONARY CIRCULATION

The fetal pulmonary circulation is a high-pressure, low-flow circulation containing approximately 7% of the combined cardiac output. Immediately after birth there is a decrease in pulmonary vascular resistance and an increase in pulmonary circulation. The mechanisms for the transition from fetal to neonatal circulation are not completely understood, but are known to occur after expansion of the lungs and increase in alveolar Pao_2 and arterial oxygen tension Pao_2. The mechanisms for the transition may also be mediated by prostacyclin, leukotrienes, and thromboxanes. By in vitro study, a variety of factors and endogenous and exogenous vasoactive materials have also been shown to affect pulmonary vasculature.

PATHOGENESIS AND CAUSES

The underlying pathogenesis of PPHN probably can be classified as (1) pulmonary vascular constriction, (2) pulmonary arterial muscular hypertrophy, and (3) decreased pulmonary vascular bed. Any condition that interferes with normal oxygenation or lung expansion may cause pulmonary vascular constriction and delay the transition of fetal circulation to normal neonatal circulation. Chronic intrauterine hypoxia may cause muscular hypertrophy and new muscle formation of pulmonary vasculature. Hypoplastic lung provides an inadequate vascular bed for pulmonary blood flow, and hypertension may occur. Clinically, the causes of pulmonary hypertension in newborn infants can be classified into three groups:

1. Noncardiopulmonary causes of persistent pulmonary hypertension
   Chronic intrauterine hypoxia
   Perinatal hypoxia and acidosis
   Hypothermia
   Metabolic factors (e.g., hypoglycemia, hypocalcemia, hypomagnesemia)
   Polycythemia with hyperviscosity
   Prenatal administration of prostaglandin synthesis inhibitors (e.g., aspirin, indomethacin, ibuprofen, naproxen)
   Maternal phenytoin therapy
   Nonbacterial endocardial thrombosis
2. Respiratory disease predisposing to persistent pulmonary hypertension
   Obstructive airway disease
   Aspiration syndrome (meconium)
   Primary pulmonary hypoplasia
   Secondary pulmonary hypoplasia (diaphragmatic hernia)
   Pneumonia (group B β-hemolytic streptococci)
   Transient tachypnea of newborn
   Respiratory distress syndrome
3. Cardiac disease predisposing to pulmonary hypertension
   Pulmonary venous hypertension (pulmonary venous, left atrial, and mitral valve obstruction; left ventricular failure with cardiac lesions)
   Transient left ventricular dysfunction, myocarditis
   Large left-to-right shunting through an aortopulmonary or intraventricular communication without pulmonary stenosis

CLINICAL FEATURES AND DIAGNOSIS

The most prominent clinical features of PPHN are cyanosis and persistent hypoxemia. Based on the onset of persistent hypoxemia, this disorder can be recognized shortly after birth, as seen in infants with prenatal hypoxia and low Apgar score; can be moderately delayed (4 to 6 hours of age), as seen in infants with aspiration syndrome or group B β-hemolytic streptococcal infection; or may even present late, as seen in infants with airway disease.[10]

In those infants who do not have an underlying pulmonary disease, the clinical signs are sometimes indistinguishable from those of cyanotic congenital heart disease. For those infants who have underlying pulmonary disease, hypoxemia cannot be corrected completely by conventional mechanical ventilation with regular settings. Pao_2 in these infants fluctuates widely, with minimum changes in inspired oxygen concentration (flip-flop phenomenon). These patients also are critically sensitive to handling: very minor stimuli will trigger sudden deterioration and produce profound right-to-left shunting and hypoxemia. The following features are commonly seen with this disorder; none is specific for diagnosis.

1. Tachypnea, retraction, hypoxia, hypercarbia, acidosis
2. Tricuspid regurgitation murmur
3. Polycythemia
4. Meconium staining
5. Hypoglycemia, hypocalcemia, hypomagnesemia
6. Thrombocytopenia
7. Seizure and electrolyte imbalance
8. Congestive heart failure
9. Signs of sepsis

Pulmonary hypertension usually lasts 2 to 3 days, but clinical signs of respiratory distress may last for weeks. It is important that the following conditions be met before the diagnosis of PPHN can be made:[10] (1) normal systemic blood pressure and sustained suprasystemic pulmonary arterial pressure; (2) profound hypoxia with or without acidosis while breathing 100% oxygen; (3) normal cardiac anatomy; (4) evidence of right-to-left shunting of blood through the ductus arteriosus, patent foramen ovale, or both.

DIAGNOSTIC TESTS

Clinically, several tests are helpful for the provisional diagnosis of PPHN. These include the hyperoxia test, preductal versus postductal arterial Pao_2, and assisted ventilation with or without hyperventilation.[10] These tests are relatively noninvasive and can be done at bedside. Pao_2 responses to these tests under various clinical conditions are shown in Table 8–1.

In neonates with pulmonary hypertension, there may be a significant right-to-left shunt through the ductus arteriosus. If this ductal shunting exists, there is usually a more than 15 to 20 mm Hg difference between the preductal Pao_2 (sampled from the temporal arteries, right brachial artery, or right radial

TABLE 8–1.
Pao2 Responses to Various Tests Used to Diagnose Persistent Pulmonary Hypertension (PPHN) of Neonate*

Test	Inspired O$_2$ Concentration (%)	Ventilator Status	P$_{CO_2}$ Goal (mm Hg)	Typical P$_{O_2}$ values (mm Hg)		
				PPHN (severe, acute)	Pulmonary Parenchymal Disease	Congenital Heart Disease With Fixed Right-to-Left Shunt
Room air exposure	21	Spontaneous respirations	40	40	40	40
Hyperoxia test	100	Spontaneous respirations or mechanical ventilation	40	40	100	40
Preductal and post-ductal shunting evaluation	100	Spontaneous respirations or mechanical ventilation	40	Change >15	Change <5	Change <5
Hyperpoxia-hyperventilation test	100	Hyperventilation by manual or mechanical ventilation	20–25	>100	>150	40

*From Fox WW, Duara S: *J Pediatr* 1983; 103:505–514. Used by permission.

artery) and postductal Pao_2 (sampled from the umbilical artery or posterior tibial arteries). Transcutaneous Po_2 monitoring also can be used to demonstrate this difference between the upper part of the chest (right subclavian area) and the area below the umbilicus. If there is a right-to-left shunt through the patent foramen ovale, a Pao_2 difference between the preductal and postductal samples may not be demonstrated. Peckham and Fox[18] developed the hyperoxia-hyperventilation test based on their observation that pulmonary vasculature is sensitive to $Paco_2$. With a decrease of $Paco_2$ to a "critical level," the pulmonary arterial pressure decreases and a reversal of right-to-left shunt associated with an increase of Pao_2 may occur. This test is helpful in diagnosing PPHN; it can also be used as a guideline for therapy as well as for prediction of outcome. The test may be performed by using an anesthesia bag and an endotracheal tube, with a pressure manometer connected between them. The infant's lungs are manually hyperventilated with 100% oxygen for approximately 5 to 10 minutes, until a critical level of $Paco_2$ is achieved to produce an increase of Pao_2 to more than 100 mm Hg. The experience of Fox and Duara[10] suggests that a $Paco_2$ level less than 30 mm Hg usually is required to achieve this effect. Initial ventilation is provided at a rate of approximately 100 breaths/min and with whatever pressure is needed to decrease the $Paco_2$ to the critical level. The ventilatory rate, inflation pressure, and critical level of $Paco_2$ below which the Pao_2 increases can all be determined. This information is helpful for determination of necessary rates and inflation pressure for subsequent mechanical ventilation and can also be used to determine prognosis. An inflation pressure greater than 35 to 40 cm H_2O, a critical $Paco_2$ level of less than 20 mm Hg to achieve Pao_2 greater than 50 mm Hg, and a ventilatory rate greater than 130 breaths/min indicate a poor prognosis.

LABORATORY DATA

Laboratory tests are important to confirm the diagnosis and to exclude the possibility of cyanotic congenital heart disease. The congenital cardiac anomalies that merit consideration include total anomalous pulmonary venous return with obstruction, severe pulmonary stenosis with intact ventricular septum, and Ebstein's anomaly of the tricuspid valve.

Echocardiography

Echocardiography is helpful for early diagnosis and for sequential evaluation. Infants with pulmonary hypertension may show prolongation of the ratio of right ventricular preejection period to right ventricular ejection time (>0.50) and left ventricular preejection period to left ventricular ejection time (>0.38).[23] These echocardiographic findings may precede clinical deterioration and can therefore be used for early identification of this disorder.

Echocardiography with contrast material can demonstrate a right-to-left shunt in infants with PPHN. A dose of 0.25 to 0.5 mL/kg of 5% glucose in water can be injected through the umbilical vein or a peripheral vein from lower extremities while an echocardiogram is being obtained.[10] Simultaneous appearance of echo bubbles in the right atrium or its outflow tract and left atrium indicates a right-to-left shunt. A two-dimensional echocardiograph is imperative to exclude congenital anatomic lesions of the heart.

Catheterization

Cardiac catheterization or continuous monitoring of pulmonary arterial pressure with a pulmonary artery catheter has been used to confirm the diagnosis of PPHN. With the advanced echocardiography techniques, these invasive methods rarely are necessary in clinical practice, and are used only in cases where diagnosis is not clear.

MANAGEMENT

General Management

All infants should be kept inside the incubator and the environmental temperature should be maintained at neutral thermal range. Oxygen should be given, *warmed and humidified.* Unless indicated, the infant should not be handled excessively. Preferably all infants with PPHN should have a catheter in place in either the umbilical artery or radial artery for continuous monitoring of blood pressure and for blood gas sampling. During therapy, intake and output should be monitored. If these infants have perinatal asphyxia, fluid intake may have to be restricted and anticonvulsants for seizures may be needed. For the treatment of renal failure or cerebral edema associated with birth asphyxia, see Chapters 19 and 22, respectively.

Respiratory Therapy

The Pao_2 is often labile and hypoxic; flip-flop frequently is noted, and therefore the Pao_2 may be maintained as high as 100 to 120 mm Hg and the pH should be greater than 7.3 in the early critical period of the disease before the right-to-left shunt becomes irreversible.

The following guidelines apply during mechanical ventilation in infants with PPHN.

1. Muscle relaxants (e.g., pancuronium) may be used if there is fighting with the respirator and labile Pao_2.
2. Base deficit should be corrected to a miniumum with half-strength sodium bicarbonate.

3. Central venous pressure at 6 to 8 cm H_2O and arterial systolic pressure greater than 50 mm Hg should be maintained with either saline or 5% albumin solution if needed.

4. Once PaO_2 is stabilized, any change in fractional concentration of oxygen in inspired gas (FiO_2) or in inflation pressure should be minimized with each change. This may avoid hypoxic flip-flop.

5. Once the inflation pressure is above 35 cm H_2O, the pressure should first be decreased without changing FiO_2. Only when the inflation pressure is down to 35 cm H_2O or below, can the FiO_2 slowly be tapered.

6. Hand ventilation is usually more effective than machine ventilation to achieve desired PaO_2; therefore, if PaO_2 is labile manual ventilation can be used.

7. High continuous positive airway pressure or positive end expiratory pressure is not required unless underlying pulmonary disease is present.

For successful treatment it is essential to avoid and identify iatrogenic nursing and medical problems during ventilation therapy. The severity of underlying disease and degree of pulmonary hypertension vary from patient to patient, and each infant should be managed individually. Most infants can be managed successfully in the early course of the disease by appropriate and skillful use of a conventional ventilator. It is not uncommon to see an infant transferred to a tertiary center for extracorporeal membrane oxygenation (ECMO) therapy because of the improper management of respiratory care.

Drug Therapy

Tolazoline
The vasodilator *tolazoline hydrochloride* (Priscoline) has been used to reduce pulmonary arterial pressure in PPHN for years, yet its pharmacologic action in neonates has not been completely studied. Tolazoline has both pulmonary and systemic vasodilator effects. Tolazoline is classified pharmacologically as an α-adrenergic blocking agent. In addition, tolazoline has important actions on cardiac and smooth muscle that are described as (1) sympathomimetic, and include cardiac stimulation; (2) parasympathomimetic, and include stimulation of the gastrointestinal tract; and (3) histamine-like, and include stimulation of gastric secretion and peripheral vasodilation.[25] Goetzman and Milstein[11, 12] demonstrated that the pulmonary vasodilator action of tolazoline in newborn lambs was mediated by both histamine H1 and H2 receptors and probably not by its α-adrenergic blocking action. On the other hand, it has been shown that pulmonary vasoconstriction mechanisms, such as hypoxia and acidosis, have specific α-adrenergic activity and elicit their effects through α-adrenergic receptors in the lung.[19] Pharmacologic blockade of these receptors by tolazoline can reduce vasoconstriction to 20% of control values and theoretically should be effective in reducing right-to-

left shunt. Tolazoline has also been shown to have weak adrenergic vaso-constrictor action[2]; this effect may become prominent when the endogenous histamine stores are depleted, such as by the use of morphine or curare[5] prior to administration of tolazoline. Tolazoline is largely excreted unchanged by the organic-base transport system of the renal tubules.[25]

Little is known about the pharmacokinetics of tolazoline in newborn infants. Monin et al.[16] gave a bolus of 2 mg/kg body weight followed by continuous infusion of 2 mg/kg/hr to neonates with PPHN and suggested that:

1. The disappearance of plasma concentration followed a one-com-partment model. The half-life of elimination ranged from 3.3 to 33 hours (mean 7.7 hours, approximatley four times that in the adult).
2. The plasma level of tolazoline did not appear to correlate with its pharmacodynamic effects. The duration of the vasodilator action of tolazoline after a bolus was short; therefore continuous infusion of the drug is required.

A recent study by Ward et al.[24] recommended that after the initial loading dose an infusion of 0.16 mg/kg/hr for every 1 mg/kg loading dose should maintain a stable plasma concentration and avoid rapid accumulation.

Indications and Contraindications.—Any neonate with hypoxemia caused by high pulmonary vascular resistance and without an anatomic cardiac lesion may be administered a trial course of tolazoline, either as first-line therapy or as an adjunct to hyperventilation. It is critical that blood gases, blood pressure, and echocardiography be monitored before and after drug admin-istration.

The contraindications for tolazoline therapy include systemic hypoten-sion or shock, renal failure, and gastrointestinal or intracranial hemorrhage.

Recommended Dosage and Route of Administration.—Current dosing schedules are somewhat varied and based on clinical experience. It is gen-erally recommended that a bolus of 1 to 2 mg/kg be infused over 5 to 10 minutes through a peripheral vein, followed by continuous infusion at 1 to 2 mg/kg/hr. The maximum continuous infusion dose in one report was 6 mg/kg/hr.[3] Because Pao_2 is labile, weaning from tolazoline therapy should be gradual even with apparently good blood gas values.

The intravenous infusion should be given through the branches of the superior vena cava, because they provide the highest initial exposure of tolazoline to the pulmonary arteries by avoiding the right-to-left shunting of inferior vena cava blood across the patent foramen ovale.

Effectiveness.—Theoretically, those infants who have normally devel-oped but constricted pulmonary vasculature should have a better response to tolazoline therapy than those who have pulmonary arterial muscular hypertrophy or those who have decreased pulmonary vascular bed. The underlying pathogenesis of pulmonary hypertension cannot always be defined clinically. Therefore it is difficult to predict the response in individual infants. Clinical experiences, however, indicated that those infants who had no underlying pulmonary disease had better responses than those with associated pulmonary disease. Based on improvement in Pao_2, Goetzman et al.[12] reported a response rate of 80% in infants without apparent lung disease and 58% in infants with a variety of pulmonary disorders. In a previous review[17] of 314 infants with pulmonary hypertension of various causes given tolazoline either by bolus injection or by prolonged infusion, 59% were reported improved, with increases in Pao_2. Unfavorable response may be seen in infants with pulmonary arterial muscular hypertrophy, as seen in infants with chronic intrauterine hypoxia or prenatal exposure to prostaglandin inhibitors or phenytoin; group B β-hemolytic streptococcal infection; decreases of the pulmonary vascular bed, as seen in primary or secondary pulmonary hypoplasia; or nonbacterial endocardial thrombosis and pulmonary hypertension.

Side Effects.—The overall incidence of side effects following tolazoline therapy in neonates is approximately 70%.[17] The side effects include:

1. Gastrointestinal tract: abdominal distention, increased gastrointestinal secretion, gastrointestinal bleeding, gastric perforation
2. Cardiovascular: tachycardia, systemic hypotension
3. Renal: oliguria, hematuria, hyponatremia
4. Other: erythematous flush of skin, thrombocytopenia, seizures

Among the side effects commonly encountered with tolazoline therapy, systemic hypotension, renal failure, and gastrointestinal bleeding are the most clinically significant. Continuous monitoring of blood pressure is essential during therapy. If the systemic blood pressure drops to less than 50 mm Hg, volume expanders (saline or 5% albumin solution, 10 to 20 mL/kg, repeated as needed) or dopamine infusion (2 to 5 µg/kg/min) can be given. If blood pressure greater than 50 mm Hg cannot be maintained despite these treatment methods, tolazoline may have to be discontinued. Gastric lavage with normal saline solution may be indicated if there is excessive gastrointestinal secretion or bleeding. Cimetidine should not be used for tolazoline-induced gastric hemorrhage, because it may also antagonize tolazoline-induced pulmonary vasodilation.

Prostaglandins
Most prostaglandins produce vasodilation in both pulmonary and systemic vasculature; therefore they have no advantage over tolazoline. Among the prostaglandin compounds, PGI_2 (prostacylin) and PGD_2 have been tried in individual neonates and in lambs, with various success.[4, 15, 20] Further studies are needed before they can be generally recommended.

Dopamine

The effects of dopamine (1,2-benzenediol, 4-(2)-aminoethyl), a positive inotropic agent, on the pulmonary and systemic circulation are divergent and dose dependent. With low doses (1 to 2 μg/kg/min), dopamine produces vasodilation of the mesenteric, renal, coronary, and cerebral blood vessels, with reduction in total peripheral resistance. No effect on the cardiac system has been observed in this dose range. Medium doses (2 to 10 μg/kg/min) have a direct effect on β-adrenergic cardiac receptors, causing an increase in cardiac output. Doses greater than 10 μg/kg/min produce vasoconstriction because of α-adrenergic stimulation, and arterial blood pressure increases as total peripheral resistance increases. Although a numer of studies of dopamine have been done in newborn animal models, limited data are available in human newborn infants. DiSessa et al.[6] demonstrated that after dopamine infusion (2.5 μg/kg/min) in severely asphyxiated neonates there was a rise in systolic blood pressure, an increase in cardiac performance, and an increase in inulin clearance; the heart rate remained unchanged.

Indications.—Dopamine therapy may be indicated (1) in infants with PPHN associated with myocardial dysfunction as a common sequela of perinatal asphyxia (dopamine or a combination of dopamine and tolazoline may be given) or (2) when systemic hypotension (<50 mm Hg) occurs following tolazoline therapy.

Recommended Dosage.—Before dopamine is administered, hypovolemia should be corrected by giving saline or albumin solution or other appropriate fluid. Inasmuch as the half-life of dopamine in plasma is extremely short, continuous infusion is needed to obtain optimum effects. Based on previous reports in newborn infants, a starting dose of 2 to 5 μg/kg/min is recommended.[7] The dose may be increased to a maximum of 15 to 20 μg/kg/min if necessary.[10] Careful adjustment of dosage and frequent monitoring of vital signs are most essential.

Side Effects.—Side effects of dopamine rarely have been reported in neonates. Untoward effects due to overdosage generally are attributable to excessive sympathomimetic activity. Because dopamine has a very short half-life, most side effects may disappear quickly if the infusion is slowed or discontinued. Other side effects include ischemic blanching of infusion site, excessive diuresis, and salt wasting.

High-Frequency Jet Ventilation

High-frequency jet ventilation has recently been used in cases in which conventional mechanical ventilation fails or the underlying lung disease is complicated by air leak. The device can be used alone or in combination with intermittent mandatory ventilation. For details, the reader is referred to a recent review article by Spitzer et al.[21]

Extracorporeal Membrane Oxygenation

The concept of ECMO was first introduced by Hill et al.[14] who showed the feasibility of long-term pulmonary support with extracorporeal circulation in shock-lung syndrome. Since then it has been used in adults and older children with respiratory failure. Bartlett et al.[1] first used ECMO to treat respiratory failure in newborns as a final resuscitative measure. Subsequently this method of therapy was applied by Hardesty et al.[13] to treat PPHN in infants with diaphragmatic hernia. In the ECMO system, venous blood is diverted externally, oxygen is added, and carbon dioxide is removed with a membrane oxygenator; then blood is returned to the ascending aorta. The pulmonary circulation is thus decompressed and systemic circulation is supported, which alleviates the right-to-left shunting characteristic of PPHN.

Current unsettled issues in ECMO therapy include criteria for the selection of infants, and long-term outcome. At present this invasive measure should be tried only in those infants who fail to respond to conventional ventilation, drug therapy, and high-frequency jet ventilation.

PROGNOSIS

Because of the wide variety of underlying clinical conditions that cause PPHN and of therapeutic methods, outcome is difficult to predict. In a previous review before the application of high-frequency jet ventilation and ECMO, the overall mortality of PPHN was about 44%.[8, 22] With the use of these newer methods the survival rate could reach 90% or higher. The long-term outcome of infants with PPHN, excluding those who receive ECMO therapy, appears to be good.[21]

REFERENCES

1. Bartlett RH, et al: Extracorporeal circulation (ECMO) in neonatal respiratory failure. *J Thorac Cardiovasc Surg* 1977; 74:826–833.
2. Benfey BG, Varma DR: Vasoconstrictor action of tolazoline. *Br J Pharmacol* 1964; 22:66–71.
3. Bloss RS, et al: Tolazoline therapy for persistent pulmonary hypertension after congenital diaphragmatic hernia repair. *J Pediatr* 1980; 97:984–988.
4. Cassin S, et al: Effects of prostaglandin D2 on perinatal circulation. *Am J Physiol* 1981; 240:H755–H760.
5. Comroe JH, Dripps RD: The histamine-like action of curare as tubocurarine injected intracutaneously and intra-arterially in man. *Anesthesiology* 1946; 7:260–262.
6. DiSessa TG, et al: The cardiovascular effects of dopamine in the severely asphyxiated neonate. *J Pediatr* 1981; 99:772–776.
7. Drummond WH, Williams BJ: Effect of continuous tolazoline infusion on cardiopulmonary response to dopamine in unanesthetized newborn infant. *J Pediatr* 1983; 103:278–284.

8. Fox WW: Arterial blood gas evaluation and mechanical ventilation in the management of persistent pulmonary hypertension of the neonate. Presented at the Eighty-third Ross Conference on Pediatric Research: Cardiovascular sequelae of asphyxia in the newborn, Chatham, Mass, June 10–13, 1981.

9. Fox WW, et al: Pulmonary hypertension in perinatal aspiration syndrome. *Pediatrics* 1977; 59:1205–1211.

10. Fox WW, Duara S: Persistent pulmonary hypertension in the neonate: Diagnosis and management. *J Pediatr* 1983; 103:505–514.

11. Goetzman BW, et al: Neonatal hypoxia and pulmonary vasospasm: Response to tolazoline. *J Pediatr* 1976; 89:617–621.

12. Goetzman BW, Milstein JM: Pulmonary vasodilator action of tolazoline. *Pediatr Res* 1979; 13:943–944.

13. Hardesty RL, et al: Extracorporeal membrane oxygenation—successful treatment of persistent fetal circulation following repair of congenital diaphragmatic hernia. *J Thorac Cardiovasc Surg* 1981; 81:556–563.

14. Hill JD, et al: Prolonged extracorporeal oxygenation of acute posttraumatic respiratory failure (shock-lung syndrome). *N Engl J Med* 1972; 288:629–634.

15. Lock JE, et al: Use of prostacyclin in persistent fetal circulation. *Lancet* 1979; 1:1343.

16. Monin P, Vert P, Morselli PL: A pharmacodynamic and pharmacokinetic study of tolazoline in the neonate. *Dev Pharmacol Ther* 1982; 4(suppl 1):124–148.

17. Peckham GJ: Risk-benefit relationships of current therapeutic approaches. Presented at the Eighty-third Ross Conference on Pediatric Research: Cardiovascular sequelae of asphyxia in the newborn, Chatham, Mass, June 10–13, 1981.

18. Peckham GJ, Fox WW: Physiological factors affecting pulmonary artery pressure in infants with persistent pulmonary hypertension. *J Pediatr* 1978; 93:1005–1010.

19. Porcelli RJ, et al: Relation between pulmonary vasoconstriction, its humoral mediators and alpha-beta adrenergic receptors. *Chest* 1977; 71(suppl):249–251.

20. Soifer SJ, Morin FC III, Heymann MA: Prostaglandin D2 reverses induced pulmonary hypertension in newborn lamb. *J Pediatr* 1982; 100:458–463.

21. Spitzer AR, Davis J, Clarke WT, et al: Pulmonary hypertension and persistent fetal circulation in the newborn. *Clin Perinatol* 1988; 15:389–413.

22. Steven DC, et al: An analysis of tolazoline therapy in the critically ill neonate. *J Pediatr Surg* 1980; 15:964–970.

23. Valdes-Cruz LM, Dudell GG, Ferrara A: Utility of M-mode echocardiography for early identification of infants with persistent pulmonary hypertension of the newborn. *Pediatrics* 1981; 68:515–525.

24. Ward RM, Daniel CH, Kendig JW, et al: Oliguria and tolazoline pharmacokinetics in the newborn. *Pediatrics* 1986; 77:307–315.

25. Weiner N: Drugs that inhibit adrenergic nerves and block adrenergic receptors, in Gilman AG, Goodman LS, Gilman A (eds): *Goodman and Gilman's The Pharmacological Basis of Therapeutics,* ed 6. New York, Macmillan, 1980, pp 183–184.

9

Hypertension

Ian Carr, M.D.

Because hypertension is not a disease but a sign of disease, there is always a primary cause or causes to which this sign is secondary. The cause of systemic arterial hypertension in neonates is usually identifiable and often curable without prolonged use of antihypertensive drugs; the prolonged use of such drugs for the treatment of hypertension in neonates may therefore be a sign of a missed diagnosis.

Independently of its primary cause, hypertension can lead to encephalopathy[7, 9] and other malignant consequences, although it rarely does so in neonates. Such consequences do require treatment, both of the hypertension and of themselves, at least until the primary cause of hypertension has been identified and treated. Treatment of hypertension itself usually should be regarded as palliative.

MEASUREMENT OF BLOOD PRESSURE IN THE NEONATE

The problems of measuring neonatal blood pressure have been exhaustively discussed in the past and have been well summarized by Adelman.[2] Whatever method is used should convincingly demonstrate that the blood pressure really is elevated; among other things, this requires that the values are reproducible by independent observers using the same method.

Cuffs should be the widest that can be applied to the upper arm and should remain in close contact; for a neonate the cuff is typically 4 cm wide. If any doubt exists with this method, the blood pressure should be determined by direct intra-arterial puncture.

The chosen method should be consistently used to monitor the time course of the hypertension. When coarctation of the aorta is suspected and pressure is measured in both upper and lower halves of the body, whatever method is used for the lower half of the body should also be used for the upper half, otherwise the readings will not be comparable.

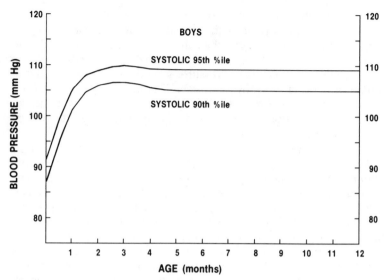

FIG 9–1.
Age-specific percentiles for systolic blood pressure in boys from birth to 12 months of age. (Data from Report of the Second Task Force on Blood Pressure Control in Children—1987. *Pediatrics* 1987; 79:1–25. Used by permission.)

HYPERTENSION

What levels of blood pressure represent hypertension in neonates? It might be more appropriate to ask, "What level of blood pressure suggests that the physician should investigate further?" There is a shortage of comprehensive normative blood pressure data in neonates, but the Task Force on Blood Pressure Control in Children[12] has published estimates of blood pressure standards for infants (Fig 9–1) and children. These estimates are based on nine reasonable well-conducted studies with assertedly compatible data. Three of the studies included blood pressure measurements beginning with the newborn age group and continuing through infancy into the older childhood age groups. However, the standards applicable to infants are still uncertain. Systolic readings seem more reliable than diastolic readings, and the data in Figure 9–1 are selected as likely to be close to the values that more definitive studies would show. The validity of the difference between infant boys and infant girls in standards provided by the Task Force is uncertain. The Task Force recognized that the spectrum of variation found in blood pressure from person to person and within the same person at different times is represented by a continuum and that there is no single, sharp dividing line below which it can be concluded that the person has normal blood pressure but above which it can be concluded that the person has hypertension. However, as indicated earlier, as a matter of practical necessity, criteria are necessary to help us decide when to investigate further, when to treat, and how vigorously to treat. The Task Force therefore did develop definitions of blood pressure as normal, high normal, and hypertensive according to percentile values. Pressures less than the 90th percentile were designated "normal." Pressures whose average was between the 90th and 95th percentiles were designated "high normal." Pressures whose average exceeded the 95th percentile were designated "hypertensive." Within the hypertensive category, pressures persistently between the 95th and 99th percentiles were designated "significant hypertension," and pressures persistently at or above the 99th percentile "severe hypertension."

These definitions, while necessarily arbitrary, represent the consensus clinical wisdom of the Task Force. When acting on such arbitrary definitions, pediatricians will be automatically labelling one in every 20 children as having "hypertension," with the risk of unnecessarily alarming parents, altering the behavior of parents toward their child, and possibly impairing the child's own attitude toward himself or herself. Care should be taken therefore to communicate this information to the parents in an appropriate perspective. This means communicating that the pediatrician is not necessarily diagnosing a disease. Rather, the pediatrician has recognized that the value of the child's blood pressure is in the range found in the top 5% of the apparently normal population, analogous to any other quantitative bodily attribute whose value is in the top 5% of the population; that this justifies a heightened vigilance in finding out whether there is an underlying disease that should be treated; and that, even if such a disease is not identified, it may be prudent as a precautionary measure to prescribe medications to bring the blood pressure into a lower range.

The most significant feature of blood pressure in infants is the normal neonatal rise in systolic blood pressure[6, 13] (see Fig 9–1). It is worth noting that a change of systolic blood pressure from 92 mm Hg at birth to 101 mm Hg at 1 month of age represents a fall from the 95th percentile to the 90th percentile. That an absolute rise actually represents a relative fall is no more of a paradox than that a change in weight from 10 lb at birth to 11 1/4 lb at 1 month of age represents a fall from the 95th percentile to the 90th percentile for age.

CAUSES AND CLINICAL FINDINGS

The causes of hypertension in neonates are listed in Table 9–1.

Adelman[1] reported that surgery may be avoidable in infants with hypertension caused by renovascular lesions because, in his experience, medical therapy usually controlled the hypertension. Nevertheless, mortality from severe uncontrolled hypertension in neonates is very high, and if medical control is not achieved within a short time, the physician should carefully reevaluate in each case whether the risk of surgery really is greater than the risk of not doing it.

TABLE 9–1.
Causes of Hypertension in Neonates

Coarctation of the thoracic aorta*
Raised intracranial pressure (including those cases
   caused by hemorrhage, edema, tumor, trauma)
Exogenous sodium overload
Renal
Renovascular*
   Renal artery thrombosis or embolism complicating
     umbilical artery catheterization
   Renal artery stenosis (including cases caused by fi-
     bromuscular dysplasia, idiopathic hypercalcemia
     syndrome, rubella syndrome, neurofibromatosis)
   Renal arteritis with or without aneurysms (including
     cases caused by Kawasaki syndrome)
   Renal arteriovenous fistula
   Renal vein thrombosis
Intrinsic*
   Hydronephrosis
   Hypoplasia
   Leiomyoma
   Trauma
   Wilms' tumor
Adrenal
   Adrenogenital syndrome
   Carcinoma
   Cushing's syndrome
   Hemorrhage
   Neuroblastoma
   Pheochromocytoma
   Primary aldosteronism
Drugs
   Phenylephrine eye drops
   Phenylephrine nose drops
   Steroids
   Vitamin D overdose
Miscellaneous
   Bronchopulmonary dysplasia*
   Burns
   Candidiasis
   Closure of abdominal wall defects
   Coarctation of abdominal aorta
   Dysgammaglobulinemia
   Ganglioneuroma
   Hepatic hemangioendothelioma
   Hyperthyroidism

*Common cause of chronic sustained hypertension in neonates.

Clinical Findings

The only sign specific to hypertension is the blood pressure level itself, and measurement of blood pressure should be included in the evaluation of all sick infants. Adelman[1] found respiratory distress in 9 of 17 neonates with hypertension; patent ductus arteriosus was diagnosed in 9; congestive heart failure in 7; and lethargy, tremors, apnea, opisthotonos, seizures, and hemiparesis in 5 of 17 hypertensive neonates. (Specificity of other signs and symptoms is related more to the underlying cause and is beyond the scope of this discussion.)

Diminished femoral pulses with elevated blood pressure restricted to the upper half of the body are reliable signs of coarctation of the aorta. Because only an aortogram will allow one to distinguish reliably between thoracic and abdominal coarctation, aortography should be performed whenever coarctation is suspected.

General clinical evaluation should always include careful palpation for abnormal masses. Abdominal murmurs rarely have been reported in newborns;[3] if a murmur was heard on auscultation of the abdomen, its significance would still be doubtful, and therefore the presence or absence of such a murmur contributes little of prospective significance.

Tests of renal function and coagulation should always be included, and renal scans are a valuable complement to aortography. The definitive diagnostic test for renovascular abnormalities is a pararenal aortogram; when renovascular disease is a reasonable possibility, delay in definitively performing such a study can have serious consequences.[4]

TREATMENT

"It is apparent that the sodium intake of children is far in excess of that required for optimal growth and development. Thus, the potential benefit of dietary sodium restriction appears to outweigh any potential risk from this form of intervention."[12]

Unless a cause for abnormal sodium loss is present, common sense suggests that sodium intake need not exceed that provided by human milk (1 mEq/kg/day, on average), which covers normal losses and growth requirements. If diuretics are being administered, however, fluid and electrolyte balance should be monitored carefully (see Chapter 19).

The decision to administer antihypertension drugs should be based on a global evaluation of the clinical circumstances and be influenced by presence of sustained and significantly high blood pressure findings, symptoms or signs related to elevated blood pressure, and evidence of target organ injury.

Drug therapy should follow the standard progressive three-step titration approach to the administration of antihypertensive drugs (Fig 9–2), always beginning with and continuing with diuretics unless a specific contraindi-

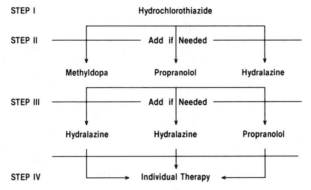

FIG 9–2.
Standard progressive titration approach to administration of antihypertensive drugs.

cation is present. Such contraindications are low body sodium concentration, excessive urinary or alimentary sodium loss, or untoward reaction to diuretic when it is administered (rare). If increasing the dosage of the diuretic to the maximum recommended daily dose (Table 9–2) is not associated with acceptable progress, a second drug should be added.

As indicated in Figure 9–1, because of the relatively large but normal rise in blood pressure during the neonatal period, the physician should take into account that an absolute rise from 92 mm Hg systolic at birth to 101 mm Hg systolic at 6 weeks of age is actually a fall from the 95th to the 90th percentile for age and indicates that the desired change in blood pressure is occurring. The physician should therefore take care to interpret blood pressure changes in neonates relative to changing age. If the clinical progress of the infant is satisfactory, even an increase in the absolute level of blood pressure, let alone an absence of change, is not in itself an indication to increase therapy. Progress must be judged globally.

Response to combined therapy (see Fig 9–2) should not be judged inadequate before both drugs have been increased to the maximum recom-

TABLE 9–2.
Dosage of Antihypertensive Drugs in Neonates*

Drug	Dosage
Hydrochlorothiazide	1–2 mg/kg/day PO
Hydralazine	0.25–9.0 mg/kg/day PO; 3–6 doses IV
Methyldopa	5–50 mg/kg/day PO; 3–4 doses IV
Propranolol	0.5–2.0 mg/kg/day PO; do not give IV
Nitroprusside	0.4–5.0 μg/kg/min IV
Diazoxide	3–5 mg/kg/day IV in divided doses

*Data from Adelman RD: *Pediatr Clin North Am* 1978; 25:99–110, and Ingelfinger JR: Hypertension in the first year of life, in *Pediatric Hypertension.* Philadelphia, WB Saunders, 1982, 229–240.

mended daily dosage without satisfactory clinical response, in which case a third-level drug should be added to the first two or, if a special reason exists, substituted for the second. Dosage of the third drug should likewise be increased to the maximum daily recommended dose before the combination is judged inadequate. The selection of drugs and the progression of their dosage should be systematic. Diuretics should be maintained at all steps in the progressive titration approach, because most of the other antihypertensive drugs produce some degree of sodium retention and their effectiveness is enhanced by diuretics. Failure to follow this approach may be the reason for reports of disappointing response to antihypertensive therapy. Similarly, physicians should try drugs that are already known to be effective in most cases and with which they are already familiar before using drugs whose effectiveness in neonates and whose freedom from side effects are less certain. A bewildering assortment of antihypertensive drugs is on the market, and it is theoretically possible to select a drug that will block virtually every link in the autonomic chain of blood pressure control; however, the theoretical appeal of selective therapy, tailor-made to block the desired link in the chain, has not been borne out in practice. For this reason Table 9–1 does not include the full range of drugs on the market. Adelman[1] reported success with the use of propranolol alone, but physicians should be aware that (1) at this writing propranolol has not been officially approved for this use in infants and (2) beta blockade can precipitate heart failure. Although there are reports of their use in neonates, spironolactone, clonidine, captopril, saralasin, guanethidine, minoxidil, prazosin, triamterene, and prostaglandins should all be regarded as experimental in this context.

In emergencies such as hypertensive encephalopathy, intravenous nitroprusside, which is continously titratable, offers the most controlled rapid intervention to lower blood pressure. A slight disadvantage of nitroprusside is the need to shield it from light. The clinician experienced with and comfortable with using diazoxide, which is also effective, may prefer it; however, because diazoxide is not continuously titratable, others should use intravenous nitroprusside. Any coexistent seizures may be treated with barbiturates.

DRUG THERAPY

Methyldopa

An article on antihypertensive drugs by Mirkin[10] includes a good review of this drug. Methyldopa is converted to methylnorepinephrine in the central nervous system. This in turn stimulates central alpha receptors and activates neurons in the vasomotor center.

Although methyldopa is absorbed from the gastrointestinal tract, the percentage absorbed is unpredictable; estimates range from 10% to 50%. Although the plasma half-life of methyldopa itself is about 2 hours, the hypotensive effect is prolonged. Although only 10% of the absorbed dose is converted to methylnorepinephrine, persistence of the latter is the probable explanation for the prolonged hypotensive effect. The other 90% of the absorbed dose is eliminated primarily by the kidney as sulfate.

The preferred route is oral (see Table 9–2). The most common side effect of methyldopa is sedation. Approximately 20% of those receiving this drug develop a positive direct Coombs' reaction, but the drug does not seem to be a significant cause of hemolysis.

As with all drugs that inhibit the sympathetic nervous system, methyldopa promotes fluid retention[11] and should not be given before diuretics have been proved ineffective on their own; methyldopa should be added to, not substituted for, the diuretics.

Propranolol

Mirkin[10] includes a good review of this drug. Propranolol is a β-adrenergic blocking agent. It crosses the blood-brain barrier and achieves high concentration in human brain tissues; therefore, central action is assumed to be an important part of its modus operandi. It probably exerts it major effect both in the vasomotor center, decreasing central sympathetic outflow, and peripherally in the juxtaglomerular apparatus of the kidney, where it inhibits renin secretion.

Propranolol is well absorbed from the gastrointestinal tract; peak concentrations in the blood are achieved 2 to 4 hours after oral administration, and serum half-life ranges between 4 and 6 hours. Approximately 70% to 75% of a given dose of propranolol is extracted by the liver during its initial pass following absorption from the gastrointestinal tract and entry into the portal system. Therefore, hepatic extraction and metabolism may keep blood levels too low in a given infant at a given oral dose. A given oral dose in different infants may be associated with blood levels varying by a factor of as much as 20.

Although an effective antihypertensive effect can be achieved in some patients receiving the drug only twice daily, the physician should be prepared to administer it more frequently as well as to increase the dosage.

Propranolol is contraindicated in infants with congestive heart failure, and it may precipitate failure in those whose cardiac function, although impaired, is not poor enough to lead to heart failure. Because of this and because of its other effects, especially its negative chronotropic and bronchospastic effects, propranolol should not be administered intravenously in the treatment of hypertension in neonates and older infants. The negative chronotropic effect of propranolol serves as a rough guide to its beta blockade effect. By analogy with the neonatal change in blood pressure, it should be remembered that the mean heart rate in the first postnatal week is about 124 beats/min, with standard deviation approximately 16 beats/minute, and at 6 weeks of age the normal mean heart rate is approximately 148 beats/min, with standard deviation about 15 beats/min.[5] Using these facts (or Davignon's very clear plot), the physician can better evaluate the chronotropic effect of propranolol. For example, if the average heart rate in the first week was 124 beats/min and was also 124 beats/min at 6 weeks of age, this would actually represent a fall of between 1 and 2 standard deviations in heart rate for age, equivalent to a fall from the 50th to the 5th percentile (a significant fall). Because of its effect on the smooth muscle of the bronchioles, propranolol exacerbates any tendency to bronchospasm.

As with all drugs that inhibit the sympathetic nervous system,[11] propranolol promotes fluid retention and should not be given before diuretics have been proved ineffective on their own; propranolol should be added to, not substituted for, the diuretic.

Sodium Nitroprusside

Inglefinger[8] has given a good review of this drug. Nitroprusside relaxes vascular smooth muscle, reduces vascular resistance, and therefore gives a lower blood pressure for a given flow. Flow itself also tends to decrease because relaxation of the venous smooth muscle increases venous capacity and diminishes right heart filling pressure. The net effect is nevertheless normally favorable.

Given intravenously, nitroprusside acts within seconds. It is metabolized to thiocyanate, which is excreted by the kidneys. When intravenous nitroprusside is discontinued, the effect on blood pressure is gone within minutes. Although thiocyanate tends to be toxic, the toxic risk with therapeutic doses is low.

This drug is ideal for managing episodes of severe hypertension, especially those with malignant consequences, such as encephalopathy. Because the effect is dose dependent, response should be closely monitored and the drip rate adjusted accordingly. Thiocyanate blood levels should be checked daily. If cardiac output is decreased because of myocardial dysfunction, nitroprusside usually increases output, and is by no means contraindicated in the presence of heart failure. Heart rate reflexly rises as blood pressure falls. The half-life of thiocyanate is 4 days; therefore renal dysfunction markedly delays elimination. Freshly made nitroprusside solution should be shielded from light to retard photodecomposition. Nitroprusside administration includes sodium, and it is prudent to prescribe a diuretic simultaneously.

Diazoxide

Diazoxide is a thiazide but also is nondiuretic and relaxes vascular smooth muscle with a mode of action similar to that of nitroprusside.

Because diazoxide reduces insulin secretion, blood sugar levels tend to rise following administration. Tubular secretion of uric acid also tends to decrease with consequent secondary hyperuricemia. These effects are usually mild.

Diazoxide causes sodium retention, and diuretics should be administered concomitantly.

Diazoxide is avidly bound by plasma proteins, and for that reason is unsuitable for continuous intravenous drip and should be given as an intravenous bolus. The effect is usually maximal within 5 minutes, and persists for up to 24 hours. If adequate effect has not been achieved within 30 minutes a second bolus may be given. Previously given antihypertensive drugs enhance the effect of diazoxide, and because the effect of a bolus is difficult to predict but will be prolonged, we normally prefer to use nitroprusside.

PROGNOSIS

Because renal artery thrombosis is the most common preventable cause of hypertension in neonates,[2] umbilical and other forms of arterial catheterization in neonates should be used only in the presence of a specific indication. This indication should include a specific therapeutic motivation.

Partly because of uncertainty of the definition of hypertension in neonates and because systemic monitoring of blood pressure is not generally practiced in neonates, little is known of the frequency of hypertension in the newborn. Although hypertension is the most common cause of heart failure in adults, little is known of the childhood antecedents of this problem, let alone the infant and neonatal antecedents. Little is known of the long-term effects of antihypertensive therapy begun in infancy. The opening statement of this chapter—that most instances of hypertension in neonates have a cause treatable, at least potentially, by means other than antihypertensive drugs—has to be tempered by our uncertainty as to what actually constitutes hypertension and therefore by the possibility that the normative data from apparently healthy infants actually include persons whose blood pressures, as yet unknown to us, already mark them as victims of hypertensive disease in later life if left untreated.

REFERENCES

1. Adelman RD: Neonatal hypertension. *Pediatr Clin North Am* 1978; 25:99–110.
2. Adelman, RD: The epidemiology of neonatal hypertension, in Giovannelli G, et al (eds): *Hypertension in Children and Adolescents.* New York, Raven Press, 1981, pp 21–30.
3. Angella JJ, Sommer LS, Poole C, et al: Neonatal hypertension associated with renal artery hypoplasia. *Pediatrics* 1968; 41:524–526.
4. Cook GT, Marshall VF, Todd JE: Malignant renovascular hypertension in a newborn. *J Urol* 1966; 96:863–966.
5. Davignon A, Rautaharju P, Boisselle E, et al: ECG standards for children. *Pediatr Cardiol* 1980; 1:133–152.

6. deSwiet M, Fayers P, Shinebourne EA: Systolic blood pressure in a population of infants in the first year of life: The Brompton study. *Pediatrics* 1980; 65:1028–1035.

7. Dimmick JE, Patterson MWH, Wu HWA: Systemic hypertension in a newborn infant. *J Pediatr* 1979; 95:321–324.

8. Ingelfinger JR: Hypertension in the first year of life, in *Pediatric Hypertension*. Philadelphia, WB Saunders, 1982, pp 229–240.

9. Mace S, Hirschfield S: Hypertensive encephalopathy. *Am J Dis Child* 1983; 137:32–33.

10. Mirkin BL: Antihypertensive drugs: Mechanisms of actions and therapeutic application in children, in Giovannelli G, et al. (eds): *Hypertension in Children and Adolescents.* New York, Raven Press, 1981, pp 222–238.

11. Nies AS: Cardiovascular disorders: I. Hypertension, in Melmon KL, Morrelli HF (eds): *Clinical Pharmacology.* New York, Macmillan, 1978, pp 186 and 196.

12. Report of the Second Task Force on Blood Pressure Control in Children— 1987. *Pediatrics* 1987; 79:1–25.

10

Pharmacologic Closure of Patent Ductus Arteriosus

Tsu F. Yeh, M.D.

Ian Carr, M.D.

Patent ductus arteriosus (PDA) has become a challenging problem to neonatologists and pediatric cardiologists in the last decade, not only because of its high prevalence among premature infants but also as a complicating factor in the diseases of such infants. With the better understanding of the pathophysiology of ductus arteriosus in recent years, several advances have taken place in diagnosis and management. This chapter presents a summary of developments and focuses on medical management for these infants.

GENERAL CHARACTERISTICS OF PATENT DUCTUS ARTERIOSUS

Incidence

Patent ductus arteriosus in premature infants can be classified as subclinical PDA (no heart murmur) and clinical PDA (with heart murmur). Clinical PDA can be nonsignificant (no cardiovascular dysfunction) or significant (with cardiovascular dysfunction). The overall incidence of clinical PDA reported in premature infants ranges from 18% to 80%,[35, 40] being a function of immaturity. The incidence of clinical and subclinical PDA detected by aortic contrast echocardiography during the first day of life in premature infants with respiratory distress syndrome (RDS) could be as high as 90%.[14] In premature infants whose birth weight was 1,500 g or less or in infants whose ductus arteriosus remained patent on the third postnatal day, the chance of the ductus to become clinically significant increases greatly.[14] Based on a prospective study from our nursery,[39] the incidence of significant PDA has a strongly positive correlation with birth weight (6.7% in infants weighing 1,501 to 2,040 g, 26.9% in *infants weighing 1,000 to 1,500 g*, and 51% in infants less than 1,000 g) and gestational age (7.3% in infants 33 to 37 weeks, 26.8%

123

TABLE 10–1.
Incidence (%) of Patent Ductus Arteriosus in Premature
Infants in Relation to Respiratory Distress Syndrome and
Birth Weight

Condition	Birth Weight (g)		
	<1,000	1,000–1,500	1,501–2,040
RDS	62.5	63.2	56.3
Type II RDS	31.1	12.2	2.2
Other	33.3	11.1	1.5

in infants 29 to 32 weeks, and 50% in infants ≤28 weeks). The presence of RDS is also associated with increased frequency of significant PDA (Table 10–1).

Physiology of the Ductus

In healthy full-term infants, closure of the ductus arteriosus occurs shortly after birth; in premature infants, the ductus may remain patent for days or weeks. Many factors may influence the constriction or relaxation of ductal smooth muscle in animals. Among these, arterial oxygen tension (PaO_2) and prostaglandin E (PGE_2) appear to be the most important. It has been hypothesized that during intrauterine life circulating PGE_2 and PGI_2 produced locally in the ductus maintain the patency of the ductus,[8, 12] and that following birth, the loss of the placenta, a source of PGE_2 production, and the spontaneous decrease in local production of PGE_2 and PGI_2 allow factors that constrict the ductus, such as the increase in oxygen tension, to act relatively unopposed, and the ductus closes. The immature ductus is more sensitive to the dilating effects of prostaglandins and less sensitive to the constricting effects of oxygen,[9] which accounts for the high incidence of PDA in premature infants. Steroids may decrease the sensitivity of the ductus to PGE.[10] Prenatal administration of steroids may decrease the incidence of PDA.[11]

Circulating prostaglandins (PGs) also may be important in maintaining the patency of the ductus arteriosus. During the acute stage of RDS, both PGE and PGF levels were elevated significantly, compared with values in infants without RDS.[15] Concomitant with the appearance of PDA there was a decrease in PGF and an increase in PGE.[15] Because the lung is an important organ for synthesis and degradation of PGs it is possible that in premature infants with RDS the synthesis and degradation may be altered and that a resultant high circulating PGE may exert an effect on the ductus.

PATHOPHYSIOLOGY

The cardiorespiratory pathophysiology in infants with RDS and PDA is shown in Figure 10–1. It is important to recognize that (1) the majority of

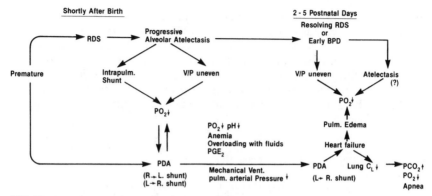

FIG 10–1.
Pathophysiology of respiratory distress syndrome *(RDS)* and patent ductus arteriosus *(PDA)*. Following the decrease in pulmonary vascular resistance, the left-to-right shunt of ductus increases, resulting in increased pulmonary flow and congestive circulatory state. This may further compromise the poor lung mechanics already present in infants with RDS. The consequent increase in ventilatory and oxygen therapy may enhance the risk for bronchopulmonary dysplasia *(BPD)* or intraventricular hemorrhage. C_L = lung compliance; *V/P* = ventilation-perfusion ratio.

premature infants may have ductus arteriosus early in life without apparent clinical symptoms; (2) multiple postnatal factors may affect the devolution of pulmonary vascular resistance and ductus constriction, which will influence the direction and size of the ductus shunt; and (3) in infants with RDS the ductus shunt may lead to aggravation of the pulmonary dysfunction and prolong the need for mechanical ventilation and oxygen therapy, with increase in the risk for bronchopulmonary dysplasia. Alterations in the dynamics of the cerebral circulation by the ductal shunt may increase the risk for intraventricular hemorrhage.[30] Increased incidence of necrotizing enterocolitis has also been reported.

CLINICAL AND LABORATORY CONSIDERATIONS

Subclinical Cases

In the absence of a ductus murmur, PDA can be diagnosed noninvasively only by contrast or Doppler echocardiography. Factors associated with high risk for PDA[13] include (1) birth weight less than 1,500 g, (2) diagnosis of RDS, (3) acute perinatal stress, and (4) need for assisted ventilation within 24 hours of birth.

Cases Without Significant Cardiovascular Distress

In infants who have no underlying lung disease the diagnosis of PDA can be easily made by the characteristic systolic or continuous murmur at the left sternal border in the second intercostal space. In infants with RDS who require assisted ventilation the diagnosis of PDA can be confounded by signs associated with the underlying respiratory condition. Temporary disconnection of the respirator may make it easier to detect the cardiac murmur. Awareness of the high prevalence of PDA in infants with RDS during the first week of life and frequent careful physical examination are the initial steps leading to the diagnosis. Diagnosis can usually be made clinically and confirmed by contrast or Doppler echocardiography.

Cases With Significant Cardiovascular Distress

Infants with PDA can have resting tachycardia, bounding peripheral pulse, hyperactive precordium, cardiomegaly on the chest radiograph, and echocardiographic changes suggesting a large left-to-right shunt. Frequent apnea, carbon dioxide retention, or unexplained deterioration of respiratory status may be seen. A clinical scoring system has been used to evaluate the cardiovascular distress (cardiovascular distress score or CVD score) (Table 10–2).[42] There is a good correlation between the CVD score and blood gases and echocardiogram. A CVD score of 3 or greater is usually associated with LA/Ao (left atrium/aortic root dimension) ≥1.3 on echocardiogram, indicating a significant ductus shunt (normal LA/Ao values 0.66 to 1.06).

Echocardiography can be used not only for the diagnosis of PDA but also for estimating the degree of ductus shunt. Increase in LA/Ao ratio (≥1.3) suggests a significant left-to-right shunt. High left ventricular function index (as shown by left ventricular shortening fraction) indicates a left-to-right shunt with high left-sided heart volume load and excludes causes of dilation of the left side of the heart associated with decreased left ventricular function, such as cardiomyopathies. The shortening fraction is expressed as $(EDD - ESD)/EDD \times 100$, where EDD is the end-diastolic dimension and ESD is the end-systolic dimension. The normal value for shortening fraction of left ventricle is $34 \pm 3\%$.

TABLE 10–2.
Cardiovascular Distress Score in Premature Infants With Patent Ductus Arteriosus*

Measure	0	1	2
Heart rate (bpm)	<160	160–180	>180
Heart murmur	None	Systolic murmur	Murmur continue to diastole
Peripheral pulse	Normal	Bounding brachial	Bounding brachial and dorsal pedis
Precordial pulsation	None	Palpable	Visible
Cardiothoracic ratio	<0.60	0.60–0.65	>0.65

*From Yeh TF, Ravel D, Luken J, et al: *Crit Care Med* 1981; 9:655–657. Used by permission.

Other echocardiographic changes include decrease in the left ventricular pre-ejection period, decrease in the ratio of LPEP to left ventricular ejection time, and diastolic pulmonary valve flutter. By using two-dimensional echocardiography, direct visualization of the PDA can be obtained, with a few false negative or false positive studies. Contrast echocardiographic technique with injection of 2 to 5 mL normal saline solution through the umbilical arterial catheter has been successful in demonstrating the left-to-right PDA shunt. Doppler echocardiography has been helpful in detecting flow patterns in the pulmonary artery suggestive of a PDA shunt.

A significant PDA can be diagnosed if there is clinical cardiovascular dysfunction (e.g., CVD score >3) or if there is an echocardiographic change suggesting a significant left-to-right ductus shunt.

MANAGEMENT

Although pharmacologic or surgical closure of the ductus may be required, PDA in some infants may close spontaneously without specific therapy. Management of subclinical PDA remains controversial. However, for infants who have clinical PDA, with or without cardiovascular dysfunction, several therapeutic methods may facilitate ductus closure or improve cardiovascular status:

1. Fluid restriction to 80–100 mL/kg/day (100 to 120 mL/kg/day if under phototherapy)
2. Maintenance of hematocrit values ≥40% with packed-cell transfusion
3. Ventilatory adjustment to keep arterial Pao_2 50 to 90 mm Hg and $Paco_2$ ≤45 mm Hg, and pH >7.25
4. Maintenance of normal electrolytes and of serum Ca ≥7.5 mg/dL
5. Treatment with furosemide (1 mg/kg IV q 12–24 hr for one or two doses) if there is evidence of fluid overloading or circulatory congestion.
6. Treatment with the prostaglandin inhibitor indomethacin if all of the above therapies fail to close the ductus in 24 hours

DRUG THERAPY

Furosemide

Mechanism and Pharmacokinetics
Furosemide (Lasix) is the diuretic most commonly chosen for use in the neonate for various reasons. Renal effects of furosemide include (1) diuresis, (2) natriuresis, (3) increased renal blood flow, and altered distribution. Fu-

TABLE 10–3.
Half-life and Clearance of Furosemide in Newborn Infants

Reference	Birth Weight (g)	Half-life* (hr)	Clearance (mL/kg/hr)	Postnatal* Age
Aranda et al.[3]	2,391 ± 289	7.7 ± 1.0 (4.5 ± 12.0)	81.6 ± 14.9 (34.3–165.6)	11.5 ± 5.9 (1–40 days)
Peterson et al.[31]	1,270 ± 169	19.9 ± 3.0 (8.7–46)	10.8 ± 7.2 (2.4–29.4)	8.5 ± 1.9 (1–20 days)
Najak et al.[29]	(700–2,560)	5–26	—	1–3 wk
Green[19]	—	26.5 ± 31.2	—	2–6 days
	—	1.79 ± 1.26		1–36 mo

*Mean ± standard error.

rosemide produces diuresis and natriuresis primarily by inhibition of active chloride reabsorption from the ascending limb of Henle's loop, resulting in a decrease in passive reabsorption of sodium. Furosemide may stimulate renal PGE synthesis[2] and renal renin secretion.[37] The hemodynamic effect of furosemide on the kidney is believed to be mediated by renal PGs.

Furosemide also has systemic vascular effects that are independent of its diuretic action. These vascular effects might be mediated by PGs because in animal experiments these effects were prevented by pretreatment with a PG inhibitor, indomethacin.[17] The mechanisms for the reduction of pulmonary edema in premature infants with PDA could be related to diuresis or the vascular effects of the drug, or both.

Various pharmacokinetic studies of furosemide in neonates have shown conflicting results (Table 10–3).[3, 19, 29, 31] Green[19] reported a half-life of 26 hours in premature infants within the first 5 days of life; Aranda et al.[3] reported a half-life of 7.7 hours in infants aged 1 to 40 days. Ross and colleagues[33] and Woo and co-workers[38] have shown that after intravenous injection a peak diuretic effect is reached within 1 to 3 hours and that this effect persists above the baseline for approximately 6 hours.

Indication
Furosemide can be recommended in infants with fluid overload whether or not they have congestive heart failure. Furosemide also can be used simultaneously with indomethacin to prevent its renal side effects.[43]

Recommended Dosage
For rapid diuresis in infants with congestive heart failure a dose of 1 to 3 mg/kg IV is adequate. For infants with fluid overload and PDA we recommend one or two doses of furosemide (1 mg/kg) in 12- to 24-hour intervals.

Side Effects
The two potential side effects of short-term furosemide therapy in neo-

nates are ototoxicity and displacement of bilirubin from albumin binding sites. Ototoxicity appears to be related to serum concentration of furosemide, but has not been reported in neonates.[20] Similarly, the displacement of bilirubin from albumin binding sites has not been reported to cause any significant problem in neonates.[20] Controversies remain as to whether furosemide promotes patency of the ductus.[21, 46]

Indomethacin

Mechanism and Pharmacokinetics

PGE is synthesized in the wall of the ductus arteriosus, and circulating PGE may play an important role in maintaining patency of the ductus during fetal and early extrauterine life. Indomethacin, a PG synthetase (cyclooxygenase) inhibitor, has been used to promote ductus closure.[16, 22]

The pharmacokinetic data on orally or intravenously administered indomethacin reported by various authors are shown in Table 10–4[5, 36, 39] and appear to be consistent with each other. Studies from our nursery[36] showed a mean plasma half-life of 20.7 hours, which is three times longer than reported in adults. The plasma clearance of indomethacin was positively correlated with postnatal age: the "older" the infant the faster the clearance. However, the relationship between plasma clearance of indomethacin and birth weight or gestational age was inconsistent among various studies.[4, 36] Indomethacin has been shown in adults undergoing demethylation, deacylation, and conjugation with glucuronic acid. Very little work has been reported on indomethacin metabolism in neonates. Variability in hepatic metabolism, renal excretion, and enterohepatic recirculation could contribute to differences in pharmacokinetics.[36] Indomethacin has also been shown to bind with albumin, and in theory can compete with bilirubin for protein binding.

TABLE 10–4.
Half-life and Clearance of Indomethacin in Newborn Infants

Reference	Route of Administration	Mean Postnatal Age (days)	Mean Birth Weight (g)	Mean Half-life (hr)	Mean Clearance
Thalji et al.[36]	IV	10.8	1,253	20.7	13.0 mL/kg/hr
Yaffe et al.[39]	IV	<2	—	17.7	14.4 mL/hr
		2–7	—	21.4	13.8 mL/hr
		>7	—	12.2	25.2 mL/hr
			<1,000	20.7	9.6 mL/hr
			>1,000	15.4	22.8 mL/hr
Bianchetti et al.[5]	PO	10–15	1,020–1,650	30–90	4.5–20.1 mL/kg/hr
Bhat et al.[4]	PO	12.0	1,490	16.0	NA

The ductus response to indomethacin correlated significantly with plasma concentration. Brash et al.[6] have shown that the ductus response to indomethacin is related to plasma concentration at 24 hours after the dose is given; failure of the ductus to respond was often associated with a plasma level less than 250 ng/mL. Yeh et al.[45] reported that small premature infants (<1,000 g) had lower plasma levels because of their higher volume of distribution, as compared to larger premature infants (>1,000 g), when indomethacin was given based on body weight. Small premature infants may therefore require more doses or higher dosage than a large premature infant in order to achieve good response. Combined administration of indomethacin and betamethasone may enhance ductus closure.[28] A recent study from our nursery[49] demonstrated that ductus response to indomethacin correlated significantly with plasma levels at 12 hours after intravenous dosing; with a blood level of 600 ng/mL or more there is a 50% or greater chance that ductus will close; when the blood levels reach 1,400 ng/mL there is a 75% chance that ductus will close. Because renal side effects were commonly observed in these infants, the safe therapeutic ranges of plasma indomethacin levels for ductus closure appear to be narrow (Fig 10–2). In other words, to reach the therapeutic level for ductus closure, a majority of the infants would also experience some degree of renal dysfunction. The renal side effects are transient and usually do not last for more than 72 hours after discontinuance of the drug.

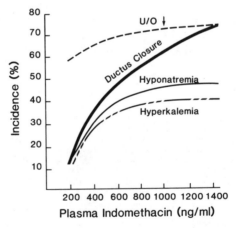

FIG 10–2.
Incidence of ductus closure, decreased urine output *(U/O)*, hyponatremia, and hyperkalemia, as a function of plasma indomethacin concentration at 12 hours after a single dose. (Modified from Yeh TF, Achanti B, Patel H, et al: *Dev Pharmacol Ther* 1989; 12:169–178.)

Indications

Indomethacin may be used for prophylaxis or for treatment of PDA. However, routine prophylactic therapy for very low birth weight infants is not recommended at present because of the lack of complete study of the side effects and long-term outcome. In infants with subclinical PDA, administration of indomethacin may close the ductus and prevent subsequent development of symptomatic PDA. For infants who have clinical PDA with or without significant cardiovascular dysfunction, administration of indomethacin will reduce the ductus shunt or close the ductus and improve cardiorespiratory distress.

Contraindications

The tentative contraindications for indomethacin therapy are (1) serum indirect bilirubin levels greater than 10 mg/dL, (2) blood urea nitrogen levels exceeding 20 mg/dL, (3) shock, (4) intracranial hemorrhage, (5) necrotizing enterocolitis, (6) hemorrhagic disease, and (7) platelet count less than 50,000/ mm.[3]

Ductus Closure Following Indomethacin Therapy

Reports of the use of intravenous indomethacin have been favorable, but indomethacin has not been shown to be beneficial in all cases. Some trials have suggested that indomethacin may have been less effective in small, premature infants of very low birth weight, of very low gestational age, of higher postnatal age, and in those of higher postconceptional age. Our approach to the use of indomethacin in the treatment of PDA is based on the results of a double-blind controlled study from our nursery.[40] In this study indomethacin (0.3 mg/kg) was administered intravenously to 28 infants (mean postnatal age 8.9 days), and saline placebo was given to 27. The same dosage was repeated at 24-hour intervals for a maximum of three doses, unless the ductus closed. The results of the study are shown in Figure 10–3. Successful response with improvement in clinical condition and echocardiogram was seen in 89.2% (25/28) of infants who received indomethacin and in 22.2% (6/27) who received placebo. When adjustments were made for the number of infants expected to improve spontaneously, indomethacin was successful in closing the ductus in 86% of the infants. This success rate was consistent with the later report from the National Collaborative study.[18]

In our study, after one dose (0.3 mg/kg) of indomethacin, 50% of the infants experienced ductus closure; after two doses (in 24 hours) closure was achieved in 75%; after three doses (in another 24 hours) 89% had ductus closure. After one dose, 14% of the respondent infants had return of ductus murmur; after two doses, 9.5%; and after three doses, 8%.

Side Effects

The possible side effects of indomethacin therapy are:

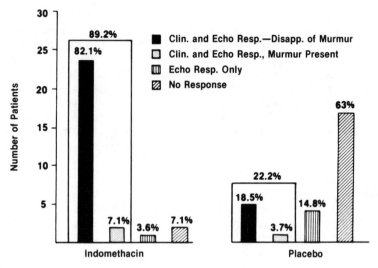

FIG 10–3.
Clinical, echocardiographic, and murmur changes evaluated approximately 24 hours after the last dose of indomethacin or placebo. These changes were divided into four categories. "Success" was achieved if both positive clinical and echocardiographic responses were observed. (From Yeh TF: *Neonatal Lett* 1982; 1:1. Used by permission.)

1. Transient renal dysfunction
2. Hyponatremia
3. Transient decrease in plasma glucose
4. Decreased platelet aggregation
5. Increased risk for gastrointestinal hemorrhage
6. Increased risk for necrotizing enterocolitis
7. Gastric perforation
8. Increased risk for retinopathy of prematurity
9. Displacement of bilirubin from binding sites

Among these side effects, the most significant recognizable complication is transient renal dysfunction.

Renal Complications

A transient decrease in urine output and in fractional excretion of sodium and chloride and in osmolar and free water clearance is observed following indomethacin administration. All of these renal functions return to normal within 72 hours after discontinuance of medication. Indomethacin may decrease the glomerular filtration rate.[7]

There was no apparent correlation between the plasma indomethacin levels and renal side effects. Seyberth et al.[34] have demonstrated an adverse effect on renal function in infants during prolonged indomethacin therapy in which plasma indomethacin levels were maintained between 150 and 750 ng/mL. A recent study from our nursery[48] indicated that when plasma indomethacin levels reach 170 ng/mL, a majority of infants have decreased urine output.

The renal side effects of indomethacin may be prevented by simultaneous administration of furosemide.[43] Furosemide may induce renal PG synthesis.[2] Simultaneous administration of furosemide (1 mg/kg) promotes free water clearance and osmolar clearance, which otherwise would be reduced if indomethacin was used alone (Fig 10–4). Although furosemide has been shown to enhance ductus patency,[21] we did not observe any significant changes in the efficacy of indomethacin on the closure of PDA with simultaneous administration of furosemide. Simultaneous administration of indomethacin and furosemide also can be used in premature infants who have congestive heart failure and oliguria.[47]

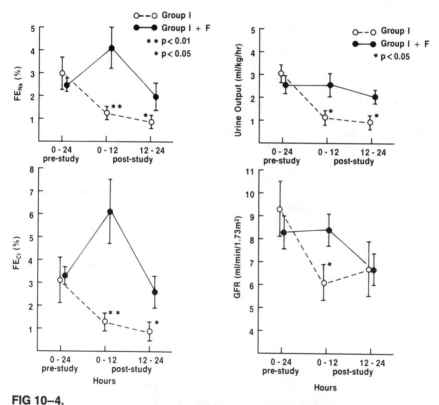

FIG 10–4.
Comparison of fractional excretion of sodium (FE_{Na}) and chloride (FE_{Cl}), glomerular filtration rate *(GFR)*, and urine output in infants who received indomethacin alone (group I) with those who received indomethacin and furosemide simultaneously (group I + F). Infants in group I + F had significantly higher FE_{Na}, FE_{Cl}, GFR, and urine output than infants in group I.

Recommended Dosage

Current dosing schedules are somewhat variable, depending on the therapeutic purposes and the postnatal age of the infant. The following recommendations are based on published literatures.

1. For infants who have symptomatic PDA, dosage should be adjusted based on postnatal age. For infants 48 hours of age or younger, an initial dose of 0.2 mg/kg followed by 0.1 mg/kg every 24 hours for two doses can be given. For infants older than 48 hours but 4 weeks of age or younger, 0.2 mg/kg every 12 hours or 0.3 mg/kg every 24 hours for a total of three doses can be recommended. For infants over 4 weeks of age, 0.3 mg/kg every 12 hours can be given. Infants whose postnatal age is over 6 weeks are usually not responsive to indomethacin[1] regardless of higher dosage or more doses.

2. To prevent reopening of the ductus, prolonged indomethacin therapy has been given to infants weighing less than 1,500 g who have subclinical PDA.[32] Doses were given as follows: 0.15 mg/kg every 12 hours for two doses initially, then 0.1 mg/kg/day as maintenance for 5 days. This therapeutic regimen, however, does not improve mortality or morbidity.[32] Further studies are needed before it can be generally recommended.

3. Because of the high prevalence of PDA in very low birth weight infants, indomethacin has been given during the first day of extrauterine life for prevention of subsequent development of symptomatic PDA. Three doses were given: 0.2 mg/kg as first dose, and then 0.1 mg/kg given at 12 hours and 48 hours later. Again there was no apparent improvement in morbidity or mortality with this therapeutic regimen.[24]

Outcome and Long-Term Follow-up

There has been no solid evidence to demonstrate that the presence of PDA contributes significantly to the development of bronchopulmonary dysplasia. Similarly, there has been no concrete evidence of decreases in incidence of BPD following surgical or indomethacin closure of the ductus arteriosus. However, indomethacin closure of the ductus does decrease the incidence of surgical ligation and the need for assisted ventilation.[40, 41]

The use of indomethacin did not show long-term adverse effects, incidence of recurrent respiratory infection, neurologic defects (major and minor), or abnormal electroencephalogram[44] when the infants were examined at 1 year[26] and at preschool age.[27]

Digoxin

The use of digoxin for PDA has been questioned by many pediatric cardiologists and neonatologists. A control study by McGrath[25] failed to show any advantage of using digoxin in premature infants with PDA. Furthermore, premature infants treated with digoxin have a high incidence of arrhythmias and subendocardial ischema.[25] The poor elimination of the drug may result in high levels in the serum, leading to toxicity. Thus digoxin should be reserved only for infants in whom indomethacin is contraindicated, such as those with necrotizing enterocolitis or renal failure. Because of the prolonged half-life when indomethacin is added to digoxin therapy, the digoxin dosage should be reduced by 50% until urine output and digoxin serum level can be better assessed.[23] The relevant action of digoxin is the positive inotropic action. This action is applicable only when there is ventricular myocardial dysfunction. Unless echocardiography demonstrates dysfunction, digoxin is not indicated.

Aspirin

The experience of using aspirin (acetylsalicylic acid) for the closure of PDA has been very limited. Aspirin was given by nasogastric tube to three premature infants with PDA by Heymann et al.[22] The ductus closed permanently in one infant; in another it was partially constricted; the third infant did not respond. Aspirin did not appear to be as effective as indomethacin in the closure of PDA.[22] The apparently more dramatic effect with indomethacin may be explained by the fact that different PG inhibitors affect various tissues to different degrees.

The therapeutic serum level of aspirin for the closure of PDA is not known. The recommended dose is 20 mg/kg every 6 hours for three to four doses.[22] Because aspirin may displace the bilirubin from albumin binding sites, the large doses administered may increase the risk of kernicterus in jaundiced infants. Other side effects of aspirin include interference with platelet aggregation, bleeding, and gastrointestinal tract irritation. All of these side effects are also side effects of indomethacin.

PERSPECTIVE

Clinical experience indicates that in about 25% of infants significant PDA may undergo spontaneous closure. Administration of indomethacin may enhance closure of the ductus in nearly 90% of the infants. The resultant improvement in lung mechanics after ductus closure may facilitate extubation and decrease the need for assisted ventilation. Our earlier study suggested that if indomethacin is to be effective in improving bronchopulmonary dysplasia morbidity, it might have to be administered very early in postnatal life. Recent studies have shown that when indomethacin was administered early during the first day of life and the therapy was prolonged for 5 days[32] the incidence of symptomatic PDA or ductus reopening was significantly reduced. Whether this therapeutic regimen would improve mortality or decrease BPD morbidity remains to be answered.

REFERENCES

1. Achanti B, Yeh TF, Pildes RS: Indomethacin therapy in infants with advanced postnatal age and patent ductus arteriosus. *Clin Invest Med* 1986; 9:250–253.
2. Ahallah AA: Interaction of prostaglandins with diuretics. *Prostaglandins* 1979; 18:369–375.
3. Aranda JV, et al: Pharmacokinetic disposition and protein binding of furosemide in newborn life. *J Pediatr* 1978; 93:507–511.
4. Bhat R, et al: Pharmacokinetics of oral and intravenous indomethacin in premature infants. *Dev Pharmacol Ther* 1980; 1:101–110.
5. Bianchetti G, et al: Pharmacokinetics of indomethacin in the premature infant. *Dev Pharmacol Ther* 1980; 1:111–124.
6. Brash AR, et al: Pharmacokinetics of indomethacin in the neonates. Relation of plasma indomethacin levels to response of ductus arteriosus. *N Engl J Med* 1981; 305:67–71.
7. Cifuentes RF, et al: Indomethacin and renal function in premature infants with persistent patent ductus arteriosus. *J Pediatr* 1979; 95:583–587.
8. Clyman RI: Ontogeny of the ductus arteriosus response to prostaglandins and inhibitors of their synthesis. *Semin Perinatol* 1980; 4:115–124.
9. Clyman RI, Heymann MA: Pharmacology of the ductus arteriosus. *Pediatr Clin North Am* 1981; 28:77–93.
10. Clyman RI, et al: Glucocorticoids alter the sensitivity of the lamb ductus arteriosus to prostaglandin E. *J Pediatr* 1981; 98:126–128.
11. Clyman RI, et al: Prenatal administration of betamethasone for prevention of patent ductus arteriosus. *J Pediatr* 1981; 98:123–126.
12. Coceani F, Olley PM: Role of prostaglandins, prostacyclin and thromboxanes in the control of prenatal patency and postnatal closure of the ductus arteriosus. *Semin Perinatol* 1980; 4:109–113.
13. Cotton RB, Lindstrom DP, Stahlman M: Early prediction of symptomatic patent ductus arteriosus from perinatal risk factors: Discriminant analysis model. *Acta Paediatr Scand* 1981; 70:723–727.
14. Dudell GG, Gersony WM: Patent ductus arteriosus in neonates with severe respiratory distress. *J Pediatr* 1984; 104:915–920.
15. Friedman WF: In Session II, Physiology and pharmacology of the ductus arteriosus: Studies of the responses of the ductus arteriosus. Presented at the Seventy-fifth Ross Conference on Pediatric Research: The Ductus Arteriosus, Florida, December 4–7, 1977.
16. Friedman WF, et al: Pharmacologic closure of patent ductus arteriosus in the premature infant. *New Engl J Med* 1976; 295:526–529.
17. Gerber JG, Nies AS: Furosemide induced vasodilatation: Importance of the state of hydration and filtration. *Kidney Int* 1980; 18:454–459.
18. Gersony WM, et al: Effects of indomethacin in premature infants with patent ductus arteriosus: Results of a national collaborative study. *J Pediatr* 1983; 102:895–906.
19. Green TP: Influence of biological maturation on the determinants of response to furosemide (abstract). *Pediatr Res* 1981; 15:495.
20. Green TP: The use of diuretics in infants with the respiratory distress syndrome. *Semin Perinatol* 1982; 6:172–180.
21. Green TP, et al: Furosemide promotes patent ductus arteriosus in premature infants with the respiratory distress syndrome. *N Engl J Med* 1983; 308:743–749.

22. Heymann MA, Rudolph AM, Silverman NH: Closure of the ductus arteriosus in premature infants by inhibition of prostaglandin synthesis. *N Engl J Med* 1976; 295:530–533.

23. Koren G, Zarfin Y, Perlman M, et al: Effects of indomethacin on digoxin pharmacokinetics in premature infants. *Pediatr Pharmacol* 1984; 4:25–30.

24. Mahony L, et al: Prophylactic indomethacin therapy for patent ductus arteriosus in very low birth weight infants. *N Engl J Med* 1982; 306:506–510.

25. McGrath RL: In General Discussion, Session III: Persistent patency of ductus arteriosus in premature infants, in Heymann MA, Rudolph AM (eds): *The Ductus Arteriosus: Report of the Seventy-fifth Ross Conference on Pediatric Research*. Columbus, Ohio, Ross Laboratories, 1978, p 92.

26. Merritt TA, et al: Patent ductus arteriosus treated with ligation or indomethacin: A follow-up study. *J Pediatr* 1979; 95:588–594.

27. Merritt TA, et al: Pre-school assessment of infants with a patent arteriosus. Comparison of ligation and indomethacin therapy. *Am J Dis Child* 1982; 136:507–512.

28. Momma K, Takao A: Increased constriction of the ductus arteriosus with combined administration of indomethacin and betamethasone in fetal rats. *Pediatr Res* 1989; 25:69–75.

29. Najak A, et al: Furosemide pharmacokinetics and drug renal excretion in premature infants on chronic therapy (abstract). *Pediatr Res* 1981; 15:498.

30. Perlman JM, Hill A, Volpe JJ: The effect of patent ductus arteriosus on flow velocity in the anterior cerebral arteriosus: Ductual steal in the premature newborn infant. *J Pediatr* 1981; 99:767–771.

31. Peterson RG, et al: Pharmacology of furosemide in the premature newborn infant. *J Pediatr* 1980; 97:139–143.

32. Rhodes PG, Ferguson MG, Reddy NS, et al: Effects of prolonged versus acute indomethacin therapy in very low birth-weight infants with patent ductus arteriosus. *Eur J Pediatr* 1988; 147:481–484.

33. Ross BS, Pollak A, Oh W: The pharmacologic effects of furosemide therapy in the low birth weight infant. *J Pediatr* 1978; 92:149–152.

34. Seyberth HW, Rascher W, Hackenthal R, et al: Effect of prolonged indomethacin therapy on renal function and selected vasoactive hormone in very low birth weight infants with symptomatic patent ductus arteriosus. *J Pediatr* 1983; 103:979–984.

35. Siassi B, et al: Incidence and clinical features of patent ductus arteriosus in low birth weight infants: A prospective analysis of 150 consecutively born infants. *Pediatrics* 1976; 57:347–351.

36. Thalji A, et al: Pharmacokinetics of intravenously administered indomethacin in premature infants. *J Pediatr* 1980; 97:995–1000.

37. Weber PC, Scherer B, Larsson C: Increase of free arachidonic acid by furosemide in man as a cause of prostaglandin and renin release. *Eur J Pharmacol* 1977; 41:329–332.

38. Woo WCR, Dupont C, Collinge J, et al: Effect of furosemide in the newborn. *Clin Pharmacol* 1978; 23:266–271.

39. Yaffe SJ, et al: The disposition of indomethacin in premature babies. *J Pediatr* 1980; 97:1001–1006.

40. Yeh TF, et al: Intravenous indomethacin therapy in premature infants with persistent ductus arteriosus: A double-blind controlled study. *J Pediatr* 1981; 98:136–145.

41. Yeh TF, et al: Improved lung compliance following indomethacin therapy in premature infants with presistent ductus arteriosus. *Chest* 1981; 80:698–700.
42. Yeh TF, Raval D, Luken J, et al: Clinical evaluation of premature infants with patent ductus arteriosus: A scoring system with echocardiogram, acid-base, and blood gas correlations. *Crit Care Med* 1981; 9:655–657.
43. Yeh TF, et al: Furosemide prevents the renal side effects of indomethacin therapy in premature infants with patent ductus arteriosus. *J Pediatr* 1982; 101:433–437.
44. Yeh TF, et al: Intravenous indomethacin therapy in premature infants with patent ductus arteriosus: Causes of death and one-year follow-up. *Am J Dis Child* 1982; 136:803–807.
45. Yeh TF, et al: Indomethacin treatment in small versus large premature infants with ductus arteriosus: Comparison of plasma indomethacin concentration and clinical response. *Br Heart J* 1983; 50:27–30.
46. Yeh TF, Shibli A, Leu ST, et al: Early furosemide therapy in premature infants with RDS—a randomized study. *J Pediatr* 1984; 105:603–609.
47. Yeh TF, Wilks A, Luken J, et al: Indomethacin therapy in premature infants with patent arteriosus and oliguria. *Dev Pharmacol Ther* 1986; 9:369–374.
48. Yeh TF, Achanti B, Patel H, et al: Indomethacin therapy in premature infants with patent ductus arteriosus—determination of therapeutic levels. *Dev Pharmacol Ther* 1989; 12:169–178.

11

Prostaglandin Therapy of Congenital Heart Disease

Julie A. Luken, M.D.

Recent advances in the understanding of the role of prostaglandins (PGs) in the regulation of pulmonary vasculature and ductus arteriosus have led to the use of PGs in ductus-dependent congenital heart disease and a trial of use in persistent pulmonary hypertension (PPH). In this chapter we discuss the use of PGs to maintain ductal patency in infants with ductus-dependent cardiac lesions; PPH is discussed in Chapter 8.

PROSTAGLANDINS

The PGs are naturally occurring substances in the human body that are derived from essential saturated fatty acids. Linoleic acid is the immediate precursor from which arachidonic acid, a polyunsaturated fatty acid, is formed. The endoperoxides (PGG_2, PGH_2) are then formed by way of the enzyme cyclooxygenase. These endoperoxides are unstable but highly biologically active intermediate compounds. Once formed in the body, they are quickly metabolized to more stable end products that are far less potent in biologic activity. These end products—PGE_2, PGF_2, PGD_2, prostacyclin (PGI_2), and thromboxanes (TXA_2, TXB_2)—have been identified in various tissues throughout the body, including the umbilical artery, placenta, fetal membranes, lung, brain, aorta, platelets, stomach, and ductus arteriosus. They have been implicated in a wide variety of bodily functions, including platelet aggregation, inflammatory response, uterine contractions, regulation of body temperature, convulsions, and vasoconstriction and vasodilation of pulmonary and systemic arteries, including the umbilical arteries and the ductus arteriosus.[18]

PROSTAGLANDINS AND DUCTUS ARTERIOSUS

Much research has been performed in fetal and neonatal lambs. This work has shown that the prostaglandin PGE_2 and prostacyclin (PGI_2) are synthesized in the wall of the ductus arteriosus.[7, 10] These products cause relaxation of the ductus arteriosus, and it is believed they are responsible for maintaining ductal patency in the fetus. High levels of circulating PGE_2 have been found in fetal lambs; the concentration of PGE_2 fell shortly after birth in neonatal lambs.[6] Neonatal lambs with respiratory distress syndrome had higher concentrations of PGE_2; in these lambs the ductus arteriosus was widely patent.[6] There is an age-dependent sensitivity of the lamb ductus arteriosus to PGs. The PGs cause the most marked relaxation of the ductus arteriosus early in gestation, and as the lamb fetus advances in gestation the sensitivity of the ductus to PG decreases.[5]

Observation of the effect of PGs on the lamb ductus arteriosus led to the use of PGs in the human neonate with ductus-dependent congenital heart disease.

THERAPY OF CONGENITAL HEART DISEASE

Alprostadil

Pharmacology

Alprostadil, or PGE_1 (prost-13-en-1-oic acid, 11,15-dihydroxy-9-oxo-, [$11\alpha,3E,15S$]), has molecular weight of 354.49. It is a white to off-white crystalline powder with a melting point of 110° to 116° C. The solubility at 35° C is 8,000 mg/dL double-distilled water. Alprostadil is metabolized very rapidly: 80% of the drug may be metabolized in one pass through the lungs, primarily by beta and omega oxidation.[17] The metabolites of alprostadil are excreted by the kidney, usually within 24 hours after administration is stopped. Because of its rapid metabolism, alprostadil must be given as a continuous infusion. There are no absolute contraindications for the concomitant use of alprostadil and standard drugs used to treat ductus-dependent congenital heart disease (i.e., digoxin, diuretics, dopamine, isoproterenol, antibiotics).

Alprostadil (Prostin VR Pediatric Sterile Solution) is available in packages of five 1 mL ampules. Each milliliter contains 500 µg alprostadil in dehydrated alcohol. It must be diluted prior to usage with either sterile sodium chloride injection USP or sterile dextrose injection USP. The dilute solution can be used for only 24 hours, then should be discarded and a fresh solution made. The solution must be stored in the refrigerator at 2° to 8° C.

Indications and Contraindications

Alprostadil is to be used in infants with the following ductus-dependent congenital heart lesions:

1. Cyanotic group
   Tetralogy of Fallot
   Pulmonary atresia with ventricular septal defect
   Pulmonary atresia with intact ventricular septum
   Tricuspid atresia with pulmonary stenosis or pulmonary atresia
   Transposition of great arteries
   Ebstein's anomaly with pulmonary stenosis or pulmonary atresia
2. Left ventricular obstructed group
   Interrupted aortic arch
   Coarctation of aorta
   Hypoplastic left-heart syndrome
   Critical aortic valvular stenosis

In addition to these cardiac lesions, alprostadil may be beneficial in the treatment of obstructed total anomalous pulmonary venous connection to the portal system by maintaining the patency of the ductus venosus as well as the ductus arteriosus.[3]

It is desirable to exclude other causes of hypoxia in the newborn, such as respiratory distress syndrome, pulmonary disease, sepsis, or intracerebral hemorrhage, before initiating alprostadil therapy. In these infants alprostadil might be detrimental by causing respiratory depression or systemic hypotension. It is no longer necessary to perform cardiac catheterization and angiography before initiating alprostadil therapy. Ductus-dependent congenital heart disease can be identified by clinical examination, analysis of arterial blood gas pattern, chest radiograph, electrocardiogram, and a complete echocardiogram (including two-dimensional pulsed Doppler and color-flow Doppler studies, where available). Alprostadil therapy should be begun as soon as the diagnosis is available. Alprostadil therapy has been successfully initiated in primary care centers in ductus-dependent infants before transfer to a definitive tertiary care unit.[9, 13] The infant will then be in the best clinical condition to withstand cardiac catheterization and cineangiography, if necessary, and then surgical intervention.

Route of Administration and Dosage

Alprostadil is available only for infusion. The preferred route of infusion is into a peripheral vein, although the umbilical vein or artery can be used. When using the umbilical artery, care must be taken to place the catheter tip at or above the level of the ductus arteriosus. It is best to use an infusion pump to provide a constant infusion rate. The maximum infusion rate of alprostadil is 0.1 μg/kg/min. Initial infusion rates of 0.005 to 0.01 μg/kg/min have been successfully used.[13, 26] Once ductal patency has been established (by continuous murmur, increased Pao_2, increased oxygen saturation, increased pH, palpable femoral pulses) the infusion rate can be reduced, if the maximum infusion rate was initially administered. If prolonged infusion of alprostadil is necessary, further reduction in infusion concentration can be

/

TABLE 11–1.
Dilution Instructions for Alprostadil*

Add 1 Ampule (500 μg) Alprostadil to Sterile Solution (mL)	Approximate Concentration of Resulting Solution (μg/mL)	Infusion Rate (mL/kg/min)
250	2	0.05
100	5	0.02
50	10	0.01
25	20	0.005

*Reprinted with permission of the Upjohn Company (8887-69), 1981.

made. Long-term low-dose infusion of alprostadil has been successfully used to maintain ductal patency.[8, 24] Alprostadil therapy should be discontinued as soon as feasible to avoid the long-term side effects (discussed later in this chapter). If bradycardia, systemic hypotension, or apnea occur, the infusion rate of alprostadil can be reduced, or it may be necessary temporarily to discontinue the infusion until vital signs are stable. Temperature elevation is not an indication to discontinue alprostadil therapy. It may be wise to obtain appropriate cultures and then to administer appropriate antibiotics. The latter would also be wise in view of the multiple invasive procedures performed on the critically ill infant with ductus-dependent congenital heart disease.

It is most important to calculate and deliver the appropriate concentration and rate of infusion of alprostadil based on the infant's body weight in kilograms. It is suggested that one intravenous bottle and tubing be used solely for alprostadil infusion. The designated intravenous setup should be labeled with the appropriate alprostadil infusion rate, and this rate should not be altered to deliver other medications or provide intravenous fluids.

An example of appropriate calculation and infusion rate of alprostadil that will provide 0.1 μg/kg/min to a 2.5-kg infant is as follows:

Step 1: Place 1 ampule (500 μg) alprostadil in 100 mL sterile saline or dextrose solution (final concentration 5 μg/mL)
Step 2: 0.1 μg/kg/min × 2.5 kg = 0.25 μg/min
Step 3: 0.25 μg/min × 60 min = 15 μg/hr
Step 4: 15 μg/hr ÷ 5 μg/mL = 3 mL/hr

Thus an infusion of 500 μg alprostadil in a 100 mL solution at a rate of 3 mL/hr would deliver 0.1 μg/kg/min alprostadil to a 2.5 kg infant. Dilution instructions are listed in Table 11–1. The dosage schedules for the appropriate concentration and infusion rate of alprostadil are given in Tables 11–2 and 11–3.

PGE_2 is available in some countries for use in the ductus-dependent infant. It can be administered either by the intravenous or oral route. The beneficial effects of both short-term and long-term use of PGE_2 therapy in these infants has been established.[2, 23] Some infants have, in fact, been discharged from the hospital to receive long-term oral PGE_2 therapy.[23]

TABLE 11–2.
Dosage Schedules for Concentration (0.1 µg/kg/min) and Infusion Rate of Alprostadil*

Alprostadil	Weight of neonate (kg)										
	0.5	1.0	1.5	2.0	2.5	3.0	3.5	4.0	4.5	5.0	5.5
µg/min	0.05	0.10	0.15	0.20	0.25	0.30	0.35	0.40	0.45	0.50	0.55
µg/hr	3.0	6.0	9.0	12.0	15.0	18.0	21.0	24.0	27.0	30.0	33
5 µg (mL/hr)	0.6	1.2	1.8	2.4	3.0	3.6	4.2	4.8	5.4	6.0	6.6

*Reprinted with permission of the Upjohn Company (8887–69), 1981.

TABLE 11–3.
Dosage Schedules for Concentration (0.05 µg/kg/min) and Infusion Rate of Alprostadil*

Alprostadil	Weight of neonate (kg)										
	0.5	1.0	1.5	2.0	2.5	3.0	3.5	4.0	4.5	5.0	5.5
µg/min	0.025	0.050	0.075	0.100	0.125	0.150	0.175	0.200	0.225	0.250	0.275
µg/hr	1.5	3.0	4.5	6.0	7.5	9.0	10.5	12.0	13.5	15.0	16.5
5 µg (mL/hr)	0.3	0.6	0.9	1.2	1.5	1.8	2.1	2.4	2.7	3.0	3.3

*Reprinted with permission of the Upjohn Company (8887–69), 1981.

Side Effects and Complications

Alprostadil infusion is not without side effects and complications. In a study by Lewis et al.[16] 43% (237/492) of infants receiving alprostadil infusion experienced at least one side effect. The cardiovascular side effects of cutaneous vasodilation or edema, arrhythmias, and hypotension appear to be the most common and were present in 18% (90) of these infants; they were more common in the cyanotic group. In this group of infants intra-arterial alprostadil infusion was more likely to be used, and the side effect of peripheral cutaneous vasodilation is much more common with intra-arterial infusion of alprostadil. The CNS side effects of seizure activity and temperature elevation were the next most common, occurring in 16% (81) of the infants, and were not influenced by the site of alprostadil infusion. Hypoventilation or apnea was the next most common side effect, noted in 12% (58) of the infants, and was not related to the site of alprostadil infusion, but was seen most often in the low birth weight infants and was not necessarily related to the alprostadil infusion. These side effects have been noted by others.[2, 13, 20] Other side effects reported included hypoglycemia, hypocalcemia, sepsis, diarrhea, renal failure, thrombocytopenia, hemorrhage, disseminated intravascular coagulation, wound infection, and necrotizing enterocolitis. Thus far no deaths have been attributed to alprostadil therapy.

Longer duration of alprostadil therapy is associated with other side effects. Reversible cortical hyperostosis and periostitis have been noted.[22, 25] Apparent widening of the cranial sutures, also reversible, has been reported.[1, 15]

Histologic studies of the ductus arteriosus and the pulmonary vasculature have been performed in infants who have received alprostadil therapy. Within the wall of the ductus arteriosus there is marked disruption of the internal elastic lamella, disarray of muscle fibers, with increased elastic tissue in the media, and thickening with infiltration of mononuclear cells within the adventitia. In addition there is an increase in mucopolysaccharides throughout the ductal wall.[8, 11, 19] Histologic features of hemorrhage, thrombosis, edema, and interruption of the internal elastic lamina in the ductal wall have not been found to be specific for alprostadil-treated ductus arteriosus by others.[4, 21] In a recent study and review by Gittenberger-de-Groot and Strengers[12] ductus arteriosus exposed to PGE$_1$ treatment had a marked, but nonspecific, increase in histopathologic findings. These histologic changes within the wall of the ductus arteriosus are disturbing in that they might result in aneurysmal dilation, with eventual rupture of the ductus arteriosus. In a study of eight infants receiving alprostadil therapy for 30 hours to 12 days, changes in the pulmonary vasculature consisted of edema within the wall of the muscular and partially muscular arteries, with breaks in the outer elastic lamina. The media appeared less compact than normal; aneurysmal dilation of the large muscular arteries and reduction in the amount of pulmonary arterial smooth muscle were noted.[14] These findings in the pulmonary arteries would increase permeability of the vessels.

CONCLUSION

The efficacy and beneficial use of both short-term and long-term alprostadil (PGE_1) and PGE_2 therapy has been well established in infants with ductus-dependent congenital heart disease. In view of the side effects noted, alprostadil and PGE_2 therapy should be restricted to those infants in whom surgical intervention is feasible but not immediately advisable.

REFERENCES

1. Beitzke A, Stein J: Pseudo-widening of cranial sutures as a feature of long-term prostaglandin E_1 therapy. *Pediatr Radiol* 1986; 16:57–58.
2. Beitzke A, Suppan CH: Use of prostaglandin E_2 in management of transposition of great arteries before balloon atrial septostomy. *Br Heart J* 1983; 49:341–344.
3. Bullaboy CA, Johnson DH, Hormoz A, et al: Total anomalous pulmonary venous connection to portal system: A new therapeutic role for prostaglandin E_1? *Pediatr Cardiol* 1984; 5:115–116.
4. Calder AL, Kirker JA, Neutze JM, et al: Pathology of the ductus arteriosus treated with prostaglandins: Comparisons with untreated cases. *Pediatr Cardiol* 1984; 5:85–92.
5. Clyman RI, Mauray F, Rudolph AM, et al: Age-dependent sensitivity of the lamb ductus arteriosus to indomethacin and prostaglandins. *J Pediatr* 1980; 96:94–98.
6. Clyman RI, Mauray F, Roman C, et al: Circulating prostaglandin E_2 concentrations and patent ductus arteriosus in fetal and neonatal lambs. *J Pediatr* 1980; 97:455–461.
7. Coceani F: Prostaglandins and patency of the ductus arteriosus, in Heymann MA, Rudolph AM (eds): *The Ductus Arteriosus: Report of the Seventy-Fifth Ross Conference on Pediatric Research.* Columbus, Ohio, Ross Laboratories, 1978, pp 28–31.
8. Cole RB, Abman S, Aziz KU, et al: Prolonged prostaglandin E_1 infusion: Histologic effects on the patent ductus arteriosus. *Pediatrics* 1981; 67:816–819.
9. Danford DA, Gutgesell HP, McNamara DG: Application of information theory to decision analysis in potentially prostaglandin-responsive neonates. *J Am Coll Cardiol* 1986; 8:1125–1130.
10. Friedman WF: Studies of the responses of the ductus arteriosus in intact animals, in Heymann MA, Rudolph AM (eds): *The Ductus Arteriosus: Report of the Seventy-Fifth Ross Conference on Pediatric Research.* Columbus, Ohio, Ross Laboratories, 1978, pp 35–43.
11. Gittenberger-de-Groot AC, Moulaert AJ, Harinick E, et al: Histopathology of the ductus arteriosus after prostaglandin E_1 administration in ductus-dependent cardiac anomalies. *Br Heart J* 1978; 40:215–220.
12. Gittenberger-de-Groot AC, Strengers JLM: Histopathology of the arterial duct (ductus arteriosus) with and without treatment with prostaglandin E_1. *Int J Cardiol* 1988; 19:153–166.
13. Hallidie-Smith KA: Prostaglandin E_1 in suspected ductus dependent cardiac malformations. *Arch Dis Child* 1984; 59:1020–1026.
14. Haworth SG, Sauer U, Buhlmeyer K: Effect of prostaglandin E_1 on pulmonary circulation in pulmonary atresia. A quantitative morphologic study. *Br Heart J* 1980; 43:306–314.

15. Hoevels-Guerich H, Haferkorn L, Persigehl M, et al: Widening of cranial sutures after long-term prostaglandin E_2 therapy in two newborns. *J Pediatr* 1984; 105:72–74.

16. Lewis AB, Freed MD, Heymann MA, et al: Side effects of therapy with prostaglandin E_1 in infants with critical congenital heart disease. *Circulation* 1981; 64:893–898.

17. Mathe AA, Hedqvist P, Standberg K, et al: Aspects of prostaglandin function in the lung. *N Engl J Med* 1977; 296:850–855.

18. Moskowitz MA, Coughlin SR: Basic properties of prostaglandins. *Curr Concepts Cerebral Disease* 1981; 16:5–10.

19. Moulaert AJ, Gittenberger AC, Harnick E: Prostaglandin and damage to ductus arteriosus. *Lancet* 1977; 1:703–704.

20. O'Hara T, Ogata H, Fujiyama JI, et al: Effects of prostaglandin E_1 infusion in the pre-operative management of critical congenital heart disease. *Tohoku J Exp Med* 1985; 146:237–249.

21. Park I, Nihill MR, Titus JL: Morphologic features of the ductus arteriosus after prostaglandin E_1 administration for ductus-dependent congenital heart defects. *J Am Coll Cardiol* 1983; 1:471–475.

22. Ringel RE, Haney PJ, Brenner JI, et al: Periosteal changes secondary to prostaglandin administration. *J Pediatr* 1983; 103:251–253.

23. Silove ED, Roberts DGV, DeGiovanni JV: Evaluation of oral and low dose intravenous prostaglandin E_2 in management of ductus dependent congenital heart disease. *Arch Dis Child* 1985; 60:1025–1030.

24. Teixeira OHP, Carpenter B, MacMurray SB, et al: Long-term prostaglandin E_1 therapy in congenital heart defects. *J Am Coll Cardiol* 1984; 3:838–843.

25. Ueda K, Saito A, Nakano H, et al: Cortical hyperostosis following long-term administration of prostaglandin E_1 in infants with cyanotic congenital heart disease. *J Pediatr* 1980; 97:834–836.

26. Yakota M, Muraoka R, Aoshima M, et al: Modified Blalock-Taussig shunt following long-term administration of prostaglandin E_1 for ductus-dependent neonates with cyanotic congenital heart disease. *J Thorac Cardiovasc Surg* 1985; 90:399–403.

12

Congestive Heart Failure

Maria Serratto, M.D.

Heart failure results when an acute or chronic stress to the myocardium impairs cardiac function to such a degree that the requirements of the body cannot be fulfilled. In the newborn and infant this syndrome is usually brought about by a congenital cardiovascular malformation, or less frequently by myocardial damage, or by a combination of these. Recently, birth asphyxia has been recognized as the underlying cause of cardiac failure in various perinatal syndromes (Table 12–1).

PATHOPHYSIOLOGY

The pathophysiology of heart failure has been discussed in depth in recent reviews.[6, 28] The heart can best be characterized as a muscular pump that must supply nutrients to the metabolizing tissues on a moment-to-moment basis. The performance of the heart depends on its ability to contract, which is constantly modified in relation to the variable needs of the body by the following major hemodynamic factors:

1. Inotropic state, which governs the rate and force of contraction
2. Preload, or ventricular filling load, which regulates myocardial contraction according to the Frank-Starling mechanism, whereby increasing the stretch of a striated muscle fiber increases the strength of contraction
3. Afterload, or the load the ventricle meets during ejection
4. Heart rate

Tachycardia produces a variable increase in the contractile state. Chronic increase in afterload produces hypertrophy; chronic increase in preload produces dilation and hypertrophy. The hypertrophied myocardium is capable of stronger contractions at the expense, however, of its distensibility and of

TABLE 12–1.
Age-related Causes of Heart Failure*

Fetus and newborn	Birth to 2 weeks
Antenatal closure of foramen ovale	Aortic or pulmonary atresia or severe
Hypoplastic left heart syndrome	stenosis
Birth Asphyxia	Coarctation of aorta
Hypoxemia with	Transposition of great arteries
Tricuspid or mitral regurgitation	Total anomalous pulmonary venous
Pulmonary or systemic hypertension	drainage
Acidemia and systemic hypotension	
(cardiogenic shock)	2 to 8 weeks
Pulmonary regurgitation	Left-to-right shunts
Systemic arteriovenous fistula	Ventricular septal defect
Hypoglycemia	Patent ductus arteriosus
Adrenal gland disorders	Atrioventricular canal
Anemia	
Polycythemia	3 months to 1 year
Sepsis	Myocardial disease
Myocarditis	Myocarditis
	Endocardial fibroelastosis syndrome
	Anomalous left coronary artery
	Pompe's disease (Cori type II)

*Heart failure may occur in any of these age groups after heart surgery and with severe dysrhythmias.

the oxygen available to the contracting myocytes. Tachycardia as well reduces oxygen availability to the myocardium, because it shortens diastole. Tachycardia, the inotropic state, dilation, and hypertrophy have been called the cardiac reserve, because they come into play with increased demands. When demands become excessive, these mechanisms are exhausted and cardiac failure ensues. Because of the intrinsic characteristics of the neonatal myocardium,[14] the newborn has very limited cardiac reserve; therefore, cardiac decompensation develops readily and progresses rapidly. Heart failure in the newborn infant is a medical emergency that requires prompt recognition and management.

CLINICAL AND LABORATORY FINDINGS

Symptoms and Signs

Cardiomegaly and hepatomegaly may be the only diagnostic clues in the clinical picture of shock produced by the fulminant form of cardiac decompensation. When cardiac decompensation develops at a slower pace, the clinical picture of congestive heart failure is the common finding. This is in contrast to the older pediatric population, in whom left ventricular failure or right ventricular failure usually present distinct findings. This different behavior may be related to the age-dependent properties of the heart (Table 12–1). Respiratory system manifestations are prominent and consist of tachypnea, dyspnea, wheezing, grunting, flaring of the alae nasi, and retraction of the ribs. The baby also shows excessive sweating, irritability or apathy, feeding difficulties, and failure to thrive. Tachycardia, gallop rhythm, splenomegaly, peripheral cyanosis, and a cold and moist skin are other common findings. The peripheral pulses are weak except when high output failure is present, as with systemic arteriovenous fistula and anemia. Rales and facial edema usually signify advanced failure. Thrills and murmurs may be absent when there is marked impairment of cardiac output and they may appear with improvement of cardiac function.

Laboratory Findings

The chest radiograph will show cardiomegaly and pulmonary congestion. Associated features often present before they become clinically apparent are pulmonary edema, atelectasis, and pulmonary infections. The electrocardiogram is not helpful in confirming the diagnosis of heart failure, but aids in the diagnosis of the disease entity responsible for the failure.

Doppler echocardiography has supplanted cardiac catheterization-angiocardiographic studies to clarify the cause of cardiac failure and to provide information on cardiac performance. Fetal echocardiography is a useful tool for the diagnosis of cardiac failure in utero. Determinations of serum sodium, chloride, potassium, calcium, and glucose levels and of blood gases and acid-base balance are useful in the evaluation of the cardiac status and of the effect of medical therapy. Correction of anemia is important because it increases cardiac output and decreases oxygen delivery to the tissues. In the newborn, placenta or twin-to-twin transfusion can result in acute anemia or volume overload and cardiac decompensation. Leukopenia is associated with viral myocarditis. Leukocytosis may indicate infection, but it may be a result of the cardiac failure. Urinary output may decrease, and urine may contain proteins, hyaline casts, white blood cells, and red blood cells. Renal failure may ensue, with severe and prolonged heart failure.

DIFFERENTIAL DIAGNOSIS

Clinical findings may mimic those of sepsis, meningitis, or primary pulmonary disorders, such as bronchiolitis, pneumonia, or alterations in the pulmonary circulation. Of great importance is the differential diagnosis between congestion of the circulation and cardiac decompensation, in view of recent studies indicating that in symptomatic infants with large left-to-right shunts, myocardial contractility is seemingly normal.

Thus the clinical picture is produced by circulatory congestion rather than true myocardial failure. However, myocardial contractility may be depressed when there is associated hypoxia, metabolic disturbances, or infections, as is often the case.

TREATMENT

The treatment of heart failure is addressed to improve myocardial function. Digitalis is still the drug most commonly used in the medical management of the syndrome, even though in recent years new drugs and mechanical and electrical aids have become available to support the failing heart. It should be pointed out that in many congenital malformations definitive treatment is obtained by surgical correction of the lesion.

Digitalis Glycosides

Mechanism of Action

Digitalis glycosides improve contractility of the failing myocardium. This positive inotropic action is exercised directly on the contractile elements of the myocardium through a transient increase in intracellular free calcium following membrane depolarization. Whether this is accomplished by the well-demonstrated inhibition of the $Na^+,K^+,ATPase$ pump or by a direct reversible alteration of calcium binding or translocation is still uncertain. In either case, the end result is transient augmentation in intracellular Ca^{++}, producing a positive inotropic effect by interaction with the contractile proteins. Thus the pharmacologic actions of digitalis seem to result from surface interaction in the sarcolemma and do not correlate with total tissue uptake of the drug.[25] In congestive heart failure the effects of digitalis on the peripheral circulation are related to improved myocardial contraction. As digitalis relieves congestive heart failure, sympathetic support is withdrawn and reflex vasoconstriction is abolished, with decrease in afterload and further increase in cardiac output.

Effects on Electrocardiogram

Digitalis glycosides modify conduction, refractoriness, excitability, and automaticity of the myocardium, both by direct effect and by acting on the autonomic nervous system. Digitalis increases central parasympathetic activity and vagal tone. The effect on sympathetic activity is dose related. At low doses sympathetic outflow is diminished; at higher doses there is an increase in sympathetic activity, which may foster the development of digitalis-related dysrhythmias. At therapeutic doses digitalis may cause decreased amplitude of the T wave, sagging of the ST segment, and shortening of the QT interval. None of these electrocardiographic effects is an index of adequate digitalization or of digitalis toxicity. In patients with sinus rhythm, slowing of the heart rate results from sympathetic withdrawal caused by improved myocardial performance and heightened vagal tone. However, heart rates less than 100 beats per minute in infants is considered presumptive evidence of early digitalis toxicity.

Prolongation of the PR interval is produced by neural and direct depressant effect on the atrioventricular (AV) node, and usually occurs with higher doses. Prolongation of the PR interval has been indicated to be a useful early warning sign of digitalis toxicity in the premature infant.[19] Advanced toxicity may manifest with (1) high degrees of AV block, resulting in bradycardia or AV dissociation due primarily to depressed conduction, and supraventricular or ventricular tachycardia, or (2) multifocal premature beats related to increased automaticity. Combinations of depressed conduction and increased automaticity result in paroxysmal atrial tachycardia with block and nonparoxysmal junctional tachycardia. Ventricular fibrillation may be preceded by any of these conditions. Ventricular premature contractions in the form of bigemini, a frequent early warning sign in older children, are rare in neonates and small infants, in whom depression of sinus and AV nodal function prevails.

In conclusion, in this age group the most common signs are sinus bradycardia or arrest, and prolonged PR interval in early toxicity and second-degree and higher AV block in more advanced toxicity.

Bioavailability and Route of Administration

Digoxin is a water-insoluble glycoside obtained from *Digitalis lanata*. Bioavailability is 100% with intravenous administration. After oral administration digitalis is absorbed mostly in the upper part of the small intestine. Absorption of digoxin elixir administered to neonates and infants with heart failure averages 72% (range, 52% to 79%), and peak serum concentrations are reached in 30 to 90 minutes. Food intake seems to alter only the rate of absorption. Several drugs interfere with digitalis bioavailability. The clinical importance of these interferences is not well established for the pediatric population. Only a few of the drugs investigated are used in the age group under consideration: neomycin and phenytoin decrease absorption; atropine enhances absorption.[7] The results obtained with digoxin tablets may not apply to digoxin in the form of elixir.[22] Studies conducted in adults have shown that clinical conditions such as celiac disease and hyperthyroidism impair intestinal absorption, but severe congestive heart failure does not seem to have a significant negative effect. Digoxin is no longer administered by intramuscular injection, because of erratic absorption and the possibility of local tissue necrosis.

Distribution and Elimination

The distribution of digoxin in the body can be approximated by a linear, two-compartment, open model. The drug is largely distributed to extravascular sites. This implies that plasma protein binding is low for digoxin, because only the unbound drug can distribute to tissue and be pharmacologically active. In fact, only approximately 21% of digoxin is bound to plasma proteins in both newborns and adults. Several authors[4, 23] have found that the apparent volume of distribution of digoxin in infants is much greater than in adults. Thus, at identical serum concentrations, tissue concentrations are higher in infancy.[1] Digoxin concentration in the kidney of premature newborns is much lower than in full-term newborns and in children.[20] The great majority of digoxin is excreted unchanged by the kidney by glomerular filtration. Small amounts undergo renal tubular secretion and reabsorption. In adults, digoxin clearance equals creatinine clearance. In infancy, renal clearance of digoxin is low in the first weeks of life, and adult values are reached at approximately 5 months of age. In adults the liver excretes the remaining digoxin. Moderate liver disease and drugs inducing hepatic microsomal enzymes do not seem to modify hepatic metabolism of digoxin. In infants and children, digoxin metabolites are absent or present in small quantities in urine and stool. The highest values for elimination half-life of digoxin are found in premature (mean 57 hours and 72 hours) and in full-term newborns (mean 35 hours, 44 hours, 69 hours), and the lowest in infants more than 1 month old (mean 37 hours).[15] High digoxin plasma levels seem to shorten plasma half-life.[23] Total body clearance is low in premature and full-term neonates because of the relative immaturity of liver and kidney function. Infants from 1 month to 1 year of age show adult levels or higher. Infants with high clearance rates are usually older than 3 months.[23]

Other Factors Affecting Digoxin Pharmacokinetics

Renal failure diminishes excretion of digoxin. Hyperkalemia decreases and hypokalemia increases Na^+, K^+, and ATPase binding. Low serum levels of digoxin are present in hyperthyroidism, whereas the opposite occurs in hypothyroidism. Antiarrhythmic drugs that increase serum digoxin concentration are verapamil, quinidine, and amiodarone. Spironolactone, triamterene, and amiloride and a state of hypokalemia have similar effects. Diazepam decreases metabolism and renal clearance of digoxin. Indomethacin decreases renal clearance of digoxin. Hemodialysis, peritoneal dialysis, and exchange transfusion remove only small amounts of total body digoxin, because of its large volume of distribution. The effects of cardiopulmonary bypass vary according to whether the patient has been recently digitalized or is receiving maintenance doses of digoxin. Krasula et al.[21] found that postoperative arrhythmias occurred only in patients recently digitalized and correlated with higher myocardial digoxin concentration in the presence of hypokalemia. Digoxin is excreted in human milk at therapeutic plasma concentrations, but is not detected in the plasma of nursing infants.[13] Digoxin crosses the placenta. Chronic administration to the pregnant woman results in equivalent concentrations in maternal and cord blood serum.[27] Transplacental transfer has been used for the treatment of congestive heart failure in utero through the administration of digoxin to the mother.[16]

Digitalization

Larger doses of digoxin per unit of body weight or surface area have been customarily used in newborn infants than in adults with cardiac decompensation, because of the greater volume of distribution. Recent progress in the understanding of the elimination kinetics of digoxin and of toxic effects of digoxin has led to a recommendation of lower digoxin dosages in newborns and infants younger than 3 months of age, particularly if premature, because the clearance of digoxin is low in premature infants.[17] With these considerations in mind, the dosages depicted in Table 12–2 could be used as a guide for therapy. Oral digoxin doses are higher than parenteral doses to compensate for 70% to 80% bioavailability. For oral digitalization, the total digitalizing dosage, calculated according to the age and weight of the patient, is given over 24 hours in three divided doses: one-half, one-fourth, and one-fourth dose 8 hours apart or in three equal doses 8 hours apart. A baseline electrocardiogram is obtained before the first dose is given, and the study is repeated before each of the subsequent two doses. Before the third dose the patient should be clinically evaluated for possible signs of toxicity. For intravenous digitalization, two thirds to three fourths of the calculated oral dose is used. One half to two thirds of this reduced amount is administered as the initial dose. Within 3 to 6 hours half of the remaining drug can be administered. Clinical examination and the electrocardiogram will indicate the route of administration of the subsequent doses.

Maintenance is started 12 hours after digitalization is completed, if there are no signs of toxicity. The maintenance dose should replenish the percentage of the peak body stores excreted each day. The majority of patients maintain adequate digitalization with one fourth (one third to one fifth) of the digitalizing dose of digoxin daily. It is common that more stable serum digoxin levels and less toxicity are obtained when maintenance is divided in two doses given 12 hours apart. Because individualization of dosing seems to be the key to optimal digitalization for patients with congestive heart failure, after initial therapy the dosage should be adjusted to the needs of the patient after careful evaluation of the clinical picture. If the therapeutic response is not judged satisfactory and the serum digoxin concentration is between 1 and 2 ng/mL, the dose may be increased, with close monitoring of serum digoxin and electrolytes and of cardiac and extracardiac signs of toxicity. Normalization of heart rate and respiratory rate is the most consistent sign of satisfactory digitalization. The baby appears more comfortable, is less irritable and listless, and feeds and sleeps better. Because digitalis intoxication

TABLE 12–2.
Recommended Oral Digitalizing Doses for Digoxin in Newborns and Infants*

Age	Weight	Digitalizing Dose (μg/kg)
Premature (newborns and infants <3 mo old)	<1,500	15 (range 10–20)
	1,500–2,500 g	30 (20–40)
Term (newborns and infants <3 mo old)	>2,500 g	45 (30–60)
Infants >3 mo old	≥5 kg	60 (40–80)

*For IV therapy, two thirds to three fourths of the oral dose is used.

is more likely to develop during rapid digitalization, a loading dose is now used only for emergency digitalization. In less severe cardiac failure, digitalization is done gradually with the calculated maintenance dose. With this regimen, a steady-state level is reached in 6 days.

Duration of Digoxin Therapy

In infants who had successful corrective cardiac surgery the drug may be discontinued according to the clinical course and the reduction in heart size. In complicated malformations with heart failure where a physiologic circulation cannot be reestablished, digoxin therapy should be continued indefinitely. In endocardial fibroelastosis and myocarditis, digoxin should be continued as long as the echocardiogram shows depressed left ventricular function. Early discontinuation of digoxin may precipitate a fatal outcome even in asymptomatic patients with an improved chest radiograph and electrocardiogram.

Toxicity

Toxicity may prompt cardiac, neurologic, and gastrointestinal symptoms. Some of the cardiac and noncardiac manifestations of digitalis toxicity, such as apathy, weakness, regurgitation, vomiting, and diarrhea, may result from heart failure itself. However, persistent vomiting is usually the most common sign of digitalis toxicity in infants. Vomiting, on the other hand, cannot be relied on as a warning sign, as serious dysrhythmias may appear in its absence. Cardiac toxicity results in dysrhythmias and occasionally in aggravation of heart failure. A number of conditions may precipitate digitalis toxicity: prematurity, hypoxemia, hypokalemia, hypomagnesemia, hypercalcemia, myocarditis, severe hepatic and renal disease, hypothyroidism, severe cardiac decompensation, and surgery; concomitant administration of drugs that decrease digoxin excretion or administration of catecholamines may foster digitalis intoxication.

Determination of Serum Digoxin Level

Determinations of serum digoxin concentration are useful in controlling digitalis therapy, particularly when it is not clear whether symptoms result from over- or underdigitalization. In neonates and small infants, toxicity rarely develops with serum digoxin levels below 3.5 ng/mL. When conditions that increase myocardial sensitivity to digoxin are present, toxicity may occur at lower serum digoxin concentrations. Blood samples for serum digoxin level must be obtained after the drug has achieved equilibrium in the body, or 6 to 8 hours after its administration. It is important to realize that digoxin radioimmunoassays are fraught with technical pitfalls that may result in falsely high levels of digoxin serum concentration, particularly in the neonatal period, when there are significant amounts of an endogenous substance that cross-react with digoxin antibodies of the commercial radioimmunoassay kits.[29] Thus, in this age group it is useful to obtain a serum sample for baseline values before digoxin therapy is initiated.

Treatment for Digoxin Toxicity

Often digoxin toxicity can be treated by discontinuing the drug; however, some dysrhythmias pose immediate danger to the patient and should be actively treated. Ventricular ectopy is best treated initially with *lidocaine,* which has practically no effect on AV conduction, has rapid onset of action, and can be easily titrated. *Potassium* is commonly used to treat ectopy, particularly when hypokalemia is present, provided there is no depression of AV conduction and no impairment of renal function. Potassium is given intravenously under close electrocardiographic monitoring, and the patient's serum potassium level should not exceed 5.5 mEq/L. The injection should be stopped when ectopy disappears or when signs of hyperpotassemia (tall, pointed T waves) become evident. *Phenytoin* is also helpful to treat ectopy, especially when there is AV block, since it rarely depresses AV conduction. *Propranolol* may effectively control atrial and ventricular tachyarrhythmias; side effects include depression of AV conduction and of myocardial contractility. *Quinidine* and *procainamide* are effective in controlling ventricular ectopy but have an even greater depressant effect on AV conduction. Quinidine may actually increase digoxin toxicity, and intravenous administration is contraindicated because it induces severe hypotension. *Bretylium* and phenytoin are used for ventricular fibrillation. Sinus node depression and second- and third-degree AV block may respond to *atropine,* but a *temporary pacemaker* may be needed. *Ventricular overdrive pacing* or *cardioversion* should be used when tachydysrhythmias present an immediate threat to life and do not respond to appropriate drug therapy. The lowest energy level necessary to achieve cardioversion should be used, to avoid serious complications. All treatments described are supportive until the excess digitalis has been excreted or metabolized. Potentially life-threatening digoxin intoxication should be treated with the *Fab portion of digoxin-specific antibodies.*[24,31] Digoxin immune Fab is nonantigenic, is eliminated in the urine even when bound to digoxin, and rapidly reverses digoxin toxicity. Improvement of toxic signs and symptoms usually begins within one-half hour of administration. Dosages for these drugs are given in Table 12–3.

Other Inotropic Agents

Sympathomimetic amines are powerful positive inotropic agents used for short-term treatment of severe heart failure in newborn infants, particularly when it has caused circulatory shock. Beneficial effects include augmentation in myocardial contractility and moderate cardioacceleration (β_1 receptors) and a decrease in peripheral vascular resistance (β_2 receptors), which all contribute to a significant increase in cardiac output. Catecholamines with strong α-adrenergic activity are less desirable because of their vasoconstrictive action; on the other hand, sympathomimetic amines producing marked peripheral vasodilation may aggravate hypotension. Sympathomimetic amines increase oxygen consumption more than digoxin for an equivalent increase

TABLE 12–3.
Treatment of Digoxin Toxicity

Drug	Route of Administration	Dosage
Atropine sulfate	IV bolus	10–40 μg/kg; maximum dose 0.4 mg (small infant dose)
Bretylium tosylate	Slow IV	5 mg/kg/dose; TSL 0.5–1.5 μg/mL (small infant dose)
DC cardioversion or defibrillation	Start at 0.5 J/kg; increase stepwise by 0.5 J/kg	Maximum 2 J/kg
Fab fraction of specific digoxin antibody (Digibind)	Slow IV	Equimolar amount (60 mg Fab/1 mg digoxin) 10 mg/mL solution in isotonic saline or sorbitol solution
Lidocaine (Xylocaine)	IV bolus	0.5–1.0 mg/kg; may be repeated × 3 doses
	IV infusion	1/mg/kg/hr; TSL 2–6 μg/mL (small infant dose)
Phenytoin sodium (Dilantin)	Slow IV push Precipitated by dilution with IV fluids	1 mg/kg; may be repeated × 15 doses given over 1–2 hr (small infant dose); TSL 10–20 μg/mL
Potassium chloride	IV infusion; ECG and serum potassium monitor	0.5 mEq K^+/kg/hr; TSL 3.5–5.5 mEq/L
Procainamide (Pronestyl)	IV infusion; ECG and BP monitor; PO	7 mg/kg/hr; × 1 dose only 7–12 mg/kg/6 hr (small infant dose)
Propranolol (Inderal)	Slow IV; standby ventricular pacing PO	0.025 mg/kg/10 min; may be repeated × 4 doses 0.5 mg/kg/6 hr; may be increased stepwise (small infant dose)
Quinidine sulfate	PO	4–12 mg/kg/6 hr (small infant dose)
Inotropic agents		
Amrinone (Inocor)	IV infusion; ECG and BP monitor	5–10 μg/kg/min
Dobutamine (Dobutrex)	IV infusion; ECG and BP monitor	2–10 μg/kg/min; maximum 40 μg/kg/min (small infant dose)
Dopamine (Intropin)	IV infusion; ECG and BP monitor Inactivated by alkali	2–20 μg/kg/min; maximum, 50μg/kg/min (small infant dose)
Epinephrine 1:10,000 (Adrenalin)	IV infusion; ECG and BP monitor	0.05–1.0 μg/kg/min (small infant dose)
Isoproterenol (Isuprel)	IV infusion; ECG and BP monitor	0.05–0.50 μg/kg/min (small infant dose)
Norepinephrine (Levophed)	IV infusion; ECG and BP monitor; extravasation will produce slough	0.05–0.50 μg/kg/min

Vasodilators

Captopril (Capoten)	PO	0.1–1.0 mg/kg/6–8 hr; maximum, 4/ mg/kg/24 hr (small infant dose)
Enalapril (Vasotec)	PO	80 μg/kg/12–24 hr
Hydralazine (Apresoline)	IV bolus	0.1–0.5 mg/kg/6–8 hr
	PO	0.25–1.0 mg/kg/6–8 hr; increase to maximum oral dose of 7.0 mg/kg/ 24 hr over 3–4 wk
Nitroglycerin	IV; light sensitive; absorbed by plastic tubing	0.5–20 μg/kg/min; maximum, 60 μg/kg/min
Prazosin (Minipress)	PO	0.01–0.05 mg/kg/6–8 hr; maximum 0.10 mg/kg/6–8 hr
Sodium nitroprusside (Nipride)	IV infusion; titrate with BP, light sensitive	0.5–6 μg/kg/min (small infant dose)
Diuretics		
Chlorothiazide (Diuril)	PO	20–40 mg/kg/24 hr divided in two doses
Furosemide (Lasix)	IV	1–2 mg/kg/dose
	PO	1–3 mg/kg/dose
Hydrochlorothiazide (Hydrodiuril)	PO	2–5 mg/kg/24 hr divided in two doses

TSL = therapeutic serum levels.

in myocardial contractility. The positive inotropic effect of catecholamines seems to be related to activation of adenylate cyclase, with increase in intracellular levels of cyclic adenosine monophosphate (cAMP), followed by activation of cAMP-dependent protein kinase and subsequent delivery of Ca^{++} to cardiac contractile proteins. Sympathomimetic amines are administered by intravenous infusion through a calibrated pump. During the infusion, electrocardiographic monitoring must be used, because the amines can induce serious dysrhythmia; central venous, arterial, and pulmonary wedge pressure and urinary output should also be monitored. The naturally occurring *epinephrine* and *norepinephrine* are seldom used in the treatment of heart failure in newborn infants.

Isoproterenol, a synthetic substance, is structurally related to epinephrine but acts almost exclusively on beta receptors. Although isoproterenol has been used to improve tissue perfusion because of its inotropic and peripheral effects, this drug actually decreases renal perfusion through redistribution of blood flow to skeletal muscle. The usefulness of isoproterenol is limited by its tachycardiac, dysrhythmic, and peripheral vascular effect; the latter may aggravate hypotension. Isoproterenol increases venous return to the heart and decreases pulmonary vascular resistance.

Dopamine, an endogenous catecholamine, is both a direct and indirect β-adrenergic receptor agonist weaker than epinephrine or norepinephrine. Dopamine also releases norepinephrine from sympathetic nerve terminals, and it has the property to selectively dilate renal, mesenteric, cerebral, and coronary vessels by bonding with dopamine receptors. This effect is not blocked by beta blockers. Dopamine produces less tachycardia and myocardial oxygen consumption than isoproterenol. The excretion products of dopamine are various metabolites that are rapidly excreted in the urine, with approximately 80% of the administered dose recovered in the urine in 24 hours. Small amounts of dopamine are converted to norepinephrine and epinephrine. Dopamine dose-effect data obtained in adults can be summarized as follows:

1. Low doses (2.5 μg/kg/min) augment renal cortical blood flow, thus promoting diuresis, with minor effects on heart rate, blood pressure, and myocardial contractility.
2. Moderate doses (5–15 μg/kg/min) increase renal cortical blood flow, heart rate, blood pressure, myocardial contractility, and cardiac output
3. High doses (20 μg/kg/min) may depress renal blood flow and urine output; heart rate may increase or decrease; both blood pressure and peripheral resistance increase

The effects of dopamine on pulmonary arterial pressure and resistance are controversial. In the neonate, dopamine has been found effective at low dosage in the treatment of myocardial failure due to perinatal asphyxia and persistent transitional circulation.[10, 12] In these studies cardiac performance, systemic arterial pressure, and renal function improved with dopamine infused at a dose of 2.0–8.0 μg/kg/min. In infants in cardiocirculatory shock, larger doses (mean 9.3–15 μg/kg/min) were usually required to obtain a favorable hemodynamic response.[11]

Dobutamine is a synthetic catecholamine with powerful positive inotropic effects that acts on β- and α-adrenergic receptors. Dobutamine induces much less vasoconstriction than norepinephrine and much less change in heart rate and rhythm than isoproterenol, for an equivalent increase in myocardial contractility.[26] Dobutamine has a plasma half-life of 2 minutes; onset of action is 1 to 2 minutes after beginning of the infusion, with peak action within 10 minutes. Elimination is through liver metabolism. Dobutamine has been used in the treatment of cardiocirculatory shock with significant improvement in cardiac performance and no change in heart rate. However, in infants dobutamine produces significant decrease in systemic arteriolar resistance and increase in pulmonary wedge pressure. Adverse effects can be encountered at doses greater than 7.5 μg/kg/min.[26]

Amrinone and *milrinone* belong to a new category of nonglycosidic nonsympathomimetic positive inotropic compounds with vasodilator properties that has become available for the management of severe cardiac decompensation refractory to conventional treatment. The positive inotropic effect of these agents is mediated through selective inhibition of myocardial phosphodiesterase F-III with accumulation of intracellular cAMP. This results in increased delivery of calcium to the contractile system. Vasodilation is produced by direct relaxation of vascular smooth muscle, with reduction of venous hypertension and systemic resistance. Heart rate remains generally unchanged. Unlike catecholamines, these drugs usually increase cardiac output without increase in myocardial oxygen consumption in congestive heart failure.[8] Recently amrinone has been used in the short-term management of severe cardiac decompensation in the newborn infant,[30] and is replacing the dobutamine-nitroprusside combination in postoperative low-output states. Amrinone cannot be given orally because of its narrow therapeutic-toxic ratio by this route. With intravenous administration, the hemodynamic changes are maintained for several hours after continuous infusion. Adverse effects are thrombocytopenia and hepatic toxicity.

Milrinone, a second-generation phosphodiesterase inhibitor, is about 15 times more potent than amrinone and has very similar hemodynamic effects. Milrinone can be administered both intravenously and orally. The clinical pharmacology of amrinone and milrinone in newborn infants has not yet been investigated. Dosages for isoproterenol, dopamine, dobutamine, and amrinone are shown in Table 13–3. Milrinone dosages are not well established for newborn infants.

Vasodilators

Vasodilators are an effective addition to the management of cardiogenic shock, acute pump failure associated with cardiac surgery, and chronic pump failure that has become unresponsive to conventional treatment.[2, 9] Vasodilators in general have no direct positive inotropic properties. The primary effect of these drugs is related to their ability to relax the smooth muscle in the arteriolar and venous wall. The premise of vasodilator therapy in low-output heart failure is based on the fact that in severe cardiac decompensation there is generalized vasoconstriction that adversely affects ventricular pump function. By inducing dilation of the arterioles, these vasoactive drugs reduce afterload, with improvement in cardiac output. By promoting dilation of the veins, preload is reduced. The reduction in ventricular filling volume and pressure decreases pulmonary and systemic venous congestion. The lack of a direct positive inotropic and chronotropic effect in most vasodilators contributes to the overall diminution in myocardial oxygen requirements. Vasodilators have been classified as venodilators, such as nitroglycerin, arterial dilators such as hydralazine, and balanced vasodilators such as nitroprusside, prazosin, captopril, and enalapril. None of the currently used vasodilators have pure arteriolar or venodilator activity. In recent years nitroglycerine, sodium nitroprusside, hydralazine, prazosin, and captopril have been used as an adjunct to conventional therapy in newborns and infants with acute or chronic severe heart failure of various causes.[2, 3, 9]

Nitroglycerin induces direct relaxation of smooth muscle mediated by an increase in intracellular cyclic guanosine monophosphate. The predominant site of action is on the venous bed and on the pulmonary arterial bed and to a lesser extent on the systemic arterioles. Its principal application is in the relief of systemic and pulmonary venous congestion. The drug is extensively and rapidly metabolized in the liver into compounds that are largely devoid of vasodilator properties; thus nitroglycerin is ineffective by the oral route. Nitroglycerin is widely distributed in the body and is bound to plasma proteins. Experience with this drug in the pediatric population is limited to its use after heart surgery.[5, 18] Careful monitoring should be exercised during intravenous administration, because overdosing may produce hypotension, tachycardia, and hypoxemia.[3]

Hydralazine relaxes the arteriolar wall directly, increasing cardiac output with negligible effect on ventricular filling. Hydralazine does not dilate all resistance vessels equally; renal, coronary, cerebral, and splanchnic vascular beds are preferentially affected. Hydralazine is effective both intravenously and orally; however, as it undergoes extensive first-pass clearance by the intestine and the liver, oral doses must be twice the intravenous dose. Metabolism of the drug is through enzymatic and nonenzymatic processes. Hemodynamic effects are noted within 10 minutes of intravenous administration and 30 to 60 minutes after being given orally; peak effects occur, respectively, at 30 minutes and 2 hours. Duration of action is approximately 6 hours. The most important side effects are tachycardia, vomiting, fever, rash, fluid retention, and a systemic lupus erythematous–like syndrome that occurs in approximately 15% of adults requiring high doses and has been described in infancy.[3] Tolerance to the drug may develop in some patients during maintenance therapy. This phenomenon has not yet been reported in the pediatric literature.

Prazosin has both arterial and venodilating properties. Although the primary pharmacologic activity is due to postsynaptic α-adrenergic blockade, direct relaxation of vascular smooth muscle also occurs. After oral administration, plasma concentrations reach a peak at about 3 hours, with a plasma half-life of 2 to 3 hours, but the pharmacologic effect may last up to 6 hours. Prazosin is extensively metabolized and excreted mainly by way of bile and feces. The circulatory effects of prazosin are comparable to those of nitroprusside, but prazosin can be given orally. In small doses prazosin increases hepatic blood flow. The most important side effect is the possible occurrence of severe hypotension following administration of the first dose. The tachyphylaxis reported in adults with chronic use of the drug has not yet been demonstrated in the pediatric population.[9] In premature infants and in neonates, smaller doses or less frequent administration should be used because of the immaturity of hepatic glucuronidase with lower hepatic clearance.[14]

Captopril is an orally effective angiotensin converting enzyme inhibitor that induces a significant drop in systemic vascular resistance and augmentation of cardiac output, with initial slowing of heart rate. Captopril increases venous capacitance with diminution in right atrial, pulmonary artery, and wedge pressure and pulmonary vascular resistance. Renal blood flow is usually increased. Peak plasma level occurs 1 hour after oral administration, and the effect lasts approximately 8 hours. The presence of food in the gastrointestinal tract impairs absorption. Nearly all of the absorbed dose is excreted in the urine within 24 hours, half as unchanged drug. One fourth of circulating captopril is bound to plasma protein. The apparent elimination half-life is less than 3 hours. Maintenance therapy seems to afford sustained improvement in ventricular performance in chronic heart failure. Fluid retention is extremely rare. Serum potassium levels tend to rise. Severe hypotension has been reported to occur after the first dose. If given in small initial doses with titration this complication of the drug may be avoided. White blood cells should be closely monitored; neutropenia may occur and require cessation of therapy. Nephrotic syndrome may occur with chronic use of captopril, but seems to be reversible on discontinuation of the drug. Blood urea nitrogen levels, serum electrolytes, and urinary protein should be checked closely, particular in the premature infant and neonate and in any patient with impaired renal function.

Enalapril, another angiotensin converting enzyme inhibitor, is effective orally. The presence of food in the intestine does not decrease absorption. Its actions are similar to those of captopril, but are slower in onset and longer in duration (12 to 24 hours). The protracted duration of action allows administration only once or twice a day. Enalapril is hydrolyzed to the active compound enalaprilat. Enalaprilat is poorly absorbed, but can be administered intravenously. Experience with both compounds in the newborn infant is still limited.

Sodium nitroprusside is discussed in Chapter 9.

Dosages of the most commonly used vasodilators are given in Table 13–3.

Diuretics

The inadequate renal perfusion present in heart failure promotes sodium and water retention, a compensatory phenomenon to maintain intravascular volume. Sodium and water retention increases venous return and ventricular end-diastolic volume, with potential improvement in ventricular contraction through the Frank-Starling mechanism. However, this compensatory phenomenon eventually leads to excessive filling volumes, with pulmonary or systemic venous congestion. Diuretics, by inducing urinary excretion of salt and water, diminish venous congestion (see Chapters 5, 9, 19, and 20).

Drug Treatment of Underlying and Associated Pathologic Conditions

In young infants heart failure is often precipitated or complicated by respiratory tract infections. Antipyretics to decrease oxygen requirements and antibiotics should be added to the therapeutic regimen. In acute myocarditis of viral origin, steroids are indicated. Prednisone, the drug of choice, is started at 2 mg/kg/day and subsequently adjusted according to clinical response. As soon as heart failure is controlled, the drug is discontinued by stepwise decrease, usually over 1 week. When anemia, hypertension, or metabolic or endocrine diseases originate or aggravate heart failure, the appropriate treatment for each entity should be applied in addition to the heart failure therapy.

PROGNOSIS

Heart failure in this age group requires prompt diagnosis and vigorous management. It is important to remember that the newborn infant with structural heart disease and cardiac failure should be regarded as a potential candidate for surgery. Thus, if after a short period of vigorous medical therapy no significant improvement occurs, surgical intervention should be considered. This attitude, together with improvements in diagnostic technique, available drugs, and surgical procedures, has contributed to the decrease in mortality from cardiac failure in the newborn.

REFERENCES

1. Andersson KE, Bertler A, Wettrell G: Post-mortem distribution and tissue concentrations of digoxin in infants and adults. *Acta Paediatr Scand* 1975; 64:497–504.
2. Appelbaum A, et al: Afterload reduction and cardiac output in infants early after intracardiac surgery. *Am J Cardiol* 1977; 39:444–451.
3. Artman M, Graham TP Jr: Guidelines for vasodilator therapy of congestive heart failure in infants and children. *Am Heart J* 1987; 113:994–1005.
4. Assael BM, et al: Digoxin pharmacokinetics during human development. Presented at the International Symposium on Perinatal Pharmacology, Milan, Italy, June 1974.
5. Benson LN, Bohn D, Edmonds JP: Nitroglycerin therapy in children with low cardiac index after heart surgery. *Cardiovasc Med* 1979; 4:207–215.
6. Braunwald E: Pathophysiology of heart failure, in Braunwald E (ed): *Heart Disease,* ed 3. Philadelphia, WB Saunders, 1988, pp 426–448.
7. Brown DD, Juhl RP: Altered bioavailability of digoxin produced by gastro-intestinal medications (abstract). *Abstr Clin Res* 1979; 27:610A.
8. Colucci WS, Wright RF, Braunwald E: New positive inotropic agents in the treatment of congestive heart failure. Second of two parts. *N Engl J Med* 1986; 314:349–358.
9. Dillon TR, et al: Vasodilator therapy for congestive heart failure. *J Pediatr* 1980; 96:623–629.
10. DiSessa TG, et al: The cardiovascular effects of dopamine in the severely asphyxiated neonate. *J Pediatr* 1981; 99:772–776.
11. Driscoll EJ, Gillette PC, McNamara DG: The use of dopamine in children. *J Pediatr* 1978; 92:309–314.
12. Fiddler GI, et al: Dopamine infusion for the treatment of myocardial dysfunction associated with persistent transitional circulation. *Arch Dis Child* 1980; 55:194–198.
13. Finley JP, et al: Digoxin excretion in human milk. *J Pediatr* 1979; 94:339–340.

14. Friedman WF, George BL: Treatment of congestive heart failure by altering the loading conditions of the heart. *J Pediatr* 1985; 106:697–706.
15. Gorodischer R: Cardiac drugs, in Yaffe SJ (ed): *Pediatric Pharmacology— Therapeutic Principles in Practice.* New York, Grune & Stratton, 1980, pp 281–301.
16. Harrigan JT, et al: Successful treatment of fetal congestive heart failure secondary to tachycardia. *N Engl J Med* 1981; 304:1527–1529.
17. Hastreiter AR, et al: Digoxin pharmacokinetics in premature infants. *Pediatr Pharmacol* 1982; 2:23–31.
18. Ilbawi MN, Idriss FS, DeLeon SY, et al: Hemodynamic effects of intravenous nitroglycerin in pediatric patients after heart surgery. *Circulation* 1985; 72(suppl II):II-101, II-107.
19. Johnson GL, et al: Complications associated with digoxin therapy in low birth weight infants. *Pediatrics* 1982; 69:463–465.
20. Kim WP, et al: Post-mortem tissue digoxin concentration in infants and children. *Circulation* 1975; 52:1128–1131.
21. Krasula RW, et al: Serum, atrial, and urinary digoxin levels during cardiopulmonary bypass in children. *Circulation* 1974; 49:1047–1052.
22. Manninen V, et al: Altered absorption of digoxin in patients given propantheline and metoclopranide. *Lancet* 1973; 1:398–400.
23. Morselli PL, et al: Digoxin pharmacokinetics during human development, in Morselli PL, Garattini S, Sereni F (eds): *Basic and Therapeutic Aspects of Perinatal Pharmacology.* New York, Raven Press, 1975, pp 377–392.
24. Murphy DJ, et al: Massive digoxin poisoning treated with fab fragments of digoxin–specific antibody. *Pediatrics* 1982; 70:472–473.
25. Okarma TB, Tramell P, Kalman SM: The surface interaction between digoxin and cultured heart cells. *J Pharmacol Exp Ther* 1972; 183:559–576.
26. Perkin RM, et al: Dobutamine: A hemodynamic evaluation in children with shock. *J Pediatr* 1982; 100:977–983.
27. Rogers MC, et al: Serum digoxin concentrations in the human fetus, neonate, and infant. *N Engl J Med* 1972; 287:1010–1013.
28. Talner NS: Heart failure, in Adams FH, Emmanouilides GC, Riemenschneider TA (eds): *Moss' Heart Disease In Infants, Children, and Adolescents,* ed 4. Baltimore, Williams & Wilkins Co, 1989, pp 890–911.
29. Valdes R, et al: Endogenous substance in newborn infants causing false positive digoxin measurements. *J Pediatr* 1983; 102:947–950.
30. Walker PC, Perry BL, Shankaran S: Safety of amrinone for treating congestive heart failure in a premature neonate. *Clin Pharm* 1987; 6:327–331.
31. Zucker AR, et al: Fab fragments of digoxin–specific antibodies used to reverse ventricular fibrillation induced by digoxin ingestion in a child. *Pediatrics* 1982; 70:468–471.

13

Arrhythmias

Ronald Grifka, M.D.
Arthur Garson, Jr., M.D.

Arrhythmias in the fetus and neonate are being discussed more frequently, as a result of the increased number of fetal ultrasound examinations and the increased use of monitoring in the newborn nursery. Statistically, the heart rates of patients with arrhythmias in this age group are much faster than those of older children and adults, and entirely different criteria are necessary for their recognition. In addition, the QRS duration in newborns is normally so narrow that "wide" QRS tachycardia in a newborn would be "narrow" by adult standards.

Arrhythmias are relatively common in healthy newborn infants. We begin with a discussion of the range of normal heart rates, progress through the various arrhythmias in terms of their identification and need for treatment, and finish with the properties of antiarrhythmic drugs used in newborn infants. Criteria for arrhythmias are given here; a more detailed description of arrhythmias in the infant can be found elsewhere.[3, 4]

HEART RATE: RANGE OF NORMAL

When analyzing arrhythmias in the fetus and newborn, an understanding of the variations in normal heart rate is required. The normal fetal heart rate during the late second and third trimesters is 120 to 160 beats/min. A heart rate between 160 and 200 beats/min is usually associated with fever, infection, fetal distress, or maternal drug ingestion. In general, fetal tachycardia is diagnosed when the heart rate is more than 200 beats/min.

To ascertain heart rate in the newborn, Southall et al.[11] studied neonates with 24-hour electrocardiograms. They found that over the 24 hours the lowest heart rate taken over six beats averaged 87 beats/min with a standard deviation of 12. The lower limit of normal therefore was 63 beats/min. At this low heart rate, 80% of the infants had sinus rhythm; 20% of these healthy infants had junctional rhythm with a transient rate in the range of 60 to 70 beats/min. The highest heart rate in 24 hours averaged 179 beats/min with a standard deviation of 19. Therefore the upper limit of normal in a newborn is 217 beats/min.

The incidence of fetal and neonatal arrhythmias on a routine ECG has also been studied by the same group.[11] With respect to the fetus, they found that in 3,383 routine ultrasound examinations during the third trimester, three patients had fetal tachycardia (0.09%). With respect to the neonate, 31 patients (0.9%) had an arrhythmia on routine ECG taken within the first 4 days of life. This incidence is approximately the same as that found in structural congenital heart disease, which is 0.8%. The most common neonatal arrhythmia in this study was premature atrial contractions, followed by premature ventricular contractions, supraventricular tachycardia, and atrial flutter. In this series no patient had complete atrioventricular (AV) block or ventricular tachycardia. Wolff-Parkinson-White syndrome was diagnosed in two of these asymptomatic normal newborns (0.06%).

COMPLETE ATRIOVENTRICULAR BLOCK

Criteria

The criteria for complete AV block are (1) no evidence of AV conduction and (2) complete AV dissociation. By no evidence of AV conduction, we mean that P waves, which should conduct to the ventricles, do not conduct. There is a certain normal period after AV conduction when the AV conduction system recovers; this is known as the "refractory period" of the AV conduction system. In healthy infants and children, this period is approximately 0.3 to 0.4 seconds ($1^{1}/_{2}$ to two "big boxes" on the surface ECG). After a QRS complex, if a P wave falls within the next 0.3 to 0.4 seconds, it would normally not conduct to the ventricles. If a P wave occurs 0.3 to 0.4 seconds after the preceding QRS complex, it should conduct to the ventricles, making another QRS complex. On the surface ECG the T wave extends for approximately 0.3 or 0.4 seconds after the QRS complex. Although the T wave has nothing to do with the refractory period of the AV conduction system, it does provide a convenient marker for the period extending 0.3 to 0.4 seconds after the QRS complex. Therefore, if a P wave falls on a T wave, in general we would not expect this P wave to conduct. If a P wave falls beyond the end of a T wave, it should conduct to the ventricles.

Clinical Situations

In the patient with congenital complete AV block, several associated conditions must be evaluated. The first is structural congenital heart disease. Michaelsson and Engle[8] directed a large, cooperative international study on patients with congenital complete AV block and found a 30% incidence of associated structural heart disease. Pinsky and associates[10] in Houston found a 40% incidence of congenital heart disease of which 79% had ventricular inversion with L-transposition of the great arteries.

Collagen disease in the mothers of children with congenital complete AV block was first reported by McCue et al.[7] In their study 64% of babies with congenital complete AV block had mothers with collagen disease, and 36% of these mothers were asymptomatic. With newer tests (anti–SS-A and anti–SS-B) as many as 90% of such infants with otherwise normal hearts appear to have mothers with collagen disease. Therefore, the mother of a child with congenital complete AV block should be thoroughly evaluated for collagen disease.

Course and Management

The course of the patient with congenital complete AV block as determined by the Michaelsson and Engle[8] study depends largely on the presence or absence of congenital heart disease and on ventricular rate. In their study only 34% of the patients were diagnosed by 1 week of age. They defined congenital complete AV block as block that occurred at an early age and without history of an infection that might cause acquired complete AV block. With 5 to 10 years follow-up, they found a much higher mortality (29%) in the patients with congenital heart disease than in those without (8%). The majority of these deaths occurred by the age of 5 years.

The heart rate during complete AV block also had prognostic significance. For those patients with a ventricular rate greater than 55 beats/min and an atrial rate less than 140 beats/min there was 4% mortality; patients with a ventricular rate less than or equal to 55 beats/min and an atrial rate greater than or equal to 140 beats/min had 29% mortality. We have not found the atrial rate to be as prognostic as the ventricular rate. Our data on ventricular rate are similar to those of Michaelsson and Engle.[8] We found a high association of symptoms with a ventricular rate less than 50 beats/min.

In infants with congenital complete AV block, an absolute indication for a pacemaker is a ventricular rate less than 50 beats/min taken over five beats. A heart rate of 50 beats/min is used whether the patient is awake or asleep; in these infants the ventricular rate has little variation. A pacemaker is placed if the infant has clinical evidence of congestive heart failure, especially if there is coexistent congenital heart disease. Any patient with congenital complete AV block who has a wide QRS complex should have a pacemaker because the site of the escape pacemaker is likely to be below the bundle of His, and such pacemakers may slow or stop unexpectedly. Finally, congenital complete AV block with a long QT_c requires pacemaker placement because of the higher incidence of sudden death. A ventricular (single chamber) pacing system with an epicardial lead is used.

In the past 8 years we have inserted 16 pacemakers in infants younger than 1 month of age because of complete AV block. One infant developed a pacemaker "pocket" infection, necessitating removal. The pacemaker was relocated to another site and the infant has done well. Four patients, all of whom had complex congenital heart disease in addition to complete AV block, died of causes other than AV block.

Complete congenital AV block may be diagnosed prenatally. Most often these fetuses do well. Rarely a fetus may be severely hydropic due to fetal bradycardia, resulting in inadequate cardiac output. Administering isoproterenol or terbutaline to the mother rarely increases the fetal ventricular rate. Hydropic infants may develop pleural, pericardial, and peritoneal effusions.

Using ultrasound guidance, we placed a transuterine transthoracic fetal pacing catheter into the right ventricle in a 24-week-gestation fetus with severe hydrops secondary to complete AV block.[1] An external pulse generator was used for pacing. For several hours the fetal myocardium responded well, but ventricular capture was abruptly lost, asystole occurred, and death ensued.

PREMATURE ATRIAL CONTRACTIONS

Criteria

The primary criterion for a premature atrial contraction is a premature P wave. A premature atrial contraction either conducts normally, affording a premature P wave followed by a premature normal QRS complex, or it conducts aberrantly. This aberrancy may simulate a premature ventricular contraction, especially if the preceding P wave is not noticed. Finally, the atrial contraction may not conduct at all, which simulates sinus bradycardia if the premature P wave is not noted.

Clinical Findings

Premature atrial contractions most often occur in infants whose hearts are otherwise normal. Occasionally an infant with premature atrial contractions may have atrial enlargement as a result of congenital heart disease or cardiomyopathy or may have mechanical stimulation of the atrium because of a central venous catheter. Administration of sympathomimetic amines such as isoproterenol or dopamine may produce premature atrial contractions or premature ventricular contractions.

Course and Management

Prognosis for the infant with premature atrial contractions is generally excellent. Southall et al.[11] found in their large group of newborns that 15 of the 3,300 patients had premature atrial contractions on routine ECG. Of the 15, seven had a 24-hour ECG, and on this more extended tracing two of the seven had episodes of supraventricular tachycardia. Therefore, premature atrial contractions in newborns may be associated with short asymptomatic periods of supraventricular tachycardia. In follow-up of the 15 patients, 13 (87%) had the premature atrial contractions resolve within 3 months, and there were no episodes of symptomatic tachyarrhythmias.

In the infant with premature atrial contractions, it is reasonable to obtain a chest x-ray study and possibly an echocardiogram to rule out coexistent congenital heart disease or cardiomyopathy. We recommend observing these infants for 2 to 3 days. If there are no episodes of tachyarrhythmia, we do not treat the premature atrial contractions, but may reevaluate the child in 1 month. If at any time supraventricular tachycardia or atrial flutter is found, these arrhythmias are treated.

INTRAUTERINE SUPRAVENTRICULAR TACHYCARDIA

Diagnosis

If the fetal heart rate is 200 beats/min or greater without any variation in the rate, the diagnosis of intrauterine tachycardia should be made. In most types of supraventricular tachycardia, the atrial rate (the A wave on the AV valve tracing in the echocardiogram) is the same as the ventricular rate (ventricular contraction). Intrauterine atrial flutter is likely if the atrial rate is greater than the ventricular rate and the atrial rate is more than 200 beats/min. Both supraventricular tachycardia and atrial flutter may occasionally exist in the same patient.

We have seen two children with elevated fetal heart rate in whom the diagnosis of ventricular tachycardia was made postnatally. In one infant the ventricular rate was quite rapid and the atrial rate was slow with AV dissociation; ventricular tachycardia was suspected. In the other infant, both the ventricular and atrial rates were the same, and the patient was thought to have supraventricular tachycardia.

Course

More cases of intrauterine supraventricular tachycardia are being reported. This is most likely the result of advances in prenatal diagnosis, not increased incidence. Intrauterine supraventricular tachycardia may be intermittent or incessant and is usually diagnosed between week 28 of gestation and term, although earlier diagnosis has been reported. Some infants tolerate the tachycardia well; others have severe nonimmune fetal hydrops.

Kleinman and colleagues[6] reported 16 infants with intrauterine supraventricular tachycardia, 15 of whom had hydrops. Fifteen were successfully converted to sinus rhythm with administration of digoxin to the mother— alone or in combination with either propranolol or verapamil. The infants continued to receive the antiarrhythmic medication postnatally, and no arrhythmias were reported with follow-up from 2 weeks to 53 months.

Postnatally, we have noted a significant percentage of patients with intra-uterine supraventricular tachycardia to have evidence of Wolff-Parkinson-White syndrome on the surface ECG. Wolff-Parkinson-White syndrome was not apparent at birth in several of these patients, but appeared within 1 to 2 weeks. Therefore, these children should be observed closely for at least 1 month after birth for the presence of Wolff-Parkinson-White syndrome. The majority of patients with intrauterine supraventricular tachycardia had an otherwise normal heart; 11% had structural heart disease in one study.

Management

The diagnosis of sustained intrauterine supraventricular tachycardia should be considered a medical emergency, especially in the presence of hydrops. The mother should be admitted and close monitoring of the mother and fetus initiated. We would begin therapy with oral digoxin. Digoxin concentration in fetal cord blood may vary from half the maternal serum level to an equivalent level. Since newborns have a higher required serum digoxin concentration than older patients, an effective maternal digoxin serum concentration may be ineffective in the fetus; therefore, the maximum tolerable maternal digoxin dosage should be given. Several mothers have tolerated 0.75 mg/day without clinical evidence of digoxin toxicity; maternal serum digoxin levels up to 2.2 ng/mL. Digoxin may be given with caution intravenously, but the oral route is preferred.

If digoxin alone does not control supraventricular tachycardia, we would add verapamil. If digoxin and verapamil are unsuccessful, we would consider the combination of digoxin plus propranolol. Verapamil and propranolol should never be used together.

Although propranolol is readily metabolized in the liver ("first-pass effect") a wide dosage range is tolerated, and adequate fetal serum levels are obtained. Maternal dosage up to 500 mg/day orally has been well tolerated. A good therapeutic end point is to observe some evidence of beta blockade such as a slight decrease in the maternal heart rate. A child born to a mother taking propranolol may have hypoglycemia and bradycardia; these factors should be monitored postnatally.

Verapamil is being used more frequently, alone or more commonly with digoxin, in the treatment of intrauterine supraventricular tachycardia. Verapamil crosses the placenta poorly; fetal cord blood serum concentrations are one-sixth the maternal serum concentration. Oral verapamil therapy often is successful. In one case, verapamil administered intravenously to the mother was followed by fetal asystole and death. In neonates, intravenous verapamil may severely reduce contractility. Thus verapamil should be given with caution to the fetus. Maternal doses up to 160 mg orally every 6 hours have been well tolerated.

Recently, flecainide (100 to 150 mg orally every 12 hours to the mother) has been used with a high success rate and no observed ill effects. Further trials will be necessary.

The postnatal management of intrauterine supraventricular tachycardia is basically the same as for supraventricular tachycardia (discussed in the following section). It is important to expect recurrence of tachycardia in these patients. Several hydropic infants died postnatally from what appeared to be digoxin toxicity. If a hydropic infant receives digoxin at a dose appropriate for its edematous weight but the weight is rapidly reduced by diuresis, the digoxin serum concentration can become quite elevated and result in AV block or ventricular fibrillation.

NEONATAL SUPRAVENTRICULAR TACHYCARDIA

Criteria

Supraventricular tachycardia is defined as tachycardia resulting from an abnormal mechanism that requires structures in the heart proximal to the bundle of His for its perpetuation and does not have the morphology of atrial flutter on the surface ECG. In the infant younger than 1 month with supraventricular tachycardia, the QRS complex is regular and narrow. In the infant with "wide" QRS tachycardia (greater than 0.06 seconds), the diagnosis is usually ventricular tachycardia. It is extremely important to differentiate between these two arrhythmias, because if a patient with ventricular tachycardia is given digoxin, the resultant rhythm may be ventricular fibrillation. In our patients with supraventricular tachycardia appearing at less than 1 month of age, the rate of tachycardia varied from 210 to 310 beats/min, with a mean of 275 beats/min. During the tachycardia, the presence of P waves and the P wave axis is also important to determine; P waves were visible in 59% of our patients during supraventricular tachycardia, and only 15% had a normal P wave axis (normal P wave axis defined as upright P waves in leads I and aVF).

Differential Diagnosis

The major differential diagnosis of supraventricular tachycardia in an infant is sinus tachycardia. Similar to supraventricular tachycardia, sinus tachycardia has a regular, narrow QRS complex. In sinus tachycardia, however, the rate is almost always less than 230 beats/min. We have seen only three infants with sinus tachycardia at rates greater than 230 beats/min (245 to 265 beats/min); all three were extremely ill with sepsis. In contrast, the infant with supraventricular tachycardia usually has no symptoms.

Therefore, if the rate is less than 230 beats/min and there are positive P waves in leads I and aVF, sinus tachycardia is more likely. If the rate is over 230 beats/min and the P waves are either not visible or not positive in I and aVF, supraventricular tachycardia is likely.

Management

The management of supraventricular tachycardia is somewhat controversial because several treatment methods may be effective. In most centers each treatment might be used; the major difference is the order in which they are chosen. Our perspective is that, in an infant with supraventricular tachycardia, it is important to stop the tachycardia. Because it is quite difficult to assess the degree of compensatory mechanisms used by an infant, the infant may be much more hemodynamically compromised than can be assessed by clinical examination.

Our recommendation for the acute management of supraventricular tachycardia is to apply a washcloth filled with ice to the infant's face to elicit the "diving reflex." This reflex involves not only vagal stimulation but also sympathetic withdrawal. The washcloth should be left in place for 10 to 20 seconds if necessary. The infant should have ECG monitoring and intravenous catheter in place throughout the time of application of the washcloth, because asystole or ventricular fibrillation can occur after this procedure. Other vagal maneuvers, such as carotid sinus massage, modified Valsalva maneuver (elicited by "gagging" the child with a nasogastric tube or abdominal compression), or ocular compression, are rarely successful in newborns. The latter method may dislodge the infant's lens, and is not recommended.

If the diving reflex procedure is unsuccessful, the next method of choice is overdrive pacing through the esophagus. The esophagus lies just posterior to the atrium, providing a convenient location for pacing. The problem with esophageal overdrive pacing is that it requires a special stimulator unit with a 10-msec pulse duration. If such a stimulator is available, a 4 F pacing catheter is easily placed through the infant's nose into the esophagus to overdrive pace the atrium. The pacing rate is set slightly faster than the tachycardia rate. Pacing lasts for approximately 5 seconds, then is abruptly stopped, with the resultant rhythm usually sinus. If the infant appears well compensated, digoxin may be used at this point (discussed later). Intravenous edrophonium or phenylephrine has been used in the past, but more modern methods have generally supplanted these measures.

If none of these methods is successful, our next treatment is DC electrical cardioversion. We have found no morbidity from cardioversion if administered correctly. Cardioversion of supraventricular tachycardia should be synchronized to the QRS complex and should be delivered in a proper dose of 0.25 to 1.0 Wt-sec/kg (1 watt-second = 1 Joule). Infants receiving digoxin who require DC cardioversion should be given lidocaine, 1 mg/kg intravenously, prior to cardioversion.

In the vast majority of cases the previously discussed methods are effective in stopping supraventricular tachycardia, but it may recur several seconds, minutes, or hours later. If the infant is hemodynamically stable, oral or intravenous medical therapy should be initiated. The treatment of choice for infants and children with supraventricular tachycardia has been digoxin; it is the most commonly used drug. Intravenous propranolol may cause acutely decreased cardiac output and severe bradycardia, and should be used only if ventricular pacing is immediately available.

There has been much discussion concerning the use of intravenous verapamil for supraventricular tachycardia in infants and children. While certain centers use intravenous verapamil in infants, we do not. We have had personal experience with several infants in whom the cardiac output was severely reduced after administration of verapamil, and we would prefer to avoid its use. One particularly dangerous side effect in infants is apnea. If the infant is given verapamil there should be standby calcium chloride and isoproterenol available to counteract the hemodynamic effects of verapamil. One of the most important points to remember from this discussion is that verapamil should never be used if an infant has received propranolol, and vice versa.

Intravenous procainamide has been used successfully for short-term treatment of supraventricular tachycardia. However, the oral preparation has a half-life of only $1\frac{1}{2}$ hours; five to six doses per day must be given.

In Europe, the treatment of choice for acute termination of supraventricular tachycardia is adenosine. This may soon be available in the United States.

Management of the infant with chronic supraventricular tachycardia depends on whether the child has Wolff-Parkinson-White syndrome. If Wolff-Parkinson-White syndrome is not present, we begin oral therapy with digoxin; if this is not effective, we add oral propranolol. Patients given propranolol should be observed for signs of congestive heart failure, bradycardia, or decreased shortening fraction. Flecainide may be effective in treating infants with supraventricular tachycardia. There has been concern about proarrhythmia with this drug, and further studies will be necessary to define its exact place in treatment.

In patients with Wolff-Parkinson-White syndrome, propranolol is the drug of choice, followed by flecainide. Some centers still use digoxin for supraventricular tachycardia in neonates with Wolff-Parkinson-White syndrome, but we prefer to avoid this practice, because in rare cases digoxin has been associated with sudden death in infants with this syndrome.[2]

ATRIAL FLUTTER

Criteria

The diagnosis of atrial flutter depends on the presence of flutter waves on the ECG. Classically, these waves are regular sawtooth undulations in the baseline that are larger than P waves. Atrial flutter in infants may occur at heart rates between 350 and 600 beats/min. The ventricular rate is most often irregular because of changes in AV conduction. Occasionally the ventricular rate is regular, with 2:1 AV conduction. In infancy, the AV node may conduct atrial flutter 1:1, resulting in an extremely rapid ventricular rate.

Clinical Findings

Atrial flutter usually occurs in a patient with an otherwise normal heart.

It seems to be slightly more common in patients who have had intrauterine supraventricular tachycardia. Occasionally atrial flutter is found in patients with atrial enlargement due to congenital heart disease, especially endocardial fibroelastosis or cardiomyopathy. It may also be found in patients with an atrial tumor or aneurysm of the atrial septum.

Course and Management

The course of atrial flutter is quite variable. Moller and associates[9] reported 24 cases of atrial flutter in infants younger than 1 week of age. In 22 of the 24, digoxin was used for initial treatment, and 11 converted to sinus rhythm. In the other 11, atrial flutter continued. Of the 11 with chronic atrial flutter five died, and the others continued to have atrial flutter for a median duration of 6 months. Digoxin was not effective in either of the two patients with associated atrial fibrillation. The mortality with atrial flutter was increased if there was associated congenital heart disease. If there was neither atrial fibrillation nor congenital heart disease, the mortality was still 11%. This indicates that continuing atrial flutter in an infant is associated with a high mortality and that flutter should be controlled.

We recommend DC cardioversion with 0.5 to 1.0 Wt-sec/kg when atrial flutter is recognized. Esophageal overdrive pacing may be used, but it is more difficult to overdrive pace atrial flutter than supraventricular tachycardia. Once the atrial flutter has stopped, we use digoxin unless the patient has Wolff-Parkinson-White syndrome. If digoxin alone is ineffective, we add propranolol. If this combination is unsuccessful we try either amiodarone or flecainide. Amiodarone or flecainide may become the treatment of choice for atrial flutter in the future. As flutter in the infant usually continues for approximately only 6 months, we generally stop therapy 6 months after the patient's last episode of atrial flutter, but continue to observe the child closely.

PREMATURE VENTRICULAR CONTRACTIONS

Criteria

The criterion for a premature ventricular contraction is a premature QRS complex not preceded by a premature P wave. It is important to examine the preceding T wave closely to rule out the presence of a premature P wave, which indicates a premature atrial contraction. In a premature ventricular contraction, the QRS configuration is different from the sinus QRS, although the QRS of a premature ventricular contraction is not necessarily "absolutely wide" (i.e., it may be 0.04 to 0.06 seconds wide). The final criterion of a premature ventricular contraction is a *fusion complex,* defined as having the morphology of both a sinus beat and a premature ventricular contraction; it is an intermediate morphology.

Clinical Findings

Premature ventricular contractions are usually found in a newborn with an otherwise normal heart; however, they may also be found in abnormal hearts. In any patient with premature ventricular contractions, it is important to measure the QT interval of normal QRS complexes. Prolonged QT intervals may be found in an idiopathic familial form, but may also result from hypocalcemia or asphyxia. Premature ventricular contractions may be associated with acidosis, hypoxia, hypoglycemia, or in heart abnormalities such as myocarditis, severe ventricular hypertrophy, or ventricular tumor. Premature ventricular contractions may also be caused by the mechanical stimulation of a catheter against the ventricular wall, especially a Swan-Ganz catheter in the pulmonary artery with a loop of the catheter touching the ventricle. Finally, premature ventricular contractions may be associated with drug intoxication (digoxin), sympathomimetic amines (isoproterenol, dopamine, dobutamine), or anesthetics (halothane).

Course

The prognosis for the infant with premature ventricular contractions depends significantly on whether the heart is normal. Southall et al.,[11] in their large study of 3,300 newborns with normal-appearing hearts, found that 11 (0.33%) had premature ventricular contractions on routine ECG. Of these 11, seven underwent 24-hour ECG in the newborn period, and three of the seven had short episodes of ventricular tachycardia. None of these infants was treated, and in 10 of the 11 with premature ventricular contractions, the arrhythmia completely disappeared by the age of 3 months.

Management

Our suggested management of the infant with premature ventricular contractions is to obtain a chest x-ray film and an echocardiogram to establish that the patient's heart is normal. Occasionally, one may unsuspectedly discover a cardiomyopathy, arrhythmogenic right ventricle, or ventricular tumor. We do not treat patients with a normal heart and uniform premature ventricular contractions. We do treat any patient with multiform premature ventricular contractions or couplets, whether the heart is normal or abnormal.

If the patient has long QT syndrome a beta blocker is the drug of choice, with propranolol most commonly used. In patients with a long QT interval, we avoid quinidine, disopyramide, procainamide, and amiodarone, as these drugs further prolong the QT interval.

The treatment for multiform premature ventricular contractions or couplets begins with propranolol or flecainide. Quinidine seems to produce a particularly high incidence of gastrointestinal side effects in infants and children, and also may occasionally worsen ventricular tachycardia.

VENTRICULAR TACHYCARDIA

Criteria

Ventricular tachycardia is defined as three or more consecutive excitations that originate from the ventricle at a rate of more than 120 beats/min. The most rapid ventricular tachycardia we have documented in a newborn was 500 beats/min. The ECG reveals a QRS complex different from sinus rhythm but not absolutely wide (up to 0.11 seconds in duration). In the diagnosis of ventricular tachycardia, AV dissociation is extremely helpful; the P waves and the QRS complexes are not related. This may not always be seen in patients with ventricular tachycardia. The presence of fusion beats is diagnostic of ventricular tachycardia for the same reason that the presence of a fusion beat proves the presence of a premature ventricular contraction. A sinus capture beat is defined as the presence of a normal QRS complex preceded by a P wave during the tachycardia; this QRS complex is narrow and also has a different morphology than the tachycardia, establishing that the tachycardia is of ventricular origin.

The differential diagnosis of wide QRS tachycardia is either supraventricular tachycardia with aberration, which is very rare in children, or ventricular tachycardia. Accelerated ventricular rhythm should also be mentioned, because it resembles ventricular tachycardia except that the rate is usually less than 120 to 150 beats/min; it is a benign rhythm, often not requiring treatment.

Clinical Findings

The clinical situations in which ventricular tachycardia is found in infants are similar to those in which premature ventricular contractions are found, except that ventricular tachycardia usually does not occur in patients with normal hearts.

Course

The prognosis for the patient with ventricular tachycardia depends on whether the patient has a normal heart. In Southall's study,[11] no infant had ventricular tachycardia noted frequently enough to be present on a routine ECG. Three (0.09%) had ventricular tachycardia on 24-hour ECG, and in all three patients the tachycardia had resolved by the age of 3 months.

In our patients at Texas Children's Hospital, the ventricular tachycardia was frequent enough to be seen on a routine ECG. It resolved in the patient with a transiently prolonged QT interval associated with myocarditis, and the patient was well by 3 months of age. The patient with the congenitally prolonged QT interval is now well with propranolol 2 years later; the QT interval continues at the upper limits of normal. The patient with the ventricular tumor had continued episodes of ventricular tachycardia with no response to conventional or investigational drugs. The tumor had not been visible by echocardiography or angiography. Electrophysiologic study localized the area of tachycardia, and the patient was taken to the operating room, where a small epicardial ventricular tumor was found. The tumor was resected, and 3 years later the patient is well without ventricular arrhythmia.

Therefore, the presence of ventricular tachycardia should make one presume that the patient's heart is abnormal until proved otherwise, and a thorough cardiac evaluation, including a 24-hour ECG (for prolonged QT interval) and echocardiogram (for anatomic abnormalities), should be obtained. Hemodynamic and electrophysiologic cardiac catheterization with endomyocardial biopsy should be reserved for infants with refractory ventricular tachycardia.

Management

The management of ventricular tachycardia begins with stopping the tachycardia. As with premature ventricular contractions, ventricular tachycardia may result from electrolyte and blood gas abnormalities, from drugs, or from ventricular catheters. If the patient is in sustained tachycardia and the hemodynamic status is unacceptable, intravenous lidocaine may be given. If lidocaine is not effective, then synchronized DC cardioversion should be performed. Overdrive ventricular pacing may also be used to terminate the tachycardia. After the initial conversion to sinus rhythm, lidocaine or procainamide infusion should be started. If the patient has a prolonged QT interval, procainamide should not be used. These methods should be continued until long-term oral medication can be started, similar to that for premature ventricular contractions.

Digoxin should be avoided in patients with ventricular tachycardia; we have had three patients younger than 6 months develop ventricular fibrillation during digitalization for what was thought to be supraventricular tachycardia but which turned out to be ventricular tachycardia.

If there is recurrent life-threatening ventricular tachycardia, electrophysiologic catheterization may be able to define an arrhythmogenic focus, which can be surgically resected, eliminating the tachycardia.

NEONATAL ANTIARRHYTHMIC MEDICATIONS

Atropine is the prototypical muscarinic cholinergic antagonist. The effect of atropine on the heart is to inhibit vagal tone, resulting in an increased heart rate. However, neonates may not have much vagal tone, and the resultant chronotropic response may be less than expected. Atropine is given intravenously at a dose of 0.02 mg/kg (0.01 to 0.04 mg/kg; minimum dose of 0.1 mg). The dose may be repeated at 10-minute intervals for three total doses.

Isoproterenol, a nonselective beta$_1$ and beta$_2$ agonist, has positive inotropic and chronotropic properties in addition to decreasing systemic vascular resistance. Cardiac output and myocardial oxygen consumption are increased; diastolic blood pressure may be decreased. An intravenous infusion is started at 0.05 μg/kg/min and may be increased to 0.5 μg/kg/min.

Digoxin can be given orally or intravenously; the oral route is preferred if the patient's condition allows. Neonates require a lower dose than older children. The total oral digitalizing dose for full-term newborns is 30 μg/kg, and the intravenous dose is 80% of that amount. One half of the total digitalizing dose is given initially, that is, 15 μg/kg (0.015 mg/kg) orally or 12 μg/kg (0.012 mg/kg) intravenously (over 1 hour). The remaining half is given in two equal doses 7 μg/kg (0.007 mg/kg) orally or 6 μg/kg (0.006 mg/kg) intravenously; these two doses may be given as close as 2 hours apart, but 6 hours is much preferred if the patient's condition allows. The oral maintenance dose of digoxin is 4 μg/kg (0.004 mg/kg) every 12 hours (8 μg/kg/day). The specific amount in milligrams (or micrograms) along with the mg/kg (μg/kg) and volume in cubic centimeters should be specified. These recommended doses may seem excessively detailed, but digoxin overdosage can be fatal (this is true for most antiarrhythmic medication). Digoxin is cleared by the kidney; patients with renal impairment will require a reduced dose. Digoxin levels are not useful in neonates because serum proteins interfere with the laboratory assay. Digoxin toxicity may be treated with digoxin-specific antibody (Fab fragments), and with phenytoin or lidocaine if any arrhythmias occur.

Propranolol is a nonspecific competitive beta antagonist. Propranolol may be given intravenously at a dose of 0.025 mg/kg every 10 minutes for a total of four doses; immediate ventricular pacing may be required, and provisions for this should be enacted before administering the drug. Propranolol may be given orally at a dose ranging from 0.5 to 1.5 mg/kg/dose every 6 hours. A dosing interval of every 8 hours is inadequate. Propranolol is completely metabolized in the liver prior to its elimination, and a significant "first-pass" metabolism occurs. Atenolol and several other beta blockers with a longer half-life may soon be used in newborns.

Verapamil is the only calcium channel blocking agent we use in the treatment of arrhythmias. Intravenous verapamil should be used with extreme caution in neonates because it may cause severe bradycardia, hypotension, and apnea. The oral dose of verapamil is 2 to 4 mg/kg every 8 hours. Verapamil is also metabolized in the liver, with extensive first-pass metabolism.

Quinidine, the stereoisomer of quinine, may be administered orally in a dose of 4 to 12 mg/kg every 6 hours. Intravenous quinidine is contraindicated because it causes marked hypotension. Up to half of older children and adults experience severe nausea, vomiting, and diarrhea, and quinidine must be discontinued. Quinidine decreases digoxin clearance, and toxicity will result; the digoxin dose is decreased by half when starting quinidine.

Lidocaine is used only intravenously. A 1 mg/kg bolus is given, which may be repeated twice at 10-minute intervals. If it is effective, a lidocaine infusion at 20 to 50 μg/kg/min is started. A therapeutic lidocaine level is 2 to 5 μg/mL. Seizures are a common side effect of toxicity. An oral equivalent of lidocaine, tocainide, has been poorly tolerated in older children and is not used in neonates.

Mexiletine is similar in structure and function to lidocaine. Although most antiarrhythmic agents are also negative inotropes, mexiletine has no negative inotropic activity; therefore, it is well tolerated in patients with decreased cardiac output. Mexiletine is an excellent drug for ventricular tachycardia responsive or resistant to lidocaine. Mexiletine is available only for oral administration, at a dose of 2.2 to 5.5 mg/kg every 8 hours. The liver metabolizes 80% of the drug; the remainder is excreted in the urine.

Procainamide is also administered intravenously with a 7 mg/kg bolus over 30 minutes, followed by an infusion of 10 to 50 μg/kg/min. Up to two thirds is excreted unchanged in the urine. The remaining third is metabolized in the liver, and N-acetylprocainamide (NAPA), the predominant metabolite, also possesses some antiarrhythmic properties. A therapeutic procainamide level is 4 to 8 μg/mL. Procainamide can produce agranulocytosis, lupuslike syndrome, positive antinuclear antibody, and arthralgia. These side effects are reversible if the drug is discontinued. Oral procainamide is not used in newborns.

Amiodarone is an antiarrhythmic agent with complex electrophysiologic properties. Amiodarone is a large, very lipid, soluble molecule with avid protein and tissue binding, resulting in a half-life of several weeks. Its use to date has been only for life-threatening arrhythmias. Amiodarone has been effective in treating atrial flutter and fibrillation and has also shown promise in the treatment of ventricular tachycardia. Amiodarone is given orally, with a loading period of 10 days at 10 mg/kg/day divided into two equal doses, then a maintenance dose of 7.5 mg/kg/day once a day. The excellent results of amiodarone are tempered by occasional side effects, including thyroid dysfunction, skin photosensitivity, interstitial pneumonitis, hepatic dysfunction, and corneal microdeposits. These side effects need to be observed closely, but resolve after discontinuance of the drug.

Flecainide is another new antiarrhythmic agent with excellent results in the treatment of supraventricular tachycardia (both with and without Wolff-Parkinson-White syndrome), premature ventricular contractions, and ventricular tachycardia. Flecainide has mild negative inotropic activity. The oral dose of flecainide is 100 to 200 mg/m²/day divided into two equal doses. Flecainide levels of 200 to 800 ng/mL are therapeutic. Toxicity in older children is manifested by blurred vision, in younger children by irritability. If given with amiodarone, flecainide levels may be increased 20%.

Bretylium tosylate is an excellent drug for management of recurrent ventricular fibrillation. It is less effective for ventricular tachycardia. It is used only for short-term therapy, in a dose of 5 mg/kg intravenously. This dose may be repeated several times at 15- to 30-minute intervals. A continuous infusion may be considered. Bretylium is not metabolized, but eliminated entirely by the kidney.

Finally, cardioversion is used at 0.25 to 2.0 Wt-sec/kg. Energy doses of 5 to 6 Wt-sec/kg can result in severe myocardial burns, congestive cardiomyopathy secondary to reduced contractility, and eventual death. One must use a defibrillator with settings low enough to deliver these pediatric doses, along with the appropriate-sized paddle surface area for the neonate.

CONCLUSION

Arrhythmias in newborn infants are extremely challenging, largely because they may be difficult to diagnose. Once the diagnosis is made, treatment can proceed in an orderly fashion. There are numerous approaches to treatment and to the order in which treatment may be given. Drug therapy must be based on the principles of the reduced hepatic and renal function and the increased ratio of body surface area to body weight of the newborn. The vast majority of arrhythmias that appear in the newborn period have a good prognosis. If the arrhythmia can be controlled in the first month of life, the eventual outlook for these infants is extremely good.

REFERENCES

1. Carpenter RJ, et al: Fetal ventricular pacing for hydrops secondary to complete atrioventricular block. *J Am Coll Cardiol* 1986; 8:1434–1436.
2. Deal BJ, et al: Wolff-Parkinson-White and atrial tachycardia in infancy: Long-term follow-up. *Pediatr Cardiol* 1983; 17:111A.
3. Garson A: *The Electrocardiogram in Infants and Children: A Systemic Approach.* Philadelphia, Lea & Febiger, 1983, pp 195–375.
4. Garson A, Bricker JT, McNamara DG: *The Science and Practice of Pediatric Cardiology.* Philadelphia, Lea & Febiger, 1989.
5. Gillette PC, Rose AP: Sinus arrhythmia, wandering pacemaker, and premature atrial contractions, in Gillette PC, Garson A (eds): *Pediatric Cardiac Dysrhythmias.* New York, Grune & Stratton, 1981, pp 145–151.
6. Kleinman CS, et al: In utero diagnosis and treatment of fetal supraventricular tachycardia. *Semin Perinatol* 1985; 9:113–129.
7. McCue CM, et al: Congenital heart block in newborns of mothers with connective tissue disease. *Circulation* 1977; 56:82–89.
8. Michaelsson A, Engle MA: Congenital complete heart block: An international study of the natural history, in Brest AN, Engle MA (eds): *Cardiovascular Clinics.* Philadelphia, FA Davis Co, 1972, p 85.
9. Moller JH, Davachi F, Anderson RC: Atrial flutter in infancy. *J Pediatr* 1969; 75:643–651.
10. Pinsky WW, et al: Diagnosis, management, and long-term results of patients with congenital complete atrioventricular block. *Pediatrics* 1982; 69:728–733.
11. Southall DP, et al: Study of cardiac rhythm in healthy newborn infants. *Br Heart J* 1979; 43:14–20.

14

Antibacterial Therapy

Norman M. Jacobs, M.D.

Antibacterial agents (ABAs) are among the most effective therapeutic agents we have, but they alone do not cure disease. These agents only inhibit or kill susceptible bacteria, and then only when enough of the ABA reaches the site of infection. The decision regarding which ABA to use ultimately depends on which bacterial pathogen is thought to be causing the disease and on the site of the infection.

Occasionally the disease and the bacterial pathogen are known before treatment is initiated, but frequently one is presented only with a neonate who has signs suggestive of an infection. The disease and the bacterial pathogen therefore must then be presumed. This is much easier when the signs exhibited by the neonate suggest a specific disease (e.g., necrotizing enterocolitis or osteomyelitis) or when a local exudate can be examined for bacteria. Lacking such information one has to rely on data collected from other ill neonates with occult infections, recognizing that prevalent pathogens may differ in different locales and at different times.

It is always wise to culture the blood of a neonate suspected of having a serious bacterial infection before beginning antibacterial therapy. In such infants bacteremia is common, and in those with an occult infection the blood may be the only source that yields the pathogen. The bacterial isolate may prove to be important, because neonates can be infected with unusual bacteria or common bacteria with unusual antibacterial susceptibility profiles.

ANTIBACTERIAL SUSCEPTIBILITY

Susceptibility Testing

For practical purposes bacteria are said to be susceptible to an ABA when they are inhibited by that agent at a concentration that is both nontoxic to the patient and easily attainable in serum. Some bacteria are almost always susceptible to some ABAs; others are variably susceptible to the commonly used ABAs. For these latter, particularly enteric bacilli and staphylococci, an in vitro susceptibility test should be performed.

The standard in vitro method of establishing antibacterial susceptibility is the tube dilution susceptibility test. The test yields an MIC (minimal inhibitory concentration) value in micrograms per milliliter. This is the minimal concentration of the ABA that inhibits an invisible bacterial inoculum in broth from growing to a visible turbidity. The test can also be performed in microtiter plates or with the ABA incorporated into an agar medium. Some laboratories perform other tests (e.g., disk diffusion susceptibility test) in which the end points have been correlated with the standard tube dilution MIC values. Many laboratories will report the MIC values for a list of commonly used ABAs; other laboratories may interpret the MICs and report only "susceptible" or "resistant." These interpretations are usually based on the recommendations of the National Committee for Clinical Laboratory Standards (Table 14–1).

These in vitro tests do not discriminate between bacterial inhibition and bacterial killing. The tests by which the bactericidal activity of ABAs is measured are time-consuming and therefore expensive. Also the methods and interpretation of these tests have not been standardized.

Susceptibility Profiles

The profiles shown in Tables 14–2 through 14–5 can be looked at in either of two ways: comparing the relative susceptibility of a bacterial species to a number of ABAs or comparing the relative inhibiting effect of an ABA against a number of bacterial species. For consistency and fair comparability, the data in these Tables come from only two general sources: Neu and his colleagues at Columbia University (the newer β-lactam ABAs) and Finland and his colleagues at the Boston City Hospital (the other ABAs).

The Tables have two deficiencies if they are used as universal truth rather than general comparability. First, only the median MICs, not the range of MICs, are presented. So the MIC for a substantial number of strains could be much higher or lower; this is true for some of the enteric bacilli. Second, the distribution of susceptible and resistant strains, and therefore the median MIC, can vary from hospital to hospital, and certainly from city to city or country to country.

AVAILABLE ANTIBACTERIAL AGENTS

It is not practical to include in this chapter all currently available ABAs. Those not discussed either are not recommended for use in young children (tetracyclines, quinolones) or are rarely used to treat neonatal infections (nitrofurans, polymyxins, sulfonamides).

TABLE 14–1.
MIC Interpretive Standards for Bacterial Susceptibility*†

Antibacterial Agent	Susceptible (≤ μg/mL)	Resistant (≥ μg/mL)
β-Lactams		
Ampicillin, penicillin G‡	0.12	0.25
Ampicillin, penicillin G§	0.12	4.
Ampicillin, penicillin‖	2.	4.
Ampicillin¶	8.	32.
Nafcillin, oxacillin‡	2.	4.
Methicillin‡	8.	16.
Ticarcillin, mezlocillin¶	16.	128.
Ticarcillin, mezlocillin#	64.	256.
Imipenem	4.	16.
Cephalothin, cefazolin	8.	32.
Ceftazidime, aztreonam	8.	32.
Cefotaxime, ceftriaxone	8.	64.
Aminoglycosides		
Gentamicin, tobramycin	4.	16.
Netilmicin	8.	32.
Kanamycin, amikacin	16.	64.
Other agents		
Clindamycin	0.5	4.
Erythromycin	0.5	8.
Rifampin	1.	4.
Trimethoprim (as TMP/SMZ)	2.	4.
Vancomycin	4.	32.
Chloramphenicol	8.	32.

* Adapted from Waitz JA, et al: *Methods for Dilution Antimicrobial Susceptibility Tests for Bacteria That Grow Aerobically*, ed 2. NCCLS Document M7-T2 (Table 2). Villanova, PA, National Committee for Clinical Laboratory Standards, 1988. For explanation, see text.
† MIC = Minimal Inhibitory Concentrations. MICs between "susceptible" and "resistant" are identified as "moderately susceptible" or "intermediate" (susceptible under selected circumstances).
‡ When testing staphylococci.
§ When testing nonenterococcal streptococci; for enterococci no "susceptible" MIC is given, but "resistant" ≥16 μg/mL.
‖ When testing *Listeria*.
¶ When testing enteric bacilli.
# When testing *Pseudomonas*.

Table 14–6, which presents the currently available parenteral β-lactam and aminoglycoside ABAs, serves three purposes: it lists all agents in an understandable order, shows which agents are closely related, and notes which agents are currently approved for use in neonates. The following general comments may clarify this classification of the β-lactam ABAs. The extended-spectrum penicillins and amdinocillin are more effective against

TABLE 14–2.
Comparative Susceptibility (median MIC in µg/mL) of Nonenteric Bacteria to Various Antibacterial Agents

Agent	Staphylococcus aureus*	Streptococcus groups A, C, G†	Streptococcus group B‡	Streptococcus enterococci§	Listeria monocytogenes‡	Neisseria gonorrhoeae‖
β-Lactams						
Ampicillin	>6.3	0.02	<0.10	1.6	0.40	0.20
Penicillin G	>6.3	<0.01	<0.10	1.6	0.80	0.10
Methicillin	3.1	0.20	—	25.0	—	1.6
Nafcillin	0.40	0.02	<0.10	12.5	6.3	6.3
Cephalothin	0.80	0.10	0.20	25.0	1.6	1.6
Aminoglycosides						
Kanamycin	3.1	>100.0	—	100.0	—	6.3
Amikacin	3.1	>100.0	>100.0	100.0	37.5	6.3
Gentamicin	0.40	25.0	100.0	12.5	3.1	1.6
Other agents						
Clindamycin	0.04	0.04	—	6.3	—	0.40
Erythromycin	0.20	0.04	—	0.10	—	0.10
Rifampin	<0.01	0.10	—	0.80	—	0.04
Trimethoprim¶	0.04	0.04	—	0.04	—	0.80
Vancomycin	1.6	1.6	—	1.6	—	50.0
Chloramphenicol	3.1	6.3	6.3	6.3	12.5	0.40

* Data from Klein JO, Finland M: *N Engl J Med* 1963; 269:1019–1025; Sabath LC, et al: *Antimicrob Agents Chemother* 1976; 9:962–969.
† Data from Finland M, et al: *Antimicrob Agents Chemother* 1976; 9:11–19.
‡ Data from Dashefsky B, Klein JO: *Clin Perinatol* 1981; 8:559–577.
§ Data from Finland M, et al: *J Infect Dis* 1976; 134(suppl):S57–S96.
‖ Data from Finland M, et al: *J Am Vener Dis Assoc* 1976; 2:33–40.
¶ As trimethoprim-sulfamethoxazole.

TABLE 14–3.
Comparative Susceptibility (median MIC in µg/mL) of Nonenteric Bacteria to Newer β-Lactam Agents

Agent	Staphylococcus aureus*	Streptococcus groups A*†	Streptococcus group B†	Streptococcus enterococci*†	Listeria monocytogenes*	Neisseria gonorrhoeae†
Ampicillin	>4.0‡	0.01	0.06	0.50	0.50‡	0.06
Ampic/Sulbactam	1.0‡	0.06‡	0.12‡	0.50*	0.50‡	—
Ticarcillin	32.0	0.25	2.0	32.0	2.0	0.03
Mezlocillin	32.0	0.02	0.25	1.0	1.0	0.01
Imipenem	0.06	0.02	0.03	0.50	0.06	0.01
Cefazolin	0.50	0.25	0.50‡	>128.0	>128.0	—
Cefuroxime	0.50	0.25	0.25‡	>128.0	>128.0	0.12‡
Cefoxatin	2.0	0.50	—	>128.0	>128.0	—
Cefotaxime	2.0	0.03	0.03	32.0	>128.0	0.01
Cefoperazone	2.0	0.12	0.12	32.0	>128.0	0.03
Ceftazidime	8.0	0.12	0.12	>128.0	>128.0	0.01
Aztreonam	>128.0	>128.0	>128.0	>128.0	>128.0	0.01

* Data from Neu HC: *Rev Infect Dis* 1986; 8(suppl 3):S237–S259.
† Data from Neu HC: *Rev Infect Dis* 1983; 5(suppl 2):S319—S336.
‡ Data from Neu HC: Personal communication, Feb 1989.

TABLE 14–4.
Comparative Susceptibility (median MIC in μg/mL) of *Haemophilus* and Enteric Bacilli to Various Antibacterial Agents

Agent	Haemophilus influenzae*	Escherichia coli†	Klebsiella pneumoniae†	Enterobacter species†	Serratia marcescens†	Pseudomonas aeruginosa†
β-Lactams						
Ampicillin	0.80	3.1	100.0	>100.0	>100.0	>100.0
Penicillin G	0.40	12.5	50.0	>100.0	>100.0	>100.0
Methicillin	1.6	>100.0	>100.0	—	—	>100.0
Nafcillin	25.0	>100.0	>100.0	—	—	>100.0
Cephalothin	12.5	6.3	3.1	100.0	>100.0	>100.0
Aminoglycosides						
Kanamycin	0.80	6.3	6.3	6.3	>100.0	100.0
Amikacin	3.1	1.6	1.6	1.6	3.1	3.1
Gentamicin	0.80	0.80	0.80	1.6	3.1	6.3‡
Other agents						
Clindamycin	6.3	>100.0	>100.0	>100.0	>100.0	>100.0
Erythromycin	3.1	50.0	50.0	50.0	100.0	>100.0
Rifampin	0.40	12.5	25.0	25.0	25.0	12.5
Trimethoprim§	0.10	0.10	0.20	0.10	0.40	6.3
Vancomycin	>100.0	—	—	—	—	—
Chloramphenicol	0.80	3.1	100.0	12.5	>100.0	100.0

* Data from Finland M, et al: *Antimicrob Agents Chemother* 1976; 9:274–287.
† Data from Finland M, et al: *J Infect Dis* 1976; 134(suppl):S57–S96.
‡ Tobramycin = 0.8.
§ As trimethoprim-sulfamethoxazole.

TABLE 14–5.
Comparative Susceptibility (median MIC in µg/mL) of *Haemophilus* and Enteric Bacilli to Newer β-Lactams

Agent	*Haemophilus influenzae**†	*Escherichia coli**†	*Klebsiella pneumoniae*‡	*Enterobacter aerogenes*‡	*Serratia marcescens*‡	*Pseudomonas aeruginosa*‡
Ampicillin	0.50	4.0	>32.0§	>32.0§	>32.0§	>32.0§
Ampic/Sulbactam	0.50§	2.0§	4.0§	>16.0§	>16.0§	>16.0§
Mezlocillin	0.25	16.0	>128.0	8.0	16.0	16.0¶
Ticarcillin	0.50	16.0	>128.0	8.0	32.0	16.0
Imipenem	0.10	0.12	0.12	0.50	1.0	1.0
Cefazolin	—	4.0	4.0	>128.0	>128.0	>128.0§
Cefuroxime	0.25	1.0	4.0	64.0	>128.0	>128.0§
Cefoxatin	—	2.0	2.0	>128.0	16.0	—
Cefotaxime	0.01	0.06	0.12	0.12	0.50	16.0
Cefoperazone	0.06	0.12	0.25	0.25	8.0	4.0
Ceftazidime	0.06	0.12	0.12	0.25	0.50	2.0
Aztreonam	0.01	0.06	0.12	0.12	0.12	2.0

* Data from Neu HC: *Rev Infect Dis* 1983; 5(suppl 2):S319–S336.
† Data from Neu HC: *Pediatr Infect Dis* 1987; 6:958–962.
‡ Data from Neu HC: *Rev Infect Dis* 1986; 8(suppl 3):S237–S259.
§ Data from Neu HC: Personal communication, Feb 1989.
¶ Piperacillin = 4.0.

many more enteric bacilli than is ampicillin. Imipenem shares this extended spectrum and is also effective against staphylococci; it is only available combined with cilastatin, which inhibits an imipenem inactivator.[19] Clavulanic acid is available only combined with ticarcillin and amoxicillin, and sulbactam is combined with ampicillin; both inhibit the common β-lactamase of *Escherichia coli*, *Haemophilus influenzae*, and *Neisseria gonorrhoeae*. The antistaphylococcal first-generation cephalsporins are effective against staphylococci and some enteric bacilli. The extended-spectrum second-generation cephalosporins are effective against more enteric bacilli. And the newer, third-generation cephalosporins are effective against even more enteric bacilli, but are less effective against staphylococci (see Table 14–3). Aztreonam, a mon-

TABLE 14–6.
Currently Available Parenteral β-Lactam and Aminoglycoside Antibacterial Agents*

Penicillins	Cephalosporins
Natural penicillins	Antistaphylococcal
Penicillin G[t]	Cephalothin[4][t]
Aqueous	Cefazolin[4]
Procaine	Cephapirin[4]
Benzathine	Cephradine[4][t]
Ampicillin[t]	
Antistaphylococcal	Extended-spectrum
Methicillin[t]	Cefamandole[5]
Nafcillin[1][t]	Cefonacid[5]
Oxacillin[1][t]	Ceforanide[5]
	Cefuroxime[5]
	Cefoxitin[6]
	Cefotetan[6]
Extended-spectrum	
Carbenicillin[2][t]	Newer cephalosporins
Ticarcillin[2][t]	Cefotaxime[7][t]
Azlocillin[3]	Ceftizoxime[7]
Mezlocillin[3][t]	Ceftriaxone[7][t]
Piperacillin[3]	Cefoperazone
Beta-lactam inhibitors	Ceftazidime[t]
Clavulanic acid	Moxalactam
Sulbactam	Aminoglycosides
Other penicillins/penems	Streptomycin
Amdinocillin	Kanamycin[t]
Imipenem	Amikacin[t]
	Gentamicin[8][t]
Monobactams	Tobramycin[8][t]
Aztreonam	Netilmicin[8][t]

*Those agents with the same superscript number have almost the same antibacterial susceptibility profiles.
[t]Currently approved for use in neonates (see *Physicians' Desk Reference*, 1989).

obactam, is like ceftazidime, except that it is inactive against gram-positive cocci and anaerobes.

SELECTION OF ANTIBACTERIAL AGENTS

General Comments

For the routine antibacterial treatment of neonatal infections both ampicillin and gentamicin have been and continue to be very efficacious.[33] Whether other, especially newer, ABAs are superior is debatable. Certainly for the treatment of infections with some bacteria, as noted later, neither ampicillin nor gentamicin is the drug of choice. The newer cephalosporins are impressively efficacious in vitro against many gram-negative bacilli, and some clinicians hope they might be able to replace the aminoglycosides. But the routine use of both cefotaxime and cefuroxime in nurseries has been associated with subsequent nursery outbreaks of resistant enteric bacillary infections.[7, 39] Similar outbreaks have been reported in adult patients with other of the newer cephalosporins.[51]

Other β-lactam ABAs also look promising, including the extended-spectrum penicillins, imipenem, and the penicillinase inhibitors, but too little data are available to recommend them for routine use in neonates. Among older agents, it is unclear whether methicillin, because of interstitial nephritis reported in older children and adults, should be superseded in neonates by other antistaphylococcal penicillins. Nor is it clear whether aminoglycosides other than gentamicin offer any routine advantage. Which of these, as well as which of various other related ABAs, will be used, will be determined in large part by which ABAs are available in the hospital's formulary.

Occult Infections

Ampicillin and gentamicin are generally recommended for empiric treatment of suspected *serious* neonatal bacterial infections. But there are three exceptions: when one suspects a staphylococcal infection, when one suspects a "resistant" enteric bacillary infection during a nursery outbreak, and when one has to retreat an infant who has already received prolonged treatment with ampicillin and gentamicin. For the latter infants, it would be prudent to initiate treatment with amikacin, to which many gentamicin-resistant enteric bacilli are susceptible, and/or an extended-spectrum penicillin or newer cephalosporin.

Staphylococci

Most isolated *Staphylococcus aureus,* even those acquired outside the hospital, are penicillinase producing, and therefore penicillin resistant. Occasionally these strains have a deceptively low penicillin MIC; so any strain with an MIC more than 0.2 µg/mL should be shown not to produce penicillinase before it is presumed susceptible. One of the antistaphylococcal penicillins is usually recommended for these strains. Methicillin-resistant strains are resistant to these penicillins and also the cephalosporins, although in vitro tests may indicate susceptibility to the latter. Vancomycin is usually recommended for methicillin-resistant strains. The same comments are true for *S. epidermidis,* recognizing that they are more commonly methicillin-resistant. When attempting to cure a staphylococcal infection associated with a synthetic prosthesis or catheter that cannot be removed, some physicians recommend adding rifampin or gentamicin.

Streptococci and *Listeria*

Most streptococci are very susceptible to penicillin and ampicillin; this includes the pneumococci, the viridans group, and the β-hemolytic groups A, C, F, and G. The group B streptococci are less susceptible. Animal and in vitro studies have shown the latter are killed more rapidly when gentamicin is combined with ampicillin; although when large penicillin concentrations are used, it is killed as rapidly as the group A streptococci. Still, many recommend beginning gentamicin with penicillin or ampicillin, though theoretically one dose may be sufficient. In neutropenic infants with group B infections it would be prudent to maintain both agents.

The enterococci are even less penicillin susceptible and require the addition of an aminoglycoside, except for localized urinary tract infections where ampicillin alone is sufficient. The nonenterococcal group D streptococci, on the other hand, are very susceptible to penicillin.

Listeria monocytogenes is susceptible to penicillin and ampicillin at levels somewhere between those of the group B streptococcus and the enterococcus. Some recommend ampicillin or penicillin alone; others add gentamicin, at least initially. *Listeria,* like the enterococci, are always resistant to the cephalosporins (see Table 14–3).

Neisseria and *Haemophilus*

Most *Neisseria* and *Haemophilus* species are also susceptible to penicillin G and ampicillin. Penicillinase-producing strains of *N. gonorrhoeae* and *H. influenzae* have become increasingly more prevalent. Their prevalence varies in different communities. For such strains most recommend one of the newer cephalosporins: cefotaxime or ceftriaxone. A single dose of ceftriaxone has proved efficacious for neonatal gonococcal ophthalmia.[30] It is not generally appreciated that these organisms are also susceptible to gentamicin (see Tables 14–2 and 14–4), but not susceptible enough to treat CNS infections.

Enteric Bacilli

The *Enterobacteriaceae,* especially *Escherichia, Klebsiella, Enterobacter,* and *Serratia* species, are commonly isolated from neonates with systemic infections. These and the less commonly isolated *Citrobacter, Proteus,* and *Providencia* species have quite variable susceptibility profiles. Among these organisms, *Proteus mirabilis* and many community-acquired *E. coli* are ampicillin susceptible, but the others usually are not. Most of the other community-acquired organisms are susceptible to the aminoglycosides, the newer cephalosporins, and the extended-spectrum penicillins. But strains of these organisms, isolated from hospital-acquired infections, may be resistant to even these ABAs.

Salmonella, Shigella, and *Yersinia enterocolitica* are *Enterobacteriaceae* that may cause localized enteritis or systemic infections. Many *Salmonella* and *Shigella* strains are susceptible to ampicillin, which is the drug of choice. Most resistant strains are susceptible to trimethoprim/sulfamethoxazole (TMP/SMZ), as are most isolated *Yersinia enterocolitica.* Systemic *Yersina* infections can also be treated with gentamicin, and recent reports suggest the newer cephalosporins are effective against systemic *Salmonella* infections.[8]

Pseudomonas aeruginosa, Plesiomonas, and *Aeromonas* species are frequently susceptible to the aminoglycosides, the extended-spectrum penicillins, and the newer cephalosporins[48] (see Tables 14–4 and 14–5). *Pseudomonas aeruginosa* is the one organism for which tobramycin is consistently more effective than gentamicin. Many of the other *Pseudomonas* species, as well as *Acinetobacter* and *Flavobacterium* species, are frequently resistant to one or all of these ABAs. Unusual ABAs may be necessary to treat infections with these organisms; neonatal meningitis caused by *F. meningosepticum,* for example, has been successfully treated with rifampin.[9]

Anaerobic Bacteria

Most anaerobic bacteria, although resistant to the aminoglycosides, are susceptible to penicillin and ampicillin. This includes the anaerobic cocci, *Bacteroides, Clostridium,* and *Fusobacterium* species.[57] The notable exceptions are strains of *B. fragilis,* which are usually susceptible to metronidazole, clindamycin, and some of the newer β-lactams, especially imipenem and ampicillin/sulbactam.[6]

Other Nonenteric Bacteria

Although not commonly encountered in neonates, a number of other bacteria are very susceptible to penicillin or ampicillin. These include *Borrelia, Eikenella, Gardnerella, Kingella, Pasteurella multocida,* and *Treponema pallidum.* Unlike the treatment of other neonatal infections, congenital syphilis has been treated with a single dose of benzathine penicillin; when there is evidence of central nervous system involvement, 10 days of aqueous or procaine penicillin is recommended. Because of benzathine penicillin failure in three reported infants who did not have CNS involvement,[4] some currently recommend 10 days of penicillin for all infants with congenital syphilis.

Other bacteria are relatively or absolutely resistant to penicillin and the other β-lactams. Included are *Bordetella pertussis, Campylobacter* species, and *Chlamydia trachomatis.* All three are susceptible to erythromycin, and erythromycin-estolate appears to be more efficacious than erythromycin-ethylsuccinate, at least against pertussis.[3] Systemic *Campylobacter* infections can be treated with gentamicin, to which they are susceptible. *Chlamydia* are resistant to the aminoglucosides; although they are also susceptible to the sulfonamides, erythromycin may be more efficacious. *Mycobacteria* and *Nocardia* species are other β-lactum–resistant bacteria, but such infections in neonates must be very rare.

NEONATAL DOSAGES OF ANTIBACTERIAL AGENTS

The recommended dose for each ABA is based on the susceptibility of the infecting bacteria and the ABA's pharmacology and potential toxicity. A number of authoritative sources have produced neonatal dosage tables, but their recommended dosages vary. Table 14–7 is adapted from tables published by McCracken and Nelson[36, 41] because of their extensive work with the neonatal pharmacokinetics of ABAs.

An accepted therapeutic serum antibacterial concentration is one that is two to eight times the MIC of the infecting bacteria, assuming that this level is not toxic. Achieving and maintaining this serum antibacterial concentration, or level, depends on the distribution of the ABA and its clearance from the body. These pharmacokinetic measurements differ in neonates from values reported in adults, both because of the relatively larger volume of extracellular water and the incompletely developed renal function of the neonate. Two comparable pharmacokinetic measurements that are more easily obtained and used are the peak serum level and the serum half-life. These measurements vary with respect to the neonate's gestational and chronologic age. Although these pharmacokinetic measurements must vary as a continuum, most published recommendations divide neonates into four groups: those with lower (<2,000 g) and higher birth weights, as both younger (<7 days) and older infants (see Table 14–7). When using data from Table 14–7 one must remember to alter the dosage or dosing frequency, or both, as younger neonates pass through their first week of life, otherwise therapeutic antibacterial levels may not be maintained.

For each ABA the recommended dosage is derived from its attainable serum level, and the dosing interval is derived from its serum half-life. Doses are usually given at intervals of two to three times the serum half-life. This should result in interval therapeutic peaks without accumulation to potentially toxic levels. Another therapeutic strategy is to give an initial therapeutic loading dose, followed by smaller maintenance doses. Such maintenance

TABLE 14–7.
Dosage (mg/kg) of Antibacterial Agents for Neonates in Accordance With Birth Weight and Age*

Agent	Route of Administration	Daily Dosage (no. of doses)			
		Birth Weight <2,000 g		Birth Weight >2,000 g	
		0–7 Days	>7 Days	0–7 Days	>7 Days
Beta-lactams					
Penicillin G[†, ‡]	IV[§], IM	30[2]	45[3]	45[3]	60[4]
Ampicillin[‡]	IV[§], IM	50[2]	75[3]	75[3]	100[4]
Methicillin[‡]	IV[§], IM	50[2]	75[3]	75[3]	100[4]
Oxacillin	IV[§], IM	50[2]	100[3]	75[3]	150[4]
Nafcillin[‡]	IV[§], IM	50[2]	75[3]	50[2]	75[3]
Ticarcillin	IV[§], IM	150[2]	225[3]	225[3]	300[4]
Mezlocillin	IV[§], IM	150[2]	225[3]	150[2]	225[3]
Cephalothin	IV[§]	40[2]	60[3]	60[3]	80[4]
Cefazolin	IV[§], IM	40[2]	40[2]	40[2]	60[3]
Ceftriaxone	IV[§], IM	50[1]	50[1]	50[1]	75[1]
Cefotaxime	IV[§], IM	100[2]	150[3]	100[2]	150[3]
Ceftazidime	IV[§], IM	100[2]	150[3]	100[2]	150[3]
Aztreonam	IV[§], IM	60[2]	90[3]	90[3]	120[4]
Aminoglycosides					
Kanamycin[‖]	IM, IV[¶]	15[2]	20[3]	20[2]	30[3]
Amikacin[‖]	IM, IV[¶]	15[2]	20[3]	20[2]	30[3]
Gentamicin[‖]	IM, IV[¶]	5[2]	7½[3]	5[2]	7½[3]
Netilmicin[‖]	IM, IV[¶]	5[2]	7½[3]	5[2]	7½[3]
Tobramycin[‖]	IM, IV[¶]	4[2]	6[3]	4[2]	6[3]
Other agents					
Clindamycin	IV[§], IM, PO	10[2]	15[3]	15[3]	20[4]
Erythromycin					
Estolate	PO	20[2]	30[3]	20[2]	30[3]
Estylsuccinate	PO			40[4]	40[4]
Vancomycin[‖]	IV[#]	20[2]	30[3]	30[2]	45[3]
Chloramphenicol	IV[§], IM, PO	25[1]	25[1]	25[1]	50[2]**
Metronidazole	IV[§], PO	15[2]	15[2]	15[2]	30[2]
Colistin	PO	15[3]	20[4]	15[3]	20[4]

*Adapted from McCracken GH Jr, Nelson JD: *Antimicrobial Therapy for Newborns,* ed 2. New York, Grune & Stratton, 1983, and Nelson JD: *Pocketbook of Pediatric Antimicrobial Therapy,* ed 8. Baltimore, Williams & Wilkins Co, 1989, pp. 20–21.
†Aqueous penicillin, where 30 mg = 50,000 U. The dose of procaine penicillin is 50,000 U/kg once daily intramuscularly (IM) for all neonates.
‡With meningitis, double the dose.
§Intravenous (IV) infusion: 15–30 min. PO = oral.
‖Infants weighing <1,200 g: smaller dosages and longer intervals between doses may be advisable.
¶Intravenous infusion: 20–30 min.
#Intravenous infusion: 30–60 min.
**Infants age >14 days.

doses, for example, may be half the loading dose at intervals of approximately one half-life. This strategy reduces the period of subtherapeutic serum levels, but it does complicate dosing orders.

PHARMACOLOGY OF β-LACTAM ANTIBACTERIAL AGENTS

Serum Levels and Half-lives

The measurements of serum peak level and serum half-life following parenteral administration of various β-lactam ABAs are summarized in Table 14–8. The attainable peak serum levels for all these agents are similar. After a single intramuscular injection of 50 mg/kg, the peak serum levels are ap-

TABLE 14–8.
Peak Serum Level and Serum Half-life of β-lactam Antibacterial Agents in Neonates*

Agent	Age (days) <7	Age (days) >7	Dose (mg/kg) and Route†	C_{max}‡ LBW‖	C_{max}‡ HBW¶	$t^{1/2}$§ LBW	$t^{1/2}$§ HBW
Penicillin[36]	+		15 IM	25	20	5	$2^{1}/_{2}$
	+		15 IM	25	20	$2^{1}/_{2}$	2
Methicillin[36]	+		25 IM	60	50	3	2
		+	25 IM	60	45	3	2
Nafcillin[36]	+		20 IM	—	35	—	$4^{1}/_{2}$
	+		50 IV	160	—	4	—
Oxacillin[36]	+		50 IM	110	—	3	—
		+	50 IM	100	—	2	—
Ampicillin[28]	+		50 IM	100	80	6	$4^{1}/_{2}$
	+		100 IM	210	180	—	—
		+	50 IM	130	85	2	$2^{1}/_{2}$
Ticarcillin[42]	+		75 IM	160	140	$5^{1}/_{2}$	5
		+	100 IM	—	145	—	2
Mezlocillin[46]	+		75 IM	160	150	3	2
		+	75 IM	—	120	—	$1^{1}/_{2}$
Cefotaxime[37]	+		50 IV	95	105	$4^{1}/_{2}$	$3^{1}/_{2}$
Ceftriaxone[34]	+		50 IV	100	120	8	$7^{1}/_{2}$
		+	50 IV	120	130	$8^{1}/_{2}$	5
Ceftazidime[38]	+		50 IV	110	100	$6^{1}/_{2}$	4
		+	50 IV	120	110	4	$3^{1}/_{2}$
Aztreonam[32]	+		30 IV	80	—	$5^{1}/_{2}$	—
Imipenem[19]	+		20 IV	25#		$1^{1}/_{2}$#	
	+		10 IV	10#		$2^{1}/_{2}$#	

*Sources are as referenced in column 1. Blank cells indicate no data.
†IM = intramuscular; IV = intravenous.
‡C_{max} = peak serum level [approximate mean peak (or 30 min after IV dosage) in µg/mL].
§$t^{1/2}$ = serum half-life [approximate mean, in hrs].
‖LBW = lower-birth-weight infants [<2,000 to 2,500 g].
¶HBW = higher-birth-weight infants [>2,000 to 2,500 g].
#LBW and HBW combined.

proximately 100 μg/mL; rapid intravenous infusions produce higher peak levels. Within the therapeutic dose range of 15 to 100 mg/kg the peak serum levels appear to be arithmetically proportional to the dose administered. It should be noted that among individual infants there is considerable variation about these mean serum levels: ± 25% to 50%.

On the other hand, the mean serum half-lives of the various β-lactams do vary. They are proportional to, though longer than, those reported in adults. The one unexplainable exception is mean half-life for ceftriaxone, but in a more recent report it was found to be 19 hours for neonates in the first week of life.[53] As expected, the observed half-life is longer in younger and smaller infants, and shorter in older and larger infants.

Similar data in neonates exist for other β-lactam ABAs: carbenicillin, cephalothin, cefazolin, cefomandole, cefoperazone, cefuroxime, and moxalactam.[36]

Systemic Infections

The recommended dosages (see Table 14–7) for the various β-lactams differ, not because of their attainable serum levels but because of the susceptibility of the targeted bacterial pathogens. Thus the recommended penicillin, methicillin, ampicillin, and mezlocillin doses should produce serum levels, respectively, 5 to 10 times the MICs for group B streptococci, staphylococci, *E. coli*, and *P. aeruginosa*. The implicit assumption is that the concentration of the ABA at the local infected site is approximately the same as its serum level. For the β-lactam ABAs this assumption is probably true with two major exceptions: concentrations in the urine and in the cerebrospinal fluid (CSF).

Urine Levels and Urinary Tract Infections

Most β-lactam ABAs are excreted primarily in the urine; the exceptions are mezlocillin, nafcillin, cefoperazone, and ceftriaxone. Therefore, in infants with compromised renal function the dose or dosing frequency for most β-lactams should be reduced. On the other hand, the urinary concentrations of ampicillin are 10 to 100 times the serum concentrations[28]; presumably it would be the same for the other β-lactams excreted in the urine. So for localized urinary tract infections, half the standard dose could be used.

Cerebrospinal Fluid Levels and Meningitis

Measurable concentrations of the β-lactams in the CSF are only a fraction of the corresponding serum concentrations. Mean penicillin CSF levels of 18%, 10%, and 5% of the mean serum levels were detected in children with meningitis on the first, fifth, and tenth days of treatment, respectively.[22] In a comparable group of children with meningitis, the mean ampicillin CSF levels were approximately twice as high, or 32%, 29%, and 8% of the mean serum levels.[58] And in experimental rabbit meningitis, ampicillin entered the CSF up to four times better than penicillin.[54] Thus, for penicillin-susceptible bacteria, ampicillin would appear to be the preferable agent. Also it should be apparent that it makes no sense to decrease the dose as the patient's condition is improving. In neonates, cefotaxime appears to enter the CSF at least as well as ampicillin.[36]

In the treatment of neonatal meningitis, it is recommended that the dosages of penicillins be doubled (see Table 14–7). Recognizing that only a fraction of the serum ampicillin concentration reaches the CSF, it would appear that even higher doses may be needed to treat bacterial meningitis. Some[2] have argued for a dose of 300 to 400 mg/kg/day for group B streptococcal meningitis. It would appear to be even more prudent to use this larger ampicillin dosage in the treatment of meningitis caused by the less susceptible *E. coli* and *Salmonella*. In our hospital, doses to 400 mg/kg/day have been used in neonates without adverse effects.

Oral Administration

One finds less pharmacokinetic data for the β-lactams given orally to neonates. With doses of 20 to 30 mg/kg the achievable mean serum level for ampicillin, cloxacillin, and nafcillin is approximately half that achieved with parenteral doses.[21] This was also true for amoxicillin given orally in doses of 50 mg/kg.[62]

Adverse Effects

One also finds little data about adverse effects of β-lactam ABAs in neonates. Moxalactam has been associated with clinically important bleeding in adults because of both prothrombin and platelet abnormalities,[11] and perhaps should be avoided in neonates. Ceftriaxone, cefaperazone, and dicloxacillin have been classified as relatively high-level displacers of bilirubin from albumin.[49, 60] Although it is not clear if this is clinically important, these agents might best be avoided in neonates with jaundice. And nafcillin should be used with some caution, because subcutaneous extravasation of this agent can cause cutaneous necrosis in infants.[59]

PHARMACOLOGY OF AMINOGLYCOSIDE ANTIBACTERIAL AGENTS

Serum Levels and Half-lives

Early pharmacokinetic data for the aminoglycoside ABAs administered intramuscularly to neonates are summarized in Table 14–9. The data are essentially the same following slow intravenous administration.[36] The dosage

TABLE 14–9.
Peak Serum Level and Serum Half-life of Aminoglycoside Antibacterial Agents in Neonates*

Agent	Age (days) <7	>7	Dose (mg/kg) and Route†	C_{max}‡ LBW‖		HBW¶	$t_{1/2}$§ LBW	HBW
Kanamycin[25]	+		10 IM	26	(22–33)	21	7½	5½
		+	10 IM	22		20	5	4
	+		7½ IM	22	(13–29)	13		
		+	7½ IM	17		15		
Amikacin[36]	+		7½ IM	17		18	6½	6
		+	7½ IM	19		17	5½	5
Gentamicin[35]	+		2½ IM	4#	(2–8½)		10	5
		+	2½ IM	4#			3½#	
Tobramycin[27]	+		2 IM	5	(4–7)	5	8½	4½
		+	2 IM	5		4	6	4
Netilmicin[55]	+		3 IM	6	(3½–10)	7	4½	3½
		+	3 IM	6		—	4	—

* Sources are as referenced in column 1. Empty cells indicate no data.
† IM = intramuscular; IV = intravenous.
‡ C_{max} = peak serum level [approximate mean (range) in μg/mL].
§ $t_{1/2}$ = serum half-life [approximate mean, in hr].
‖ LBW = low birth weight [<2,000 to 2,500 g].
¶ HBW = higher birth weight [>2,000 to 2,500 g].
# LBW and HBW combined.

administered and the resulting attainable peak serum levels are considerably lower than those of the β-lactam ABAs because the aminoglycoside ABAs are much more toxic. In adults the toxic serum level is estimated to be >12 μg/mL for gentamicin, tobramycin, and netilmicin and >35 μg/mL for kanamycin and amikacin.

In adults the serum half-life for all these agents is about equal, but Table 14–9 shows considerable differences for the younger, small neonates. This is probably because these groups are heterogeneous with respect to maturity. The glomerular clearance and the serum half-life for these agents is inversely proportional to the neonate's renal maturity and therefore the neonate's gestational and chronologic age (postgestational age). Several authors have recommended lower dosages of gentamicin for very small neonates: 2.5 mg/kg once daily for those of less than 28 weeks postgestational age, and 2.5 mg/kg every 18 hours or 3 mg/kg once daily for those of 29 to 35 weeks.[12, 23] The same should be true of the other aminoglycoside ABAs. Also it may be that the tobramycin dosage in all neonates should be the same as that for gentamicin.[40]

Systemic Infections

Again one should attempt to attain a serum level in excess of the MICs but not into the toxic range. Various serum peaks are recommended by different authors; generally, these are 5 to 10 μg/mL for gentamicin, tobramycin, and netilmicin and 15 to 25 μg/mL for kanamycin and amikacin. In an ill, truly infected infant one needs to attain a therapeutic level rapidly. As neither infecting organism nor its susceptibility is known when treatment is begun, and because a maximally safe level may be needed, it would be prudent to measure the peak serum level in these infants 30 minutes after the first dose is administered. After the susceptibility of the infecting organism is known, one may be able to reduce the dosage and still maintain a serum level of two to eight times the MIC. With gentamicin, beware. Gentamicin is supplied in two concentrations: a pediatric form (10 mg/mL) and an adult form (40 mg/mL). A kindly nurse may select the adult form so as to inject a smaller intramuscular volume (0.06 mL vs. 0.25 mL for a 1-kg neonate), but much of this smaller volume may never leave the needle. The same is true for the other aminoglycoside ABAs.

Urine Levels and Urinary Tract Infections

Aminoglycoside agents are primarily excreted by the kidneys. As the urine concentrations exceed those found in serum, localized urinary tract infections can be treated with lower doses, probably half those noted in Table 14–9.[36]

Cerebrospinal Fluid Levels and Meningitis

Measurable concentrations of these agents in the CSF, even during acute meningitis, are only a fraction of those in the serum. Although not commonly appreciated, the mean CSF peak levels can reach 40% of the peak serum levels.[25, 35] Still this may be inadequate to inhibit many "susceptible" bacteria. For this reason aminoglycoside ABAs have been administered intrathecally and intraventricularly to neonates with enteric bacillary meningitis. But the former route has been ineffective, and the latter, possibly because of neurotoxicity, may be detrimental. It is recommended, even for enteric bacillary meningitis, that these agents be administered parenterally at standard dosages, along with a β-lactam ABA. If nothing else, the aminoglycoside will inhibit the nonmeningeal organisms, thus preventing an overwhelming bacteremia. It is this bacteremia that can be rapidly lethal.

Oral Administration

Oral aminoglycosides have been used to treat recognized and putative intestinal infections. Although susceptible enteric bacilli within the intestinal lumen may be eliminated, resistant organisms conceivably can replace them. In neonates it may be wiser to use oral colistin, an agent not usually used for systemic infections. Also, oral aminoglycosides can be absorbed from inflamed intestines, causing potentially toxic serum levels when these agents are simultaneously administered parenterally.

Adverse Effects

Aminoglycoside ABAs are noted for their ototoxicity and nephrotoxicity. But there are little data demonstrating that short-term use of these agents, in proper doses, causes hearing impairment in neonates; nor are there data showing that gentamicin is more ototoxic than the other agents.[1,14] It should be emphasized that the therapeutic and toxic serum levels for these agents are very close. To be assured that the ABA is not accumulating to a toxic level, one should obtain a peak level measurement after steady state has been reached (after three doses). It is even better to obtain two timed levels (a peak and a second subsequent level, which can be a trough), to calculate the serum half-life, if the peak proves to be too high. This is especially important in neonates with perinatal asphyxia, very low birth weight, or reduced renal function. It would be prudent to repeat testing of these levels weekly for the duration of therapy.

PHARMACOLOGY OF THE OTHER ANTIBACTERIAL AGENTS

Clindamycin

The clindamycin dosages recommended in Table 14–7 produce levels in infants (Table 14–10) that exceed the MIC of most *B. fragilis,* the most

TABLE 14–10.
Peak Serum Level and Serum Half-life of Other Antibacterial Agents in Neonates*

Agent	Age (days) <7	Age (days) >7	Dose (mg/kg) and Route†	C_{max}‡ LBW‖		C_{max}‡ HBW¶	$t^{1}/_{2}$§ LBW	$t^{1}/_{2}$§ HBW
Clindamycin[5$]		10**	5–7 IV	11		10	$8^{1}/_{2}$	$3^{1}/_{2}$
Erythromycin[47]								
Estolate	+		10 PO	$1^{1}/_{2}$		1	$4^{#}$	
		+	10 PO	$2^{1}/_{2}$	(2–5)	$1^{1}/_{2}$	$4^{1}/_{2}^{#}$	
Estolate		29**	10 PO	—		$1^{1}/_{2}$	—	4
Ethylsuccinate		48**	10 PO	—		1	—	$2^{1}/_{2}$
Vancomycin[52]	+		10 IV	17	(11–21)	—	10	—
	+		15 IV	25	(17–32)	30	6	$6^{1}/_{2}$
Chloramphenicol[20,24]	+		25 IV		(16–36)	—	—	—
		+	25 IV		(10–36)	—	—	—
	+		50 IV	41	(27–56)	—	24	—
		+	50 IV	30	(16–44)	—	14	—

*Sources as referenced in column 1. Blank cells indicate no data.
†IV = intravenous; PO = oral.
‡C_{max} = peak serum level [approximate mean (range) in µg/mL].
§$t^{1}/_{2}$ = serum half-life [approximate mean, in hr].
‖LBW = low birth weight [<2,000 to 2,500 g].
¶HBW = higher birth weight [>2,000 to 2,500 g].
#LBW and HBW combined.
**Mean age, in days.

resistant of the anaerobes,[57] and greatly exceed the MICs of other susceptible bacteria (see Table 14–2). Little clindamycin is excreted in the urine. Most is evidently removed by the liver,[5] and very little diffuses into the CSF.

Erythromycin

Compared with other ABAs, erythromycin is nontoxic. Although erythromycin estolate does cause cholestatic jaundice in adults, this has not been a problem in infants. There are no pharmacokinetic data for the parenteral preparations in neonates. The estolate is well absorbed orally, and unaffected by oral feeding. The ethylsuccinate preparation produces lower serum levels and has a shorter half-life (see Table 14–10). Erythromycin diffuses poorly into the CSF, but well into tears.[47]

Trimethoprim/Sulfamethoxazole

A TMP/SMZ regimen in neonates has been calculated following intravenous administration: a loading dose with 3 mg/kg TMP followed by a 12-hour maintenance dose of 1 mg/kg TMP.[56] Recognizing that SMZ does displace bilirubin from albumin, TMP/SMZ should be avoided in jaundiced neonates.[60]

Vancomycin

The recommended therapeutic levels of vancomycin are peaks of 25 to 40 μg/mL and troughs of less than 10 μg/mL. A number of studies have been reported since those noted in Table 14–10. Nelson[41] now recommends lower dosages for smaller infants (see Table 14–7). For tiny neonates, others would give a similar total daily dosage but with longer intervals between doses, but these schedules become complicated. A recent recommendation is much more practical: a dose of 15 mg/kg administered once daily for infants weighing less than 1,000 g.[31] In any case, because of variations in individual infants, one should monitor peak (30 minutes after infusion) and trough serum levels. And this agent should be administered as a slow intravenous infusion to avoid the described prolonged cutaneous eruption. Vancomycin is excreted primarily in the urine and diffuses moderately well into the CSF, attaining 15% of the concomitant serum level.[52]

Chloramphenicol

Although the serum concentration at which chloramphenicol is toxic in neonates is unknown, it probably is greater than 50 μg/mL. Recommended therapeutic levels are 10 to 20 or 25 μg/mL. These levels are attainable with a dose of 20 to 25 mg/mL. Although a once-daily dose is recommended for low-birth-weight neonates (see Table 14–10), in younger, small neonates the serum half-life may exceed 24 hours.[20] Serum levels should be measured, recognizing that in younger, small neonates the peak serum levels occur late. In spite of its attractive properties of good oral absorption and high CSF diffusion, the potential toxicity of chloramphenicol and the availability of better ABAs for enteric infections should limit its use.

Metronidazole

Therapeutic levels of metronidazole were found in the serum in neonates following an intravenous loading dose of 15 mg/mL and maintenance doses of 7.5 mg/kg every 12 hours during the first week of life.[26] Therapeutic CSF levels have been noted after oral administration, curing even meningitis due to *B. fragiiis.*[13]

Topical Antibacterial Agents

It would seem reasonable to administer topical ABAs to the neonate as one would to older infants, but this is based on conviction, not data. The potential for transcutaneous absorption through the neonate's thin skin, especially at an inflamed site, should preclude generous or extensive applications.

DURATION OF THERAPY

The recommended duration of antibacterial therapy for most neonatal infections is from 1 to 3 weeks (Table 14–11). This duration depends on several factors: the infecting bacteria, the site of infection, and the competence of the neonate's natural defenses. Some bacteria are difficult to eradicate in deep infections (e.g., treating staphylococcal osteomyelitis for less than 3 weeks results in a 19% failure rate) whereas others are rapidly eradicated from superficial sites (e.g., treating gonococcal conjunctivitis with a single dose of ceftriaxone is curative).[30] Superficial infections with avirulent bacteria (e.g., scalp monitor abscesses due to anaerobic bacteria) probably require no antibacterial therapy; and transient occult bacteremias may require less than the 7 days of antibacterial treatment that is frequently given. In general, longer periods are required for deep infections that cannot be drained, in sites with necrotic tissue or a foreign body (e.g., an intravenous catheter), and in neutropenic or otherwise compromised infants.

TABLE 14–11.
Duration (days) of Antibacterial Therapy for Neonates

Site of Infection	Streptococci*	Staphylococci	Enteric Bacilli
Cutaneous or mucosal			
Bladder, intestine, upper respiratory tract	5–10	7–14	5–10
Subcutaneous or glandular			
Lymph node, breast	5–10	7–14†	5–10
Visceral			
Kidney, liver, lung	7–14	21–28	14–21
Meningeal, osseous, or serosal			
Joint, peritoneum, pleural	7–14	21–28	14–21
Occult‡ with bacteremia	7	7–10	7–10

*And other penicillin-susceptible bacteria.
†When drained.
‡No apparent local disease site.

REFERENCES

1. Assael BM, Parini R, Rusconi F: Ototoxicity of aminoglycoside antibiotics in infants and children. *Pediatr Infect Dis* 1982; 1:357–365.
2. Baker CJ, Edwards MS: Group B streptococcal infections, in Remington JS, Klein JO (eds): *Infectious Diseases of Fetus and Newborn Infants.* Philadelphia, WB Saunders Co, 1983, pp 861–862.
3. Bass JW: Erythromycin for treatment and prevention of pertussis. *Pediatr Infect Dis* 1986; 5:154–157.
4. Beck-Sague C, Alexander ER: Failure of benzathine penicillin G treatment in early congenital syphilis. *Pediatr Infect Dis J* 1987; 6:1061–1064.
5. Bell MJ, et al: Pharmacokinetics of clindamycin phosphate in the first year of life. *J Pediatr* 1984; 105:482–486.
6. Brown WJ: National committee for clinical laboratory standards: Agar dilution susceptibility testing of anaerobic gram-negative bacteria. *Antimicrob Agents Chemother* 1988; 32:385–390.
7. Bryan CS, et al: Gentamicin vs. cefotaxime for therapy of neonatal sepsis: Relationship to drug resistance. *Am J Dis Child* 1985; 139:1086–1089.
8. Bryan JP, Rocha H, Scheld WM: Problems in salmonellosis: Rationale for clinical trials with newer beta-lactam agents and quinolones. *Rev Infect Dis* 1986; 8:189–207.
9. Conti R, Parenti F: Rifampin therapy for brucellosis, flavobacterium meningitis and cutaneous leishmaniasis. *Rev Infect Dis* 1983; 5(suppl 3):S600–S605.
10. Dashefsky B, Klein JO: The treatment of bacterial infections in the newborn infant. *Clin Perinatol* 1981; 8:559–577.
11. Donowitz GR, Mandell GL: Beta-lactam antibiotics. *N Engl J Med* 1988; 318:490–500.
12. Edwards C: Pharmacokinetics in the neonate: 3. Gentamicin. *Pharm J* 1986; 237:518–519.
13. Feldman WE: *Bacteroides fragilis* ventriculitis and meningitis. *Am J Dis Child* 1976; 130:880–883.

14. Finitzo-Hieber T, McCracken GH Jr, Brown KC: Prospective controlled evaluation of auditory function in neonates given netilmicin or amikacin. *J Pediatr* 1985; 106:129–136.

15. Finland M, et al: Susceptibility of beta-hemolytic streptococci 65 antibacterial agents. *Antimicrob Agents Chemother* 1976; 9:11–19.

16. Finland M, et al: Susceptibility of pneumococci and *Haemophilus influenzae* to antibacterial agents. *Antimicrob Agents Chemother* 1976; 9:274–287.

17. Finland M, et al: Susceptibility of "enterobacteria" to aminoglycoside antibiotics: Comparison with tetracyclines, polymyxins, chloramphenicol and spectinomycin; (and) to penicillins, cephalosporins, lincomycins, erythromycin and rifampin. *J Infect Dis* 1976; 134(suppl):S57–S74 and S75–S96.

18. Finland M, et al: Susceptibility of *Neisseria gonorrhoeae* to 66 antibacterial agents in vitro. *J Am Vener Dis Assoc* 1976; 2:33–40.

19. Freij BJ, et al: Pharmacokinetics of imipenem-cilastatin in neonates. *Antimicrob Agents Chemother* 1985; 27:431–435.

20. Glazer JP, et al: Disposition of chloramphenicol in low birth weight infants. *Pediatrics* 1980; 66:573–578.

21. Grossman M, Ticknor W: Serum levels of ampicillin, cephalothin, cloxacillin and nafcillin in the newborn infant. *Antimicrobial Agents and Chemotherapy—1965.* Ann Arbor, Mich, American Society of Microbiology, 1966, pp 214–219.

22. Hieber HP, Nelson JD: Evaluation of penicillin in children with purulent meningitis. *N Engl J Med* 1977; 297:410–413.

23. Hindmarsh KW, et al: Pharmacokinetics of gentamicin in very low birth weight preterm infants. *Eur J Clin Pharmacol* 1983; 24:649–653.

24. Hodgman JE, Burns LE: Safe and effective chloramphenicol dosages for premature infants. *Am J Dis Child* 1961; 101:140–148.

25. Howard JB, McCracken GH Jr: Reappraisal of kanamycin usage in neonates. *J Pediatr* 1975; 86:949–956.

26. Jager-Roman E, et al: Pharmacokinetics and tissue distribution of metronidazole in the newborn infant. *J Pediatr* 1982; 100:651–654.

27. Kaplan JM, et al: Clinical pharmacology of tobramycin in newborns. *Am J Dis Child* 1973; 125:656–660.

28. Kaplan JM, et al: Pharmacologic studies in neonates given large dosages of ampicillin. *J Pediatr* 1974; 84:571–577.

29. Klein JO, Finland M: The new penicillins. *N Engl J Med* 1963; 269:1019–1025.

30. Laga M, et al: Single-dose therapy of gonococcal ophthalmia neonatorum with ceftriaxone. *N Engl J Med* 1986; 315:1382–1385.

31. Leonard MB, et al: Vancomycin pharmacokinetics in very low birth weight neonates. *Pediatr Infect Dis J* 1989; 8:282–286.

32. Likitnukul S, et al: Pharmacokinetics and plasma bactericidal activity of aztreonam in low-birth-weight infants. *Antimicrob Agents Chemother* 1987; 31:81–83.

33. McCracken GH Jr: Use of third-generation cephalosporins for treatment of neonatal infections. *Am J Dis Child* 1985; 139:1079–1080.

34. McCracken GH Jr, et al: Ceftriaxone pharmacokinetics in newborn infants. *Antimicrob Agents Chemother* 1983; 23:341–343.

35. McCracken GH Jr, Chrane DF, Thomas ML: Pharmacologic evaluation of gentamicin in newborn infants. *J Infect Dis* 1971; 124(suppl):S214–S223.

36. McCracken GH Jr, Nelson JD: *Antimicrobial Therapy for Newborns,* ed 2. New York, Grune & Stratton, 1983.

37. McCracken GH Jr, Threlkeld N, Thomas ML: Pharmacokinetics of cefotaxime in newborn infants. *Antimicrob Agents Chemother* 1982; 21:683–684.
38. McCracken GH Jr, Threlkeld N, Thomas ML: Pharmacokinetics of ceftazidime in newborn infants. *Antimicrob Agents Chemother* 1984; 26:583–584.
39. Modi N, Damjanovic V, Cooke RWI: Outbreak of cephalosporin resistant *Enterobacter cloacae* infection in a neonatal intensive care unit. *Arch Dis Child* 1987; 62:148–151.
40. Nabata MC, et al: Tobramycin kinetics in newborn infants. *J Pediatr* 1983; 103:136–138.
41. Nelson JD: *Pocketbook of Pediatric Antimicrobial Therapy*, ed 8. Baltimore, Williams & Wilkins Co, 1989, pp 20–21.
42. Nelson JD, et al: Clinical pharmacology and efficacy of ticarcillin in infants and children. *Pediatrics* 1978; 61:858–863.
43. Neu HC: Structure-activity relations of new beta-lactam compounds and in vitro activity against common bacteria. *Rev Infect Dis* 1983; 5(suppl 2):S319–S336.
44. Neu HC: Beta-lactam antibiotics: Structural relationships affecting in vitro activity and pharmacologic properties. *Rev Infect Dis* 1986; 8(suppl 3):S237–S259.
45. Neu HC: In vitro activity of a new broad spectrum, beta-lactamase-stable oral cephalosporin, cefixime. *Pediatr Infect Dis J* 1987; 6:958–962.
46. Odio C, et al: Pharmacokinetics of mezlocillin in newborn infants. *Antimicrob Agents Chemother* 1984; 25:556–559.
47. Patamasucon P, et al: Pharmacokinetics of erythromycin ethylsuccinate and estolate in infants under 4 months of age. *Antimicrob Agents Chemother* 1981; 19:736–739.
48. Reinhardt JF, George WL: Comparative in vitro activities of selected antimicrobial agents against *Aeromonas* species and *Plesiomonas shigelloides*. *Antimicrob Agents Chemother* 1985; 27:643–645.
49. Robertson A, Fink S, Karp S: Effect of cephalosporins on bilirubin-albumin binding. *J Pediatr* 1988; 112:291–294.
50. Sabath LC, et al: Susceptibility of *Staphylococcus aureus* and *Staphylococcus epidermidis* to 65 antibiotics. *Antimicrob Agents Chemother* 1976; 9:962–969.
51. Sanders WE Jr, Sanders CC: Inducible beta-lactamases: Clinical and epidemiologic implications for use of newer cephalosporins. *Rev Infect Dis* 1988; 10:830–838.
52. Schaad UB, McCracken GH Jr, Nelson JD: Clinical pharmacology and efficacy of vancomycin in pediatric patients. *J Pediatr* 1980; 96:119–126.
53. Schaad UB, Hayton WL, Stoeckel K: Single-dose ceftriaxone kinetics in the newborn. *Clin Pharmacol Ther* 1985; 37:522–528.
54. Scheld WM, et al: Comparison of cefoperazone with penicillin, ampicillin, gentamicin, and chloramphenicol in the therapy of experimental meningitis. *Antimicrob Agents Chemother* 1982; 22:652–656.
55. Siegel JD, et al: Pharmacokinetic properties of netilmicin in newborn infants. *Antimicrob Agents Chemother* 1979; 15:246–253.
56. Springer C, Eyal F, Michel J: Pharmacology of trimethoprim-sulfamethoxazole in newborn infants. *J Pediatr* 1982; 100:647–650.
57. Sutter VL, Finegold SM: Susceptibility of anaerobic bacteria to 23 antimicrobial agents. *Antimicrob Agents Chemother* 1976; 10:736–752.
58. Thrupp LD, et al: Ampicillin levels in the cerebrospinal fluid during treatment of bacterial meningitis. *Antimicrobial Agents and Chemotherapy—1965*. Ann Arbor, Mich, American Society of Microbiology, 1966, pp 206–213.

59. Tilden SJ, et al: Cutaneous necrosis associated with intravenous nafcillin therapy. *Am J Dis Child* 1980; 134:146–148.

60. Wadsworth SJ, Suh B: In vitro displacement of bilirubin by antibiotics and 2-hydroxybenzolylglycine in newborns. *Antimicrob Agents Chemother* 1988; 32:1571–1575.

61. Waitz JA, et al: *Methods for Dilution Antimicrobial Susceptibility Tests for Bacteria That Grow Aerobically,* ed 2. NCCLS Document M7-T2 (Table 2). Villanova, Pa, National Committee for Clinical Laboratory Standards, 1988.

62. Weingärtner L, et al: Experience with amoxycillin in neonates and premature babies. *Int J Clin Pharmacol* 1977; 15:184–188.

15

Nonbacterial Infections

Cheng T. Cho, M.D., Ph.D.
Howard A. Fox, M.D.

FUNGAL INFECTIONS

Infection with *Candida* species, particularly *Candida albicans*, accounts for the majority of fungal infections in neonates and young infants. Several rare fungal infections, such as aspergillosis, coccidioidomycosis, cryptococcosis, histoplasmosis, phycomycosis, and dermatophytosis, will not be discussed here. This section deals specifically with *Candida albicans* infection; however, the drug treatment discussed here may be applicable to other fungal infections.

Candidiasis

Candida species, previously known as *Monilia,* exist in varying morphologic forms, depending on their growth condition: (1) blastospores, or yeast cells (2 to 5 nm in diameter), are found in skin, sputum, urine, and feces; (2) pseudomycelia (or hyphae), filamentous forms elongated from yeast cells, are found in deep-seated tissue infections; and (3) chlamydospores (7 to 17 nm in diameter) are seen occasionally in human tissue in systemic infection.

Candida albicans is the species most frequently isolated from patients with thrush, bronchopulmonary infection, and disseminated disease. Other isolates include *C. tropicalis, C. pseudotropicalis, C. parapsilosis, C. stellatoidea, C. krusei,* and *C. quilliermondii.* The greater pathogenicity of *C. albicans* probably is due to production of endotoxin, hemolysins, pyogens, or proteolytic enzyme. The common clinical cutaneous or intertriginous forms of candidiasis represent superficial invasion of the epidermis, and occasionally the dermis, by the fungus as a result of local environmental conditions that permit *Candida* growth. Such conditions are present in the macerated diaper area from continuous contact with urine. Other such areas involved are the axillae, and the skin folds of the neck.

The pulmonary colonization by *Candida* species may occur as a result of any predisposing disease of the bronchial tree. In the severely immunosuppressed host, actual parenchymal invasion may occur. Septicemia results in widespread microabscess formation. Commonly the kidneys, bones, lungs, and meninges are affected. Septicemia arises as the result of instrumentation, the common source being an indwelling catheter for intravascular infusion. The severity with which septicemia can affect the individual depends on the type and number of organisms shed into the bloodstream. Septicemia also may occur through the ulcerative lesions in the gastrointestinal tract. The susceptibility of neonates to *Candida* infection is also enhanced by the administration of antibiotics.

Clinical Findings

Thrush.—Thrush (oral candidiasis), a common oral lesion caused by *C. albicans,* usually is acquired at birth from the mother's birth canal, and may also be acquired from other infected infants or from contaminated hands or feeding facilities. The lesions usually appear within several days after birth as small white flakes or patches on the gums, palate, buccal mucosa, or tongue. Thrush is distinguished from milk curds by swabbing the infant's tongue: milk curds are easily wiped off, thrush is not.

Oral thrush is generally a mild and self-limited disease that leaves no scars. Often the candidiasis may involve other organs, such as skin or perineal or perianal region, fingernails, and gastrointestinal tract. Candidiasis of the gastrointestinal tract occurs frequently following oral candidiasis. Candidal esophagitis is associated with feeding difficulty and vomiting. Diarrhea is seen in enteritis. Persistence or recurrence of thrush with protracted skin lesions may suggest an underlying immunodeficiency state, malnutrition, prolonged antibiotic therapy, or endocrine dysfunction.

Cutaneous Candidiasis.—Cutaneous infection usually is seen in the moist intertriginous areas (skin in the perineum or the axillae) and around the umbilicus. The lesions are moist and may be papular or vesicular with an erythematous base. The rash may consist of small (a few millimeters) discrete lesions or they may coalesce, forming large areas of inflamed skin. Candidal diaper dermatitis is a common benign condition, and recurrence is frequent. The lesions are localized in the perirectal skin, inguinal folds, perineum, and lower abdomen. Fungal id reactions or sterile grouped vesicles may occur at some distance from the primary rash and represent a nonspecific response to fungal antigens.

Congenital generalized candidiasis, a rare intrauterine infection, occurs by the transplacental route or by ascending infection. The cutaneous lesions are widespread and affect the entire body. The lesions consist of scaling, erythematous moist erosions and scattered vesicles and pustules on an erythematous base. The visceral organs and oropharynx usually are not involved.

Chronic mucocutaneous candidiasis represents a generalized integumentary infection not confined to the intertriginous areas. The nails and surrounding skin are often heavily involved. Mucous membrane involvement is severe. Particularly heavy colonization of the gastrointestinal tract is common.

Disseminated Candidiasis.—Debilitated infants, particularly those undergoing operative procedures or receiving continuous intravascular infusions, prolonged total parenteral nutrition, urinary catheters, and peritoneal dialysis may develop *Candida* septicemia with involvement of visceral organs.[2, 17] Spontaneous recovery from fungemia may occur if the source of infection is removed early. Prolonged fungemia is associated with serious complications, such as pyelonephritis, meningitis and brain abscesses, endocarditis, osteomyelitis, arthritis, gastroenteritis, pneumonitis, and endophthalmitis.

Diagnosis

Clinical diagnosis of oral thrush and cutaneous candidiasis is relatively easy and can be readily confirmed by microscopic examination and by cultures of the organism. Examination of the scraping materials suspended in 20% potassium hydroxide, or Gram stains of smears, may enable one to identify the fungus. The clinical features of disseminated infection in the neonate are nonspecific, and diagnosis is often delayed. Cultures of blood, urine, cerebrospinal fluid (CSF), bronchial aspirates, or other body fluids or tissues will assist in defining the extent of the involvement. Interpretation of a positive culture from some clinical specimens (such as respiratory tract secretions or urine) may be difficult, because many of these are the result of colonization rather than infection. It is also important to recognize that positive blood cultures, transient or persistent, may be associated with infected catheters or intravenous infusions without systemic infection. Removal of the infected source usually results in clearance of the fungus from the blood. Positive blood cultures on several successive days should be considered diagnostic. Skin tests and currently available serologic tests are not helpful in confirming the diagnosis and do not add valuable information.

Treatment

Oral thrush and gastrointestinal candidiasis are treated by application of nystatin suspension (Mycostatin), 100,000 to 400,000 U (1 to 4 mL) orally four to six times, until the lesions have cleared (usually about 1 week) and for a few days afterward. Aqueous gentian violet (1%) may be used in patients who fail to respond to nystatin; it can be applied directly to the lesions four times a day with a moistened cotton swab. Systemic antibacterial therapy often contributes to the overgrowth of *Candida,* and should therefore be discontinued as soon as possible.

Cutaneous candidiasis can be treated with nystatin ointment, amphotericin B ointment, or aqueous gentian violet (1%) applied three to four times a day for 7 to 10 days. It is important to keep the area as dry as possible. Infants with diaper rash may need topical application of antifungal agent with each diaper change. The combination of a corticosteroid and an antifungal agent may be used if inflammation is severe. In some cases, secondary bacterial infection may require additional topical or systemic antibiotic therapy. Fungal id reactions, which usually resolve when the infection is controlled, may be treated with a corticosteroid preparation. If recurrences are frequent, a course of oral antifungal agent may be used to reduce the yeast population.

Systemic candidiasis should be treated with intravenous amphotericin B. In neonates the optimum schedule and duration of therapy are not known. Amphotericin B should be given in 5% dextrose and water in a concentration of less than 0.1 mg/mL; it should not be diluted in sodium chloride because precipitation will occur. On day 1 of the therapy a test dose of 0.1 mg/kg is infused over 3 to 4 hours. If the patient shows no severe adverse reactions (e.g., hypotension, anaphylactoid reaction), the first therapeutic dose (0.25 mg/kg/day) is given the same day as the test dose. Subsequent daily doses are increased by 0.1 to 0.25 mg/kg (i.e., 0.3 to 0.5 mg/kg for day 2; 0.4 to 0.75 mg/kg for day 3; and so on) until a maintenance dose of 0.5 to 1.0 mg/kg is reached. In life-threatening infections, larger increments (0.25 mg/kg) can be given successfully by 3- to 4-hour infusions, and the total daily dose of 1 mg/kg can be reached within the first 24 hours. When the infection is controlled (i.e., sterile blood or urine cultures, signs of clinical improvement, weight gain), the daily maintenance dose can be tapered to every other day. Usually treatment is continued for 4 weeks or longer.

Some infants with uncomplicated *Candida* sepsis can be treated successfully with a brief course (10 days) of therapy. Clinical response to therapy also varies greatly: some patients show excellent response to low-dose therapy (0.1 to 0.2 mg/kg); others respond poorly even at high doses (1.0 mg/kg). Usually patients demonstrate signs of favorable response to amphotericin B therapy within a few days of therapy.

Flucytosine may be added in patients with meningitis. In rare cases with persistent positive CSF cultures, intrathecal amphotericin B may be used. The initial dose is 0.01 mg, gradually increased to 0.1 mg over 5 to 7 days, given every other day or every third day.

Side effects of amphotericin B should be closely monitored (see section on amphotericin B). Hypokalemia occurs frequently and should be corrected with potassium replacement. Anemia is also common and may require blood transfusions.

Prevention

There is no ideal method to prevent *C. albicans* infections in neonates. Some clinicians administer nystatin 100,000 U (1 mL) oral suspension for 3 to 4 days to prevent oral thrush in infants born to mothers with candidal vaginitis. Nystatin is probably helpful in infants with cultures positive for *Candida,* as isolation of *C. albicans* from the mouth of a newborn often indicates an impending clinical appearance of oral thrush.

TABLE 15–1.
Antifungal Agents for Topical or Systemic Infection Caused by *Candida* and Other Fungi

Agent (Trade Name)	Route of Administration	Indications	Comments
Nystatin (Mycostatin)	Topical, PO	Mucocutaneous candidiasis	Narrow spectrum, no GI absorption, insoluble, long experience
Amphotericin B (Fungizone)	IV, topical	Candidal and most other invasive or systemic fungal infections	Broad spectrum, effective, considerable toxicity
Flucytosine (Ancobon)	PO	Cryptococcosis, candidiasis, torulopsosis, chromomycosis	Rapid emergence of resistance, often used in combination with amphotericin B, bone marrow toxicity
Griseofulvin (Grifulvin V, Grisactin) (oral)	PO	Dermatophytic infections	Skin rash, urticaria, GI symptoms, proteinuria, leukopenia
Clotrimazole (Lotrimin)	Topical, PO	Candidiasis, dermatophytic infections	GI toxicity, poor GI absorption
Miconazole (Monistat)	Topical	Candidiasis, dermatophytic infections	Few side effects, local irritations
	IV		Phlebitis, pruritus, rash, GI symptoms, anemia
Ketoconazole (Nizoral)	PO	Candidiasis, coccidioidomycosis, histoplasmosis, chromomycosis, paracoccidioidomycosis	Broad spectrum, few toxic effects, poor cerebrospinal fluid levels, hepatic dysfunction

Infants with oral thrush or cutaneous lesions do not require isolation; however, because the infection is transmissible by direct contact, handwashing should be emphasized by all personnel in contact with the patient. General guidelines used in the prevention of infections associated with catheters or intravenous therapy should be applied to the care of sick infants.

There are several useful antifungal agents for topical or systemic therapy of infections caused by *Candida* and other fungi (Table 15–1).[5, 6] Although the pharmacokinetics and toxicity of most of these agents are well established in adults, only limited information is available in neonates. Nystatin and amphotericin have been used frequently in neonates. Experience with other systemic antifungal agents in newborns and young infants is very limited; thus, routine use of these agents in small infants is not recommended at this time.

Amphotericin B.—Amphotericin B is derived from a strain of *Streptomyces nodosus*. It inhibits many species of fungi, including *Candida* species,

Histoplasma capsulatum, Coccidioides immitis, Blastomyces dermatitidis, Cryptococcus neoformans, Sporothrix schenckii, Aspergillus fumigatus, Mucor mucedo, and *Rhodotorula.* The minimal inhibitory concentrations (MIC) range from 0.03 to 1.0 μg/mL. Amphotericin B probably increases membrane permeability through binding to sterols in the fungus and permits leakage of various small molecules. It may have similar effects on human cell membranes. The drug is effective when administered topically and is not absorbed adequately in the gastrointestinal tract. Intravenous injections are needed for treatment of serious fungal infections.

The pharmacokinetics and toxicity of amphotericin B in newborns are unknown; information provided here is from studies in older children and adults. The usual daily doses (up to 0.65 mg/kg) of amphotericin B produce peak plasma levels of approximately 2 to 4 μg/mL. Approximately 5% to 10% of the plasma levels reach the CSF. The plasma half-life is approximately 24 hours. It is highly bound (90%) to plasma proteins. Amphotericin B is excreted very slowly by the kidney and can be detected in the urine 7 weeks after discontinuation of the drug.

Most patients receiving parenteral amphotericin B therapy will exhibit some intolerance, and patients may become tolerant to the drug. The adverse reactions in children and adults include fever, chills, headache, anorexia, nausea, vomiting, diarrhea, generalized pain, thrombophlebitis, and anemia. Some symptoms can be minimized by pretreatment with antipyretics, antihistamines, or corticosteroids. Renal dysfunction is the most significant side effect and includes azotemia, hypokalemia, renal tubular acidosis, and nephrocalcinosis. These effects are the result of direct renal tubular action and renal vasoconstriction. Other side effects that occur less frequently include cardiovascular toxicity, bone marrow suppression, eosinophilia, gastrointestinal bleeding, skin rash, neurologic symptoms, liver failure, flushing, and anaphylactoid reactions. Weekly monitoring of hematologic, renal, and hepatic functions as well as serum electrolyte levels is needed to detect early laboratory signs of side effects of amphotericin B. There are insufficient data available to define duration and total dosage requirements in infants.

Amphotericin B (Fungizone) is available in various formulations: 50 mg vials and 3% lotion.

Nystatin.—Nystatin, derived from *Streptomyces noursei,* is active against a wide variety of yeasts and yeastlike fungi. It is poorly absorbed after oral administration, and most of the drug is passed in the stool. It is well tolerated in neonates, and few adverse reactions have been reported. Large oral doses may produce gastrointestinal symptoms.

Nystatin (Mycostatin) is available in multiple formulations: (1) topical ointment, cream, or powder (100,000 U/g); (2) suspension (100,000 U/mL); (3) oral tablets (500,000 U); (4) vaginal tablets (100,000 U).

Flucytosine.—5-Fluorocytosine, a fluorinated pyrimidine, has antifungal activity against *Candida, Cryptococcus,* and other fungi. The drug is indicated in severe infections such as candidal sepsis, endocarditis, and urinary tract infection and cryptococcal meningitis and pneumonitis. Flucytosine is well absorbed from the gastrointestinal tract and is excreted primarily by the kidneys. The drug reaches the CSF easily; as much as 88% of serum levels can be detected in CSF. *Candida* and *Cryptococcus* often develop resistance to flucytosine during therapy; therefore, flucytosine frequently has been used in combination with amphotericin B, especially in cryptococcal meningitis. Experimental data suggest that amphotericin B and flucytosine act synergistically against *Candida* and *Cryptococcus.*

Flucytosine is given orally in a dose of 50 to 150 mg/kg/day in four divided doses for 2 to 6 weeks in older children and adults. Patients usually tolerate the drug well. Adverse reactions include nausea, vomiting, diarrhea, rash, anemia, leukopenia, thrombocytopenia, elevation of hepatic enzymes, blood urea nitrogen, and creatinine. Close monitoring of hepatic, renal, and hematopoietic functions is needed during therapy.

Flucytosine (Ancobon) is available as 250 and 500 mg capsules.

Prognosis

Oral or cutaneous candidiasis is a benign and self-limited disease in healthy infants. Spontaneous recovery usually occurs within 2 weeks to 2 months. Topical antifungal treatment enhances the recovery process, and most lesions resolve in approximately 7 days; however, relapse is common, and immunity against reinfection is absent. Persistence of infection or recurrent relapses are usually seen in malnourished infants, infants receiving antibiotic therapy, or patients with underlying defects in host defense.

Transient fungemia, especially associated with infected catheters or contaminated fluids for parenteral use, may resolve spontaneously when the infected source is removed.

Mortality is extremely high in infants with untreated disseminated candidiasis. Even with specific antifungal therapy the prognosis is guarded, especially in infants with underlying debilitating conditions. Mortality may be reduced by early recognition of the disease and early institution of antifungal therapy. Mental retardation and hydrocephalus are common in infants who survive candidal meningitis.

VIRAL INFECTIONS

The majority of viral infections in neonates and young infants are not amenable to drug therapy. However, several viral infections are now preventable or treatable, for example, hepatitis B (HBV), herpes simplex virus (HSV), varicella-zoster, respiratory syncytial virus (RSV), cytomegalovirus (CMV), and human immunodeficiency virus (HIV) (Table 15–2). Because of limited neonatal data on CMV and HIV at the present time, only infections caused by HBV, HSV, and RSV are discussed.

Herpes Simplex Virus Infections

Infections caused by HSV *(Herpesvirus hominis)* are universal and are common in children and adults. There are at least two serologically distinguishable subtypes (1 and 2) of HSV, with minor biologic, immunologic, biochemical, and epidemiologic differences between them. In general, type 1 virus (oral type) infects the mouth, eyes, skin, and central nervous system (CNS); type 2 (genital type) causes genital and neonatal infections. Type 1 infection also can involve the areas mentioned for type 2, and vice versa.

Herpes simplex virus chiefly produces subclinical infection, but it may cause a variety of clinical diseases involving localized tissues (e.g., mucous membranes, skin, eyes, and CNS), generalized systemic infection, or both. Localized infections occur primarily in healthy hosts; in contrast, disseminated infections usually occur in newborns and in patients with compromised host response.

Clinical disease caused by HSV may appear in two forms: primary or recurrent infection. Following the primary infection, HSV often becomes latent, and the disease tends to be reactivated at irregular intervals by various provocations, such as fever, trauma, emotional upsets, and gastrointestinal tract disorders.

Neonatal HSV infection is one of the few viral infections amenable to antiviral therapy. Therefore, early diagnosis and treatment of neonatal herpes are important.

Clinical Findings

Neonatal herpes usually is acquired during the infant's passage through the infected birth canal or through ascending infection from maternal genital herpes, and the majority of infants develop symptoms 3 to 7 days after birth. Infections may also be acquired postnatally through genital or nongenital routes from the infected mother or other contacts, and symptoms may occur any time during the newborn period. Because infection also may be acquired by way of intrauterine or transplacental routes, some infants have clinical disease at birth. In neonates, HSV infection may be disseminated or localized.

TABLE 15–2.
Viral Infection Therapy

Viral Infection	Prevention/Therapy
Hepatitis B virus	Hepatitis B immune globulin
	Hepatitis B vaccine
Herpes simplex virus	Acyclovir
	Vidarabine
Varicella-zoster virus	Acyclovir
	Vidarabine
Respiratory syncytial virus	Ribavirin (aerosol)
Cytomegalovirus	Ganciclovir (potential)
Human immunodeficiency virus	Azidothymidine (AZT) (potential)

Disseminated infection is seen in approximately two thirds of patients and is most useful in differentiating herpes from other congenital infections. The vesicular lesions often appear in clusters on the scalp or face, but may appear anywhere on the skin. In disseminated infection, systemic symptoms may develop within a few days after the appearance of the vesicles. The skin lesions resemble neonatal impetigo, and usually resolve spontaneously within days, but some infants have recurrent episodes of skin lesions for weeks, months, or years without other systemic symptoms.

CNS involvement occurs in approximately 50% of infected newborns, usually manifested by irritability and seizures. The CSF usually shows a moderate pleocytosis (50 to 200 white blood cells/mm) and markedly elevated protein levels.

Laboratory Diagnosis

Diagnosis of neonatal herpes is not difficult if the infant develops typical vesicular lesions during the first week of life. A history of parental genital herpes is often helpful; however, when infection involves the CNS or other internal organs in the absence of external lesions, diagnosis may be difficult. The following tests generally are used to confirm the clinical diagnosis of HSV infection.

Virus Isolation.—Isolation of HSV in cell cultures is the most reliable method for diagnosis. Swabs from the infected lesions (e.g., skin, mouth, or eye) or tissues (e.g., brain biopsy) generally show characteristic cytopathic effects in cell cultures within 1 to 3 days. Other specimens (e.g., urine, stool, and CSF) should be submitted for viral isolation to determine the extent of involvement. A cervical swab specimen from the mother may help trace the source of infection.

Cytologic or Histologic Examination.—Smears from the infected lesions or tissue sections may be stained with hematoxylin and eosin, Giemsa, or Papanicolaou (cervical smears) stains. Demonstration of characteristic multinucleated giant cells containing intranuclear eosinophilic inclusions in the smears or inclusions in tissue sections is suggestive of HSV infection. This finding should be supported by viral isolation.

Detection of HSV Antigen.—Infected cells (smears or tissue sections) containing HSV antigens can be detected rapidly within 1 to 2 hours by the fluorescent antibody staining technique.

Antibody Studies.—Determination of HSV antibodies (IgG, IgM) in serum is not helpful in the diagnosis of neonatal HSV infection, because high titers of maternally transferred HSV IgG antibodies are detected in the serum of the majority of infants, and false positive or false negative results may be obtained with the currently available tests for HSV IgM antibiotics.

Prevention

It is recommended that pregnant women with genital herpes (primary or recurrent), who have a past history of genital lesions, or have a sexual partner with genital herpetic lesions should be monitored with virologic or cytologic studies during the final 6 to 8 weeks of pregnancy. At present, isolation of HSV in cell culture is the most reliable method. The baby can be delivered vaginally if a woman is free of active lesions and viral cultures are negative on two successive examinations, with the last negative study having been obtained within 1 week of delivery. It should be pointed out that antepartum cultures may not predict asymptomatic shedding at delivery and that premature onset of labor is common in women with HSV infection. Most neonatal exposure to HSV results from excretion of virus by asymptomatic mothers at delivery. Therefore it has been suggested that weekly cultures for HSV may not be cost effective or efficacious.

Cesarean Section.—It is recommended that pregnant women with active herpetic genital lesions, active cervical herpes, or positive virus culture deliver their infants by cesarean section. It appears that if membranes are ruptured for more than 6 hours (especially more than 12 hours), the fetus probably has been exposed to the virus; therefore cesarean section would not be protective. Nahmias et al.[18] have shown that the risk of neonatal infection is increased if the baby is delivered vaginally or if there is a rupture of membranes for more than 4 hours prior to delivery. Many obstetricians elect for cesarean delivery whenever the birth canal is infected, even if membranes had previously ruptured.

Direct Contact.— Transmission of HSV may occur in the newborn nursery. Newborns should be protected from exposure to or contact with nursery personnel or family members with observable active infection, either primary or recurrent. Such precautions also should be applied to infants with open skin lesions (e.g., eczema, burns) and infants with compromised cellular immunity, although the neonatal risk of asymptomatic nursery personnel or family members with positive HSV cultures and with cold sores is unknown.

Breast-feeding is not contraindicated if the mother has no herpetic lesions on the breast and active lesions are covered. The mother should observe handwashing precautions prior to feeding and handling the infant. Rooming-in is permissible. Circumcision should be postponed if the risk of HSV infection is great (i.e., the baby is vaginally delivered by a mother with herpetic lesions).

Antiviral Therapy

Acyclovir and vidarabine are equally effective in the treatment of neonatal HSV infections. Acyclovir is the drug of choice because of lower toxicity and ease of administration.

Ara-A.—A purine nucleoside, 9-β-D-arabinofuranosyl adenine (Adenine arabinoside, Vidarabine, Vira-A), appears to inhibit viral DNA synthesis by inhibiting the DNA polymerase activity. It has a higher affinity for viral DNA inhibition than for host cell DNA.

In humans ara-A is deaminated to arabinosyl-hypoxanthine (ara-H_x), which also has antiviral activity. The pharmacokinetics and safety data are derived mostly from studies in adults. The plasma half-life of ara-A is approximately 4 hours. The active drug and its metabolites accumulate in erythrocytes over 5 to 7 days and persist as long as 3 weeks. The highest drug levels can be found in kidney, liver, and spleen, and lower levels in muscle and brain. Cerebrospinal fluid levels are approximately half the serum levels. Constant infusions of 10 to 15 mg/kg/day over 12 hours produce peak serum levels of ara-H_x of 4 to 8 μg/mL. After reaching steady state there is no significant extracellular accumulation following multiple-dose administration. The kidneys are the major sites of clearance of ara-A from the body. In patients with impaired renal function ara-H_x may accumulate in the plasma and reach potentially toxic levels. The dosage in neonates and young infants is 15 to 30 mg/kg/day given in 12-hour intravenous infusions for 10 to 14 days. Adverse reactions include anorexia, nausea, vomiting, diarrhea, tremor, dizziness, hallucinations, confusion, psychosis, ataxia, anemia, leukopenia, thrombocytopenia, and elevations of aspartate aminotransferase (AST, SGOT). These reactions are mild to moderate and rarely necessitate discontinuation of ara-A therapy.[27]

Acyclovir.—Acyclovir (acycloguanosine, Zovirax), a guanine derivative containing an acyclic side chain at the 9 position (a synthesized nucleoside analog), has potent antiviral activity with very low toxicity. This acyclic nucleoside analog is converted to a monophosphate by a virus-specified thymidine kinase and is subsequently converted to acyclovir diphosphate and triphosphate. In the uninfected host cell these phosphorylations of acyclovir occur to a very limited extent. Acyclovir triphosphate inhibits HSV DNA polymerase 10 to 30 times more effectively than cellular DNA polymerase.

The cellular half-life in patients receiving intravenous infusions ranges from 2.1 to 4.8 hours. Acyclovir or its metabolites are mostly excreted by the kidneys, and there is no evidence for acyclovir accumulation during the course of therapy. Crystalluria has been reported.

The dosage in neonates and young infants is 30 mg/kg/day in three divided doses given intravenously for 10 to 14 days. The drug is well tolerated. The reported adverse reactions include phlebitis, transient elevation of creatinine, and rash.

Determination of plasma and CSF concentrations of acyclovir indicates that neonates receiving acyclovir (10 mg/kg/dose) every 8 hours at 0 to 11 days of age had significantly higher peak (51.7 ± 13.5 μmol/L) and trough (11.6 ± 6.7 μmol/L) levels than the peak (34.6 ± 7.1 μmol/L) and trough (5.4 ± 2.1 μmol/L) levels in neonates 18 to 61 days of age. The acyclovir levels in CSF were comparable to trough levels in each respective age group. These levels were 30 to 350 times the MIC for HSV-1 (0.15 μmol/L) and 3 to 30 times the MIC for HSV-2 (1.62 μmol/L).[15]

Prognosis

In the majority of infants with primary HSV infection after the newborn period the disease is self-limited and the prognosis generally good. Death may occur in newborns and in patients with meningoencephalitis, severe eczema herpeticum, or severe malnutrition. Neurologic sequelae are common among those recovering from meningoencephalitis. Gingivostomatitis may recur frequently, causing temporary pain and inconvenience. Recurrent keratitis may result in scarring of the cornea and blindness. Recurrent HSV skin eruptions are common in infants recovered from neonatal herpes, but usually do not require additional treatment.

Mortality of neonatal herpes depends on the extent of involvement.[28] Disseminated infection with or without CNS involvement carries a mortality of 70% to 90%. Severe growth and psychomotor retardation occurs in approximately half of the patients who survive. Blindness may occur as the result of corneal scarring, chorioretinitis, cataracts, or optic atrophy. Prognosis for infants with isolated skin lesions generally is good, although some infants have developed severe psychomotor retardation and ocular sequelae in late infancy or early childhood, suggesting that CNS involvement can occur even in infants without apparent CNS symptoms and signs. Subclinical infection due to HSV has been reported in a few newborns, but its frequency is not known. Congenital malformations associated with HSV infection have also been described in a limited number of infants (e.g., with microcephaly, intracranial calcification, microphthalmus, and psychomotor retardation).[18]

Hepatitis B Virus

Hepatitis B virus (HBV) infection remains an important public health problem. Recent results with hepatitis B vaccines and hepatitis B immunoglobulin (HBIg) indicate that effective means for prevention of hepatitis B are now available. Although several antiviral agents have been tested, there is no effective drug therapy for hepatitis B at the present time.

Most available information on hepatitis in neonates concerns hepatitis B. Hepatitis A is not a major problem in neonates, and transplacental infection probably does not occur.[26] Data are incomplete concerning non-A, non-B hepatitis in newborn infants.

HBV is a DNA virus with a size of 43 nm (Dane particle) and contains three distinct antigens: hepatitis B surface antigen (HBsAg), hepatitis B core antigen (HBcAg), and hepatitis B e antigen (HBeAg). The e antigen is an integral part of the Dane particle and is closely associated with the infectious nature of hepatitis B virus infection. Infection with HBV usually is associated with the development of antibodies to the above three antigens: anti-HBs, anti-HBc, and anti-HBe. These antigens and antibodies are useful clinically and epidemiologically as markers of HBV infection in the majority of neonatal hepatitis B acquired perinatally.

Transmission

Pregnant women with positive HBsAg may transmit hepatitis B to their newborn infants. Neonates may acquire the infection from a mother who has acute hepatitis B infection or who is a symptomatic chronic carrier. Schweitzer et al.[24] demonstrated that the frequency of HBV transmission from mothers to infants is low (10%) when acute hepatitis occurs in the first 2 trimesters of pregnancy and high (76%) when it occurs in the third trimester and within 2 months after delivery. Infection may be transmitted to the infant (1) by the transplacental route, (2) by contamination during delivery, or (3) after birth by fecal-oral spread or breast milk.

Perinatal transmission of hepatitis B from asymptomatic carrier mothers to their infants is relatively common. The rate of perinatal transmission varies. It is high (40% to 73%) in Taiwan and Japan and low (0% to 14%) in the United States, Denmark, Greece, Pakistan, Thailand, and England.[8] It appears that the risk of transmission of hepatitis B from mothers to infants is increased by the presence of HBeAg. Recent studies in Taiwan indicate that when the HBsAg-positive mother is HBeAg-positive (approximately 40% of carriers), her infant will have a 90% chance of acquiring the infection and of becoming a chronic carrier. On the other hand, if the HBsAg-positive mother is HBeAg-negative, the attack rate in the infant is less than 20% and the infant is likely to recover completely and does not become a chronic carrier.

Clinical Findings

Maternal hepatitis B infection during pregnancy has not been associated with an increased risk of abortion, stillbirth, or congenital anomalies, but there is a high incidence of premature birth (35%) and low birth weight.[24] Neonatal hepatitis B infection, as demonstrated by antigenemia, may be symptomatic (icteric) or asymptomatic (anicteric). The clinical course of perinatally acquired hepatitis B is shown in Figure 15–1. The majority of infants acquiring hepatitis B infection perinatally remain anicteric and show no signs of acute illness, but often become chronic HBsAg carriers with variable transaminase elevations. A small number of infants are symptomatic, with jaundice and elevation of liver enzymes between 2 weeks to 5 months of age. These symptomatic babies may recover completely or develop hepatitis B antibodies. Death from fulminant neonatal hepatitis is rare.

The long-term effects of chronic hepatitis B infection in neonates are not fully known. There is sufficient evidence to suggest that the carrier state enhances the risk of development of serious liver disease, such as cirrhosis and hepatoma, in later life.

Prevention

There is no effective antiviral agent for hepatitis virus infections at present. However, preventive measures are available for hepatitis A (passive immunization), hepatitis B (active and passive immunizations), and possibly hepatitis non-A, non-B (passive immunization).

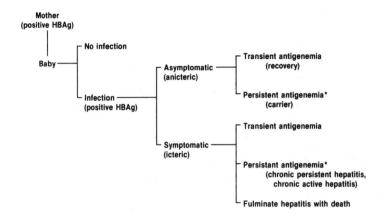

FIG 15–1.
Clinical course of perinatally acquired hepatitis B infection. HBAg = hepatitis B surface antigen. Persistent antigenemia (*) increases the risk for development of cirrhosis or hepatoma in later life.

Isolation procedures should be applied to patients with possible hepatitis virus infection. As an initial approach, all patients should be managed with precautions applicable for all hepatitis (A, B, and non-A, non-B), namely enteric plus blood precautions. Once the type of hepatitis is known, appropriate procedures may be used. Hepatitis A infection is most contagious before the onset of jaundice and early stage of clinical illness; therefore, enteric precautions for 1 week after the onset of jaundice are required for the infected young infants. Hepatitis B infection should be followed with blood precautions until HBsAg becomes negative.

Hepatitis A.—If the mother has jaundice at the time of delivery, immunoglobulin (Ig), 0.02 mL/kg intramuscularly, may be given to the baby. However, data are not available on the need for such prophylaxis.

All household contacts should be given Ig (0.02 mL/kg) as soon as possible after exposure (but not to exceed 2 weeks). Recent observations suggest that outbreaks of hepatitis A infection among infants in day care centers may occur, with transmission of the infection to staff and household contacts. Meticulous handwashing after changing diapers is essential.

Hepatitis B.—Recent studies indicate that combined use of HBIg and hepatitis B vaccine is highly effective for the prevention of hepatitis B in neonates born to hepatitis B carrier mothers. Therefore, newborns of HBsAg-positive mothers should receive (1) 0.5 mL HBIg intramuscularly within a few hours after birth and (2) hepatitis B vaccine, 0.5 mL intramuscularly at birth, and the injections should be repeated at 1 month and 6 months. The infant's serum should be tested again at 9 to 12 months to determine success or failure of the prophylaxis. A fourth dose of the vaccine may be given if the infant remains seronegative.

Detection of HBsAg-positive pregnant women is critical in preventing neonatal infection. Routine prenatal screening of all pregnant women for HBsAg is recommended. Guidelines for the care of mothers and their newborn infants at high risk for hepatitis B are listed in Figure 15–2. Recent studies indicate that breast-feeding by HBsAg-positive mothers does not increase the risk of infection in the infant.

Hepatitis non-A, non-B.—Data on prophylaxis of hepatitis non-A, non-B are not available. Until additional information becomes available, it is recommended that Ig 0.5 mL intramuscularly should be given as soon as possible after delivery and this treatment repeated at 3 and 6 months of age. The efficacy of this prophylactic regimen is not known.

Respiratory Syncytial Virus Infection

Respiratory syncytial virus (RSV) is the major cause of bronchiolitis and pneumonia in infants younger than 1 year of age. It causes significant mor-

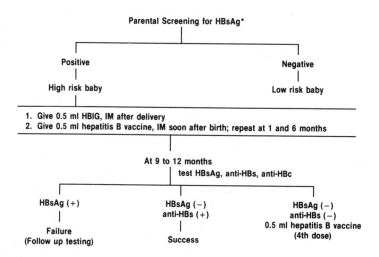

FIG 15–2.
Guidelines for the care of infants of HBsAg = positive mothers. Pregnant mothers at high risk (*) (1) have liver disease; (2) were born in Asia, Africa, the Caribbean, or South America; (3) are of Pacific Islands or native Alaskan descent; (4) are screened from giving blood; (5) work or reside in an institution for the mentally retarded; (6) work in hemodialysis unit or are receiving hemodialysis; (7) are illicit injectable drug users; (8) are hepatitis B household contacts; (9) require repeated blood transfusions (e.g., thalassemia, hemophilia); (10) have occupational exposure to blood.

bidity and mortality in infants with underlying disease, such as congenital heart disease, bronchopulmonary dysplasia, cystic fibrosis, and immunodeficiency. In addition, it is an important cause of nosocomial infection in hospitalized children.

An RNA virus, RSV has the morphologic appearance of parainfluenza virus or mumps virus (paramyxoviruses), but it contains no hemagglutinin or neuraminidase. At present its classification is undetermined (pneumoviruses). It appears that different strains of RSV contain heterogenous antigens, but this variation is not detectable with human sera. The virus behaves epidemiologically as a single serotype.

The infection is distributed worldwide. It has two epidemiologic characteristics, namely, yearly outbreaks and infection of young infants. Epidemics usually peak in January, February, or March, but may occur from December to June. The virus is usually transmitted by direct contact or droplets. The majority (over 90%) of infected infants shed virus for about 9 days (range 3 to 23 days).

During RSV epidemics the virus may be prevalent among hospital staff with upper respiratory tract symptoms. Efforts should be made to reduce the transmission of RSV from infected infants to hospital staff and from infected staff to uninfected infants. Infants with runny nose or unexplained apnea during RSV epidemics should be examined for RSV infection.

Diagnosis is usually accomplished by isolation of the virus from nasopharyngeal secretions. Rapid diagnostic techniques to identify RSV antigens are now available. Enzyme-linked immunosorbent assay or immunofluorescent antibody staining is commonly used.

Clinical Findings

Infection by RSV in older infants usually results in low-grade fever accompanied by acute respiratory symptoms, such as clear nasal discharge, cough, wheezing, tachypnea, and dyspnea. Infection in neonates may be asymptomatic or mildly symptomatic, with upper respiratory syndrome without fever, or may cause fever, with bronchiolitis or pneumonia, apnea, and cyanosis requiring ventilatory support.[7] Some infected neonates, particularly premature infants, show only nonspecific signs, such as apnea, lethargy, irritability, poor feeding, bronchiolitis, and pneumonia.

Infants older than 3 weeks have a higher incidence of lower respiratory tract symptoms. In infants younger than 3 weeks, at the time when maternal antibody is the highest, respiratory symptoms are severe. Serious infection is uncommon in infants with high titer maternal transferred RSV antibody.[16] Severe infections are usually seen in infants with underlying cardiopulmonary disorder, particularly premature infants recovering from hyaline membrane disease and bronchopulmonary dysplasia.

Treatment

The beneficial effects of ribavirin therapy in RSV infection have been reported.[11, 12, 25] Ribavirin in aerosolized form has been approved by the U.S. Food and Drug Administration for treatment of RSV infections in hospitalized children who do not require assisted ventilation. It is administered by an oxygen hood or tent and is delivered by a small-particle aerosol generator. For RSV lower respiratory tract infection, ribavirin is given over 12 to 20 hours each day for 3 to 7 days.

Ribavirin (Virazole), a synthetic neucleoside analogue, has broad-spectrum antiviral activity against RSV and other RNA and DNA viruses. It appears to interfere with the transcription of messenger RNA and to inhibit the synthesis of viral protein. In patients receiving aerosol treatment, significant concentrations of ribavirin can be detected in the respiratory secretions, with little systemic absorption. Teratogenicity has been reported in pregnant rodents. Toxic effects of ribavirin in aerosolized form have not been observed in the published studies. The long-term effects of ribavirin on pulmonary functions are being examined. Risk to caregivers exposed to aerosols is probably minimal or none. Toxicity to very low birth weight infants and pregnant women remains unknown. However, it is advised that pregnant women should not participate in the care of patients who are receiving ribavirin aerosol treatment.

The drug can precipitate and clog the ventilator line. Proper filtering devices are needed to avoid the deposition. Technical difficulties are often encountered in administering ribavirin to infants receiving assisted ventilation, and special expertise and precautions are necessary. The package insert warns against the use of this drug in infants requiring assisted ventilation.

Indications for Ribavirin Therapy

The mortality of RSV infection in normal infants is low (less than 1%); however, significant morbidity and mortality have been reported in infants with underlying disease. It has been suggested[20] that ribavirin therapy may be considered in the following groups:

1. Infants at high risk for severe or complicated RSV infection (i.e., those with congenital heart disease, bronchopulmonary dysplasia, immunodeficiency, and certain premature infants)
2. Severely ill infants with severe hypoxemia and hypercapnea
3. Infants with some increased risk of progressing to a more complicated course (i.e., multiple congenital anomalies, neurologic or metabolic disease)

Information pertaining to the efficacy and safety of ribavirin therapy in neonates is limited. It is not known whether ribavirin reduces the need for subsequent assisted ventilation. Long-term adverse effects on the neonate, especially premature infants, remain to be determined. Additional studies may be needed before accepting it as safe and efficacious.

TOXOPLASMOSIS

Congenital toxoplasmosis, caused by *Toxoplasma gondii,* is the result of a primary infection occurring in a pregnant woman. The incidence of congenital infection varies with geographic location, cooking habits, and hygiene. In Paris the risk of maternal infections is 6.3 per 100 pregnancies per year[9]; in the United States the risk is 0.15 to 0.6 per 100 pregnancies per year. The high incidence in Paris is related to the habit of eating raw or undercooked meat in an endemic area.

Toxoplasmosis in the pregnant mother usually causes no symptoms. Involvement of the fetus may lead to abortion, prematurity, stillbirth, and asymptomatic infection in the newborn. Asymptomatic infection is the most common form; some infants may develop symptoms months or even years later, with clinical presentation of CNS involvement or chorioretinitis. The classic triad of chorioretinitis, hydrocephalus, and intracranial calcification occurs only in a small number of the most severely affected infants.

T. gondii is an ubiquitous obligate intracellular protozoan. Three forms exist in nature: trophozoites, tissue cysts, and oocysts. Humans are infected by (1) tissue cysts from the meat of infected animals; (2) oocysts, which are present in soil contaminated by cat feces; or (3) trophozoites by the transplacental route.

The risk of fetal involvement by *Toxoplasma* organisms depends on the time of maternal infection in relation to gestational age. Primary infections acquired before conception do not involve the fetus. Approximately 40% of maternal infections spread to the fetus.[9] The majority (66%) of fetal infections occur during the third trimester; maternal infection during the first and second trimesters results in fetal infection in 17% and 27% of cases, respectively. Infection acquired during the first and second trimesters is associated with more severe disease, whereas infection acquired during the third trimester often results in asymptomatic toxoplasmosis.

Presence of antibodies in maternal serum is associated with immunity to fetal infection. Occurrence of infection in successive pregnancies has been reported, but is an exceptional event.

Clinical Findings

The majority of infants with congenital toxoplasmosis have no symptoms. It has been estimated that perhaps only 10% of infected infants show signs of clinical disease on routine examination; however, this figure may increase to 30% if careful eye examinations are performed.[1, 9] Symptomatic newborns have chorioretinitis, hepatosplenomegaly, lymphadenopathy, jaundice, anemia, hydromicrocephaly, and psychomotor and mental retardation.

Laboratory Diagnosis

Approximately 90% of women infected during pregnancy are asymptomatic; therefore, diagnosis must be made by laboratory tests. Laboratory methods for confirmation of congenital toxoplasmosis include (1) aerologic diagnosis (dye test, IgM fluorescent antibody test); (2) isolation of *Toxoplasma* in susceptible animals (mice, hamsters, or rabbits); (3) demonstration of the organisms in tissue sections (placenta) or smears with Giemsa or periodic acid–Schiff staining; and (4) levels of serum IgM. Serologic methods and serum IgM levels (nonspecific) are used most commonly.

Serologic diagnosis by Sabin-Feldman dye test or other methods is useful but may be difficult during the first few weeks or even months of life, because maternal IgG is transferred to the fetus. Two methods are available to differentiate maternal antibodies from antibodies synthesized by the infant: (1) demonstration of the presence of specific IgM antibodies by indirect fluorescent antibody method and (2) quantitation of the amount of antibodies persisting in the infant's serum in the early months of life (Table 15–3).

TABLE 15–3.
Serologic Diagnosis of *Toxoplasma* Infection in Pregnant Women and Newborns*

Condition	Dye Test Titer[†]	IgM-IFA Test[‡]	Infection or Risk to Baby
Pregnant a few weeks	Negative: <1:4	Negative	Susceptible
	Positive	Negative	Past infection (minimal risk to baby)
	Positive No rise in titer (in 3 weeks)	Positive	Acquired prior to pregnancy (minimal risk to baby)
	Rise in titer (in 3 weeks)		Acquired within 2 months (low risk to baby; spontaneous abortion more likely)
Pregnant a few months with suspected acute infection (lymphadenopathy)	Positive: >1:1,000	Positive	Probable infection (risk to baby)
	Positive <1:1,000 rise in titer (in 2 to 3 weeks)	Positive	Infection (risk to baby)
Newborn with suspected congenital toxoplasmosis	Positive: 1:1,200 to 1:12,000	Positive	Most often present
	Positive: 1:4,000 to 1:12,000	Negative	Often present
	Positive: 1:1,200 to 1:4,000	Negative	Seldom present
	Positive: <1:1,200	Positive	Possible[§]
	Positive: <1:1,200	Negative	Excluded

*Modified from Remington JS, Desmonts G: Toxoplasmosis, in Remington JS, Klein JO (eds): *Infectious Disease of the Fetus and Newborn Infant*, ed 2. Philadelphia, WB Saunders Co, 1983, pp 636–678.
†Dye-test titer: 300 IU/mL (1:1200), 1,000 IU/mL (1:4,000), 3,000 IU/mL (1:12,000).
‡IgM-IFA = IgM indirect fluorescent antibody test.
§Rising maternal dye test titer indicates infection; no rising titer indicates no infection.

Treatment

The suggested treatment regimen for toxoplasmosis in children and adults consists of pyrimethamine (2 mg/kg/day in two divided doses for 1 to 3 days, followed by 1 mg/kg/day in two doses, not to exceed 25 mg/kg/day) plus sulfadiazine or triple sulfonamides (120 to 150 mg/day in four divided doses). Both drugs are given orally, and the duration of therapy is approximately 4 weeks or longer. Folinic acid (leukovorin calcium), 5 to 10 mg/day, is given to reduce the antifolate effect of pyrimethamine. The use of steroids is controversial and is reserved for progressive chorioretinitis.

The drug of choice, optimal dosage schedule, and duration of therapy for congenital toxoplasmosis in newborn infants are unknown. The following treatment schedule has been used by some workers[19]:

1. Pyrimethamine plus sulfadiazine (21-day course)
   Pyrimethamine (Daraprim), 1 mg/kg/day orally (as the half-life of the drug is 1 to 5 days, the dose of 1 mg/kg can be given every 2 to 4 days) (?)
   Sulfadiazine, 50 to 100 mg/kg/day orally in two divided doses
2. Spiramycin (30- to 45-day course), 100 mg/kg/day orally in two divided doses
3. Corticosteroids (prednisone or methylprednisolone), 1 to 3 mg/kg/day orally in two divided doses, until acute inflammatory process (e.g., high CSF protein level, chorioretinitis) has subsided, then taper slowly
4. Folinic acid (calcium leucovorin), 5 mg twice weekly during pyrimethamine treatment for prevention of folic acid or folinic acid deficiency

Remington and Desmonts[19] recommend that therapy be continued for 1 year. The infant is given three to four courses of pyrimethamine plus sulfadiazine, separated by spiramycin therapy. Spiramycin, a macrolide antibiotic similar to erythromycin, has been used in Europe, Canada, and Mexico. It is not licensed in the United States but can be obtained by contacting the Centers for Disease Control in Atlanta. Others have recommended 4 to 6 weeks of therapy. Data on the need for long-term (1 year) therapy are not available at this time. Clindamycin and sulfadiazine (120 to 150 mg/kg/day) may be considered for ocular disease.

The side effects of sulfadiazine-pyrimethamine therapy (anorexia, vomiting, atrophic glossitis, bone marrow depression) are dose related. Blood counts (white blood cell, platelet, reticulocyte) should be done twice weekly to monitor the side effects of drug therapy.

Prevention

Neither active nor passive immunization against toxoplasmosis is available at the present time. Susceptible pregnant women (approximately 70% in the United States) should avoid exposure to *T. gondii,* as follows[10, 29]:

1. Avoid eating raw or undercooked meats (<66° C).
2. Avoid touching mucous membranes of the mouth and eyes while handling raw meat.
3. Wash hands carefully after handling raw meat and wash kitchen surfaces that come into contact with raw meat.
4. Wash fruits and vegetables before consumption.
5. Control flies and cockroaches.
6. Keep the household cat from hunting, and feed it only dried, canned, or cooked meat.
7. Delegate maintenance of the cat to someone other than the pregnant woman; change litterboxes daily and disinfect them with boiling water.
8. Use gloves when working in soil contaminated with cat feces.
9. Cover children's sandboxes when not in use.
10. Wash hands before meals and before touching the face.

A satisfactory means for preventing or controlling fetal infection after diagnosis of primary infection in the pregnant mother is not available. European workers have used spiramycin and sulfonamides with or without pyrimethamine with some success.[9, 19] Pyrimethamine is probably too teratogenic and therefore is not recommended for use during the first trimester. The safety of these drugs in pregnancy has not been fully evaluated. Therapeutic abortion may be considered, especially if the infection occurs during the first trimester.

Prognosis

Congenital toxoplasmosis is associated with high morbidity and mortality. The severely affected symptomatic infant may die within days or weeks or survive with high incidence (50% to 90%) of neurologic sequelae such as hydrocephalus, microcephaly, blindness, psychomotor retardation, and convulsive disorders. The efficacy of drug therapy in congenital toxoplasmosis is difficult to evaluate. Therapy may prevent further tissue damage, but regression is unlikely in the irreparable damaged tissues.

CHLAMYDIAL INFECTIONS

Chlamydiae are obligate intracellular bacteria that have the characteristics of viruses (e.g., intracellular microorganisms) and bacteria (e.g., sensitive to antibiotics). Two major species of *Chlamydia* (*C. trachomatis* and *C. psittaci*) are capable of causing diseases in humans and animals.[21–23] Clinically, *C.*

trachomatis causes localized disease in the eyes (e.g., trachoma, conjunctivitis, ophthalmia neonatorum), genitourinary tract (e.g., nongonococcal urethritis, postgonococcal urethritis, lymphogranuloma venerum), and lungs (pneumonitis of young infants); *C. psittaci* usually causes generalized disease with hematogenous dissemination and vasculitis (e.g., psittacosis, ornithosis).

Infection in newborns usually is acquired at the time of delivery from transvaginal passage in infected mothers. Transmission by direct contamination may occur in conjunctivitis. *C. trachomatis* can be found in 2% to 24% (usually 5% to 10%) of cervical cultures in pregnant women. Approximately 30% to 50% of infants whose mothers are infected develop conjunctivitis, 10% to 20% develop nasopharyngeal infections, and 3% to 18% develop pneumonia. In addition, *C. trachomatis* also can be isolated from the feces (20%) and from vaginal swabs (10% to 20%) of exposed infants.

Clinical Findings

The major clinical features of *C. trachomatis* are conjunctivitis and pneumonia; *C. trachomatis* also may cause otitis media or other forms of respiratory tract illness.

Conjunctivitis

Chlamydial conjunctivitis (inclusion blennorrhea) usually occurs at 5 to 14 days of age. The conjunctivitis is characterized by hyperemia, follicular hypertrophy, and mucopurulent exudate and may be associated with rhinitis. The organisms infect mainly the superficial epithelial cells, and the infection heals spontaneously over weeks or months.

Diagnosis can be made by examining the smears or scrapings by Giemsa or immunofluorescent staining. Giemsa stain shows bluish granular cytoplasmic inclusions in the epithelial cells. Culture for *Chlamydia* in tissue cultures can be accomplished in a specialized virology laboratory.

Chlamydial Pneumonitis

A distinctive clinical pneumonitis syndrome in infancy associated with *C. trachomatis* was described by Beem and Saxon.[3, 14] They reported a pneumonitis that developed gradually over the first 6 weeks of life with (1) nasal congestion and discharge, (2) staccato cough and tachypnea, and (3) little systemic reaction (afebrile and feeding well). The chest radiograph generally shows hyperinflation with diffuse interstitial and patchy alveolar infiltrates. Blood studies may show increased levels of IgG and IgM.

Topical erythromycin or tetracycline has been used in prophylaxis of ophthalmia neonatorum, but may not prevent nasopharyngeal colonization and does not prevent all chlamydial conjunctivitis.[13] It generally is recommended that ophthalmic ointment containing tetracycline (1%) or erythromycin (0.5%) be given as a single application, soon after delivery, into each conjunctival sac, with no rinsing of the eyes. To avoid cross-contamination, a single-use tube or ampule is preferred.

Pneumonitis of Infancy

The natural history of chlamydial pneumonia has not been well delineated. The efficacy of antibiotic therapy and optimal duration for treatment of this disease have not been established. It is suggested, however, that the infant be given oral erythromycin syrup, 40 mg/kg/day in four divided doses, for 2 to 3 weeks. It is the general impression that most infants show some improvement after 1 week of therapy and that the nasopharyngeal shedding of *C. trachomatis* is reduced. Sulfisoxazole (150 mg/kg/day) is equally effective.[4]

REFERENCES

1. Alford CA Jr, Stagno S, Reynolds DW: Congenital toxoplasmosis: Clinical, laboratory and therapeutic considerations, with special reference to subclinical disease. *Bull NY Acad Med* 1974; 50:160–181.
2. Baley JE, Kliegman RM, Fanaroff AA: Disseminated fungal infections in very low-birth-weight infants: Clinical manifestations and epidemiology. *Pediatrics* 1984; 73:144–152.
3. Beem MO, Saxon EM: Respiratory tract colonization and a distinctive pneumonia syndrome in infants with *Chlamydia trachomatis. N Engl J Med* 1977; 296:306–310.
4. Beem MO, Saxon EM, Tipple M: Treatment of chlamydia pneumonia in infancy. *Pediatrics* 1979; 63:198–203.
5. Bennett JE: Chemotherapy of systemic mycosis. Part I. *N Engl J Med* 1974; 290:30–31.
6. Bennett JE: Chemotherapy of systemic mycosis. Part II. *N Engl J Med* 1974; 290:320–321.
7. Bruhn FW, Mokrohisky ST, McIntosh K: Apnea associated with respiratory syncytial virus infection in young infants. *J Pediatr* 1977; 90:382.
8. Crumpacker CS: Hepatitis, in Remington JS, Klein JO (eds): *Infectious Disease of the Fetus and Newborn Infant,* ed 2. Philadelphia, WB Saunders Co, 1983, pp 591–618.
9. Desmonts G, Couvreru J: Congenital toxoplasmosis. A prospective study of 378 pregnancies. *N Engl J Med* 1974; 290:1110–1116.
10. Frenkel JK: Pathology and pathogenesis of congenital toxoplasmosis. *Bull NY Acad Med* 1974; 50:182–191.
11. Hall CB, McBride JT, Walsh EE, et al: Aerosolized ribavirin treatment of infants with respiratory syncytial viral infection: A randomized double-blind study. *N Engl J Med* 1983; 308:1443–1447.
12. Hall CB, McBride JT, Gala CL, et al: Ribavirin treatment of respiratory syncytial viral infection in infants with underlying cardiopulmonary disease. *JAMA* 1985; 254:3047–3051.
13. Hammerschlag MR, Cummings C, Roblin PM, et al: Efficacy of neonatal ocular prophylaxis for the prevention of chlamydial and gonococcal conjunctivitis. *N Engl J Med* 1989; 320:769–772.

14. Harrison HR, et al: *Chlamydia trachomatis* infant pneumonitis: Comparison with matched controls and other infant pneumonitis. *N Engl J Med* 1978; 298:702–708.

15. Hintz M, et al: Acyclovir pharmacokinetics in neonates with herpes simplex virus infections. *Program and Abstracts of the 23rd Interscience Conference on Antimicrobial Agents and Chemotherapy,* no. 569. Washington, D.C., American Society for Microbiology, 1983, p 187.

16. Lamprecht CL, Krause HE, Mufson MA: Role of maternal antibody in pneumonia and bronchiolitis due to respiratory syncytial virus. *J Infect Dis* 1976; 134:211.

17. Miller MJ: Fungal infections, in Remington JS, Klein JO (eds): *Infectious Disease of the Fetus and Newborn Infant,* ed 2. Philadelphia, WB Saunders Co, 1983, pp 464–506.

18. Nahmias AJ, et al: Herpes simplex, in Remington JS, Klein JO (eds): *Infectious Disease of the Fetus and Newborn Infant,* ed 2. Philadelphia, WB Saunders Co, 1983, pp 636–678.

19. Remington JS, Desmonts G: Toxoplasmosis, in Remington JS, Klein JO (eds): *Infectious Disease of the Fetus and Newborn Infant,* ed 2. Philadelphia, WB Saunders Co, 1983, pp 636–678.

20. Report of the Committee on Infectious Diseases, 21 ed. Evanston, Ill, American Academy of Pediatrics, 1988, pp 526–530.

21. Schacter J: Chlamydial infections. Part I. *N Engl J Med* 1978; 298:490–495.

22. Schacter J: Chlamydial infections. Part II. *N Engl J Med* 1978; 298:540–549.

23. Schacter J: Chlamydial infections. Part III. *N Engl J Med* 1978; 298:540–549.

24. Schweitzer IL, et al: Viral hepatitis B in neonates and infants. *Am J Med* 1973; 55:762–771.

25. Taber LH, Knight V, Gilbert BE, et al: Ribavirin aerosol treatment of bronchiolitis associated with respiratory syncytial virus infection in infants. *Pediatrics* 1983; 72:613–618.

26. Tong JJ, et al: Studies on the maternal-infant transmission of the viruses which cause acute hepatitis. *Gastroenterology* 1981; 80:999–1004.

27. Whitley RJ, et al: Vidarabine therapy of neonatal herpes simplex virus infection. *Pediatrics* 1980; 66:495–501.

28. Whitley RJ, et al: The natural history of herpes simplex virus infection of mother and newborn. *Pediatrics* 1980; 66:489–494.

29. Wilson CB, Remington JS: What can be done to prevent congenital toxoplasmosis? *Am J Obstet Gynecol* 1980; 183:357–363.

16

Immune Therapy in Neonates and Small Infants

Kwang Sik Kim, M.D.

Since the use of vaccine in the prevention of smallpox, few therapeutic methods have had as great an impact on world health problems as immunization. Conventionally, this type of immunotherapy has been directed toward the prevention of infectious diseases; however, it has been expanded to encompass the treatment or prevention of malignant neoplasms, immunologic disorders, and organ transplant rejection. In addition, with the recent development and licensure of safe preparations of human intravenous immunoglobulins (IVIg), large quantities of IgG can be administered without side effects or toxicity, and a new role for immunotherapy has been recognized (e.g., in Kawasaki disease or idiopathic thrombocytopenic purpura). In this chapter, the current concepts of active and passive immunizations in neonates and small infants are outlined.

ACTIVE IMMUNIZATION

Active immunity is the stimulation of an immune response by antigenic exposure to an infecting organism or with a modified product of all or part of the microorganism (e.g., toxoid). The success of a vaccine is assessed from the evidence of protection against the natural disease; induction of antibodies frequently is an indirect measure of protection, but in some instances the immunologic response responsible for protection is poorly understood (e.g., pertussis), and serum antibody concentrations are not always predictive of protection (e.g., *Haemophilus influenzae* type B).

Immunization Schedule

A vaccine is intended to be administered to an individual who is capable of an appropriate immunologic response and who will likely benefit from the protection afforded.

Vaccines for diphtheria toxoid, tetanus toxoid, and pertussis (DTP) and attenuated polio virus vaccines are less immunogenic in early infancy than later in infancy.[2, 21] Prorenzano et al. suggested that immunization with DTP vaccine within 24 hours of birth might produce "immune paralysis."[21] Thus a cautious approach is needed to neonatal immunization. However, in some situations (e.g., in areas of high endemicity or during epidemics) DTP and polio vaccinations can be initiated as early as 2 weeks of age.[23] Prematurely born infants should be immunized at the usual chronologic age. If an infant is still in the nursery at the time immunizations are due, only DTP should be given, to avoid cross-infection with polio virus in the nursery; the polio virus immunization can be initiated on discharge. If the infant is discharged at 2 months of age, both DTP and polio virus vaccines can be given on discharge.

The recommended doses of vaccines should not be reduced for preterm or low-birth-weight infants.[3, 23]

Immunocompromised Infants

For vaccination in immunocompromised infants and children, such as those with congenital immunodeficiencies, acquired immune deficiency syndrome, or malignancy, and recipients of immunosuppressive therapy, see the 1988 *Red Book* of The American Academy of Pediatrics.[23] In general, an inactivated vaccine is preferable to live virus vaccine.

PASSIVE IMMUNIZATION

Passive immunization entails administration of preformed antibody (rather than antigen). The following preparations are currently available.

Human Immune Serum Globulin (Intramuscular)

Human immune serum globulin for intramuscular use is a 16.5% protein solution and currently used for prophylaxis of hepatitis A and measles.

The usual dose for hepatitis A is 0.02 mL/kg, given as soon as possible after exposure, but this dose can prevent clinical disease in exposed susceptible individuals when given within 14 days of exposure. For newborn infants of mothers with hepatitis A, no special care of the infant is recommended[23] unless the mother has jaundice at the time of delivery. Neither human immune globulin nor withholding of breast-feeding is recommended. If the mother has jaundice, the infant may be given human immune globulin (0.02 mL/kg), although its efficacy in this setting has not been established. In both situations, proper hygiene should be emphasized to the mother.

Specific Human Immune Serum Globulins

Specific immune globulins (or hyperimmune globulins) are identical to human immune serum globulins except that the donor pool is derived from immunized or convalescing subjects with high titers of specific antibodies. The preparations and their indications relevant to neonates and small infants are as follows.

Newborn Infants of Mothers Infected With Hepatitis B

Neonates born to mothers who are positive for hepatitis B surface antigen should receive 0.5 mL of hepatitis B immune globulin (HBIg) as soon after birth as possible. The efficacy of HBIg given 12 to 48 hours after birth is presumed but not proved.[23] In addition to HBIg, these newborn infants should receive three doses of hepatitis B vaccine, 0.5 mL (half the adult dose). The first dose can be given at the same time as HBIg if it is given with a separate syringe at a different site. The second and third doses are given 1 and 6 months after the first. If, however, vaccine administration is delayed for as long as 3 months, a second dose of HBIg should be given.

Varicella

Varicella-zoster immune globulin (VZIg), 125 U, should be given as soon as possible after delivery to infants whose mothers have had onset of varicella within 5 days before or 2 days after delivery. For healthy full-term infants exposed 2 or more days postnatally to varicella, including those whose mother's rash developed more than 48 hours after delivery, VZIg is usually not indicated, because infants who develop varicella under these conditions are not known to be at any greater risk of complications of varicella than older children.[23] However, because of the poor transfer of immunoglobulins across the placenta early in pregnancy, all infants born before 28 weeks of gestation or all who weigh less than 1,000 g and who still require hospitalization for prematurity or related conditions and who are exposed to varicella should receive VZIg (125 units). This recommendation applies also to premature infants born after 28 weeks gestation whose mothers have a negative history of past varicella-zoster infection.[23]

Tetanus Neonatorum

In the treatment of tetanus neonatorum, tetanus immune globulin, 500 U, was shown to be efficacious, and its efficacy was equivalent to that of equine tetanus antitoxin, 10,000 U.[17]

Human Plasma

Plasma has the danger of transmission of infectious agents (e.g., hepatitis), and its use in the control of infections in neonates and small infants should be restricted.

TABLE 16–1.
Effect of Human Intravenous Immunoglobulin Preparation Methods on IgG Subclass
Distribution

Procedure	IgG Subclasses (%)			
	IgG1	IgG2	IgG3	IgG4
World Health Organization Ref. plasma pool 67/97	60.6	29.4	6.5	4.1
Enzymatically treated (e.g., plasmin)	↓↓	↑	↓↓	→
Chemically modified (e.g., β-propiolactone)	→	→	0	↓
Polyethylene glycol isolated	→	→	→	sl ↓
Nonmodified (e.g., pH4)	→	→	→	sl ↓

sl = slight.

Antibodies of Animal Origin

These products pose a special risk to the recipient (e.g., hypersensitivity), and their use should be strictly limited to certain conditions in which specific immune globulins of human origin are not available. These conditions include specific antitoxins or antivenins for prophylaxis or therapy of diphtheria, botulism (wound and foodborne, not for infant botulism), or venom exposure.

Human Immune Globulin (Intravenous)

The rationale for the use of IVIg in neonates and small infants is based on neonates' incomplete acquisition of maternal antibodies, sluggish antibody response to certain antigens, physiologic hypogammaglobulinemia (particularly in preterm or low-birth-weight infants), immature other immune mechanisms (i.e., complement, phagocytes, and reticuloendothelial systems), increased risk of infections, and ability of IVIg to achieve high levels of antibody regardless of body size or muscle mass.

To prevent serious side effects following intravenous administration, human immunoglobulins have been modified for intravenous use; modifying agents including the enzymes (e.g., plasmin) or chemicals (e.g., β-propiolactone), however, result in IVIg preparations that possess less desirable biologic characteristics (e.g., alterations in IgG subclasses or IgG molecules; Table 16–1). Therefore, IVIgs currently available in the United States have undergone pH4 treatment or precipitation procedures (e.g., polyethylene glycol) or ion exchange chromotography (Table 16–2). These IVIgs are found to be safe, contain functionally active IgG molecules, and their IgG subclasses distributions are similar to those of plasma (see Table 16–1).

Because IVIgs can provide large quantities of IgG, they may be particularly useful for reducing the morbidity and mortality associated with serious bacterial infections in neonates and small infants. However, the benefits of IVIg in the prevention and therapy of neonatal infections and immunologic disorders have not been clearly established.

In Vitro Characteristics of IVIg

Ideally, to be useful for neonatal infections, IVIg should contain sufficient amounts of functionally active antibodies against common bacterial or viral pathogens. However, not all IVIg possesses such ideal characteristics, and there is a lot-to-lot variation in the spectrum of antibacterial and antiviral activities.[15] In addition, the protective mechanism afforded by IVIg is not clearly understood. To overcome these limitations, several hyperimmune IVIg have been prepared from immunized or convalescing donors who have high titers of specific antibodies (e.g., group B streptococci). The use of such hyperimmune IVIg will further enhance the scope of immunotherapy to control serious neonatal infections.

Prevention of Infections in Preterm and Low-birth-weight Infants

Several recent studies suggest that IVIg may be beneficial in reducing sepsis in certain high-risk, low-birth-weight infants; these are summarized in Table 16–3. Haque et al.[11] gave chemically modified IVIg (i.e., using β-propiolactone), 0.12 g/kg, to one group of 50 preterm infants weighing less than 1.5 kg within 2 to 4 hours of delivery. Another group of 50 preterm infants received the additional dose of the same IVIg on day 8. The control group of 50 preterm infants received no IVIg. Culture-proved sepsis rates were significantly lower in the IVIg-treated groups (4/100 or 4%) than in the control group (8/50 or 16%). Similar beneficial effect was also reported by Chirico et al.[6] who compared preterm infants receiving 0.5 g/kg of pH4-treated IVIg weekly for 4 weeks with those receiving no IVIg. Eight (20%) of 40 control

TABLE 16–2.
Human Intravenous Immunoglobulin Preparations Available in the United States

Brand Name	Manufacturer	Procedure	Other Constituents in 5% Solution
Gamimmune-N (5% solution)	Cutter Biological, Berkeley, Calif.	pH adjustment (pH 4)	Maltose 10%
Gammagard (lyophilized)	Travenol Laboratories, Glendale, Calif.	PEG	Glucose 2% PEG 0.2% Glycine 0.3M NaCl 1%
Iveegam (lyophilized)	Immuno-U.S., Inc., Rochester, Minn.	PEG and immobilized trypsin	Glucose 5% PEG ≤0.5% NaCl 0.3%
Sandoglobulin-I (lyophilized)	Sandoz, Inc., East Hanover, N.J.	pH4 and trace amounts of pepsin	Sucrose 10% NaCl small
Venoglobulin-I (lyophilized)	Alpha Therapeutic, Los Angeles, Calif.	PEG and DEAE-Sephadox	Mannitol 2% Albumin 1% PEG ≤0.6% NaCl 0.5%

PEG = polyethylene glycol.

TABLE 16–3.
Effect of Intravenous Human Immune Globulin (IVIg) on Prevention of Sepsis in Preterm or Low-birth-weight Infants

| Source | IVIg | No. infections (%)/ Total No. (%) | | P Value[‡] |
		IVIg	No IVIg	
Haque et al., Saudi Arabia[12] (randomized)	BPL-treated, 0.12 g/kg	4/100 (4)	8/50 (16)	0.021
Chirico et al., Italy[6] (randomized)	pH4-treated, 0.5 g/kg	2/43 (5)	8/40 (20)	<0.05
Stabile et al., Italy[26] (randomized)	PEG-treated, 0.5 g/kg	5/40 (12.5)	3/40 (7.5)	NS
Clapp et al., US[7] (preliminary)	pH4-treated, 0.5–1.3 g/kg	0/41	3/37 (8)	NS
Baker et al., US[1] (randomized, double-blind)	PEG-treated, 0.5 g/kg	50/176 (28)	92/185 (50)	0.0015

BPL = β-propiolactone; PEG = polyethylene glycol; NS = not statistically significant.

infants developed culture-proved sepsis and 6 (15%) died, whereas 2 (5%) of 43 IVIg-treated infants had culture-proved sepsis and 1 (2%) died. These differences in the infection rates and mortality were significant. However, both studies reported that the organisms responsible for sepsis in IVIg-treated and control groups were similar (*Escherichia coli* and *Klebsiella* for the study of Haque et al. and *Staphylococcus aureus* and similar gram-negative bacteria for the study of Chirico et al.). These findings raise the critical question on the protective mechanisms afforded by IVIg. Unless these questions are answered, the use of certain IVIg in prevention of sepsis in low-birth-weight infants may remain controversial. In addition, Stabile et al.[26] reported that IVIg had no beneficial effect in reducing the infection rate in preterm infants using the polyethylene glycol (PEG)–treated IVIg. Preliminary reports by Clapp et al.[7] also indicated no statistically significant benefit of IVIg in the prevention of sepsis.

The most extensive study conducted to date (although only preliminary results are available at this time) was carried out by Baker et al. in a double-blind, multicenter study.[1] These investigators evaluated the effect of PEG-treated IVIg in prevention of late-onset sepsis in preterm infants. Culture-proved infection rates were 28% (50/176) in infants who received 0.5 g/kg IVIg at 3 to 7 days, 1 week later, and every 14 days for a total of five doses or until hospital discharge. By contrast, 50% (92/185) of the control infants who received placebo developed culture-proved infection (*P* = .0015). However, the organisms responsible for sepsis in both IVIg-treated and control groups were identical, and the protective mechanisms afforded by IVIg are not clear. Additional control studies are currently under way.

In conclusion, IVIg available in the United States at a dose of 0.5 g/kg appears to reduce the infection rate (particularly of late-onset sepsis) in certain preterm infants. However, the duration and interval of IVIg therapy are not clearly established. Also, almost every lot of IVIg may contain a different spectrum of opsonic antibodies against neonatal and nosocomial pathogens. Thus, unless the spectrum and functional activity of a particular lot of IVIg is known, it may be wiser to alternate several different lots (if IVIg is being used as a preventive measure against sepsis in preterm infants).

Established Bacterial Infections

Studies in animals suggest that IVIg may be effective in the treatment of certain bacterial infections in neonates. In experimental group B streptococcal infection in newborn rats, IVIg plus penicillin G was significantly more beneficial in rapidly clearing bacteria from the bloodstream than penicillin G alone.[14] Also, IVIg provided modest protection to infant rats challenged with a K1 *E. coli* strain possessing O antigen common in neonatal *E. coli* infections.[4]

Two clinical studies indicated that IVIg in conjunction with antibiotics significantly reduced mortality compared with antibiotics alone.[11, 24] However, careful analysis revealed that the differences reported in these two studies did not reach statistical significance (Table 16–4).

Thus, at present the efficacy of IVIg in treatment of neonatal bacterial disease is unknown. In addition, the optimal therapeutic dose of IVIg is not established, and the spectrum of antibacterial activity varies among different preparations or lots of IVIg. To ensure that IVIg is therapeutic, it should contain sufficient opsonic antibodies against common neonatal pathogens (group B streptococci and *E. coli*). It has been shown that not all IVIg contains sufficient opsonic antibodies against all five serotypes of group B streptococci. An attempt to restore sufficient opsonic activity through administration of large quantities of IVIg may result in detrimental effects.[15] In *E. coli*, K1-encapsulated strains are the predominant type responsible for neonatal sepsis and meningitis. K1 polysaccharide, however, is a poor immunogen (although

TABLE 16–4.
Efficacy of IVIg in Treatment of Neonatal Sepsis

Source (Reference)	IVIg	Mortality (%)		P* Value
		IVIg	No IVIg	
Sidiropoulos et al., Switzerland[24]	pH4-treated IVIg, 1 g/day for full-term;	1/7 (14)	0/6	NS
	0.5 g/day for preterm	1/13 (8)	4/9 (44)	0.13
	for 6 days overall	2/20 (10)	4/15 (27)	NS
Haque et al., Saudi Arabia[11]	IgM-enriched IVIg, 0.25 g/kg/day for preterm for 4 days	1/30 (3.3)	6/30 (20)	0.10

*By two-tailed Fisher exact test. NS = not statistically significant.

antibody to the K1 capsule is opsonic against K1 *E. coli* strains), and IVIg contains only low levels of antibody to the K1 antigen.[15] An alternative approach is the use of anti-O lipopolysaccharide antibody,[16] because antibodies to the O side chains of K1 *E. coli* possess equivalent opsonic and protective activity as the anti-K1 antibody and the number of O antigens common in neonatal *E. coli* sepsis and meningitis are limited.

Future utilization of IVIg as a therapeutic adjunct in neonatal infection may depend on the availability of IVIg possessing opsonic antibodies against common neonatal pathogens (i.e., major serotypes of group B streptococci as well as of *E. coli*). In the meantime, IVIg at a single dose of 0.5 g/kg in conjunction with antibiotics may provide some benefits in the treatment of established bacterial infections in neonates; but with significant data from control studies being unavailable, this presumption may be groundless.

Neonatal Viral Infections

IVIg may be beneficial in the treatment of neonatal viral infection. Hemming et al.[13] showed that 2 g/kg of IVIg containing high titers of respiratory syncytial virus (RSV)–neutralizing antibody resulted in significant reduction in nasal RSV shedding and in improvements in transcutaneous oximetry readings in RSV-infected infants and children. The mean duration of hospitalization was not reduced by IVIg treatment, however. These investigators noted that every lot of IVIg contained variable titers of neutralizing antibody to RSV.

Serious virus infections in newborn infants can also occur following transmission of enteroviruses (e.g., Coxsackie A and B viruses, echoviruses) from infected mothers during the perinatal period as well as from nosocomial sources after birth. Outbreaks of Coxsackie B virus and echovirus 11 infections among neonates have been associated with a high mortality.[8, 10, 20] Fatality was observed in cases where maternal illness occurred late in pregnancy to preclude development and concomitant transplantal passage of maternal IgG neutralizing antibody before delivery.[19] There is laboratory evidence that passively administered antibody protects the newborn animal from fatal Coxsackie B3 virus infections.[22] In addition, high doses of IVIg have been used successfully in the treatment of fatal echovirus infection in patients with agammaglobulinemia.[18] Thus, newborns with severe enterovirus disease may also be likely candidates for such IVIg therapy. In that case, selected IVIg should contain high titers of specific antiviral antibody and be used in high doses.

Immune-mediated Thrombocytopenia and Neutropenia of Infancy

IVIg (400 mg/kg/day for 5 days) has been shown to successfully reverse immune thrombocytopenia and neutropenia in neonates.[5, 25] Although the mechanisms responsible for these beneficial effects are not clear, high doses of IVIg may be a useful alternative in the treatment of immune-mediated thrombocytopenia and neutropenia of infancy.

ORAL HUMAN IMMUNOGLOBULIN FOR PREVENTION OF NECROTIZING ENTEROCOLITIS IN LOW-BIRTH-WEIGHT INFANTS

Necrotizing enterocolitis (NEC) is a major cause of morbidity and mortality in preterm and low-birth-weight infants. A wide range of bacterial and viral pathogens have been implicated as a contributing factor(s). A recent study suggests that human immunoglobulin may have some beneficial effect in the prevention of NEC. Eibl et al.[9] gave 0.6 g/kg/day of an oral IgA-IgG preparation as a supplement to their feeding within 12 hours of birth and daily for 3 or more doses. There was no NEC among the 88 infants receiving oral IgA-IgG, as compared with six cases (6.5%) among the 91 control infants who did not receive supplemental Ig (P = .00143). The mechanisms responsible for the protection of NEC were not clear. More control studies are needed for the potential benefit of oral human immunoglobulin in prevention of NEC in low-birth-weight infants.

ACKNOWLEDGMENT

Supported in part by Research Grant 1-1043 from the March of Dimes Birth Defects Foundation and by grants RO1-NS-26310 and RO1-AI-24420 from the National Institutes of Health.

REFERENCES

1. Baker CJ and the Neonatal IVIG Collaborative Study Group. Multicenter trial of intravenous immunoglobulin to prevent late-onset infection in preterm infants: Preliminary results (abstract 1633). *Pediatr Res* 1989; 25:275A.
2. Baraff LJ, Leake RD, Burstyn DG, et al: Immunologic response to early and routine DTP immunization in infants. *Pediatrics* 1974; 73:37–42.
3. Bernbaum J, Daft A, Samuelson J, et al: Half-dose immunization for diphtheria, tetanus, pertussis: Response of preterm infants. *Pediatrics* 1989; 83:471–476.
4. Bortolussi R, Fischer GW: Opsonic and protective activity of immunoglobulin, modified immunoglobulin, and serum against neonatal *Escherichia coli* K1 infection. *Pediatr Res* 1986; 20:175–178.
5. Bussel J, Lalezari M, Hilgartner J, et al: Reversal of neutropenia with intravenous gammaglobulin in autoimmune neutropenia of infancy. *Blood* 1983; 62:398–400.
6. Chirico G, Rondini G, Plebani A, et al: Intravenous gamma-globulin therapy for prophylaxis of infection in high-risk neonates. *J Pediatr* 1987; 110:437–442.
7. Clapp DW, Baley JE, Kliegman RM, et al: Randomized trial of IVIg to prevent nosocomial infections in preterm infants—preliminary data (abstract 1616). *Pediatr Res* 1988; 23:471A.
8. Davies DP, Hughes CA, MacVicar J, et al: Echovirus-11 infection in a special care baby unit. *Lancet* 1979; 1:96.

9. Eibl MM, Wolf HM, Furnkranz H, et al: Prevention of necrotizing enterocolitis in low-birth-weight infants by IgA-IgG feeding. *N Engl J Med* 1988; 319:1–7.
10. Gear JHS, Measroch V: Coxsackievirus infections of the newborn. *Prog Med Virol* 1973; 15:42.
11. Haque KN, Zaidi MH, Bahakim H: IgM-enriched intravenous immunoglobulin therapy in neonatal sepsis. *Am J Dis Child* 1988; 142:1293–1296.
12. Haque KN, Zaidi MH, Haque SK, et al: Intravenous immunoglobulin for prevention of sepsis in preterm and low birth weight infants. *Pediatr Infect Dis* 1986; 5:622–625.
13. Hemming VG, Rodriguez W, Kim HW, et al: Intravenous immunoglobulin treatment of respiratory syncytial virus infections in infants and young children. *Antimicrob Agents Chemother* 1987; 31:1882–1886.
14. Kim KS: Efficacy of human immunoglobulin and penicillin G in treatment of experimental group B streptococcal infection. *Pediatr Res* 1987; 21:289–292.
15. Kim KS: Use of intravenous immunoglobulin in bacterial diseases, in Stiehm ER (moderator): Intravenous immunoglobulins as therapeutic agents, pp 369–371. *Ann Intern Med* 1987; 107:367–382.
16. Kim KS, Kang JH, Cross AS, et al: Functional activities of monoclonal antibodies to the O side chain of *Escherichia coli* lipopolysaccharides in vitro and in vivo. *J Infect Dis* 1988; 157:47–53.
17. McCracken GH Jr, Dowell DL, Marshall FN: Double-blind trial of equinine antitoxin and human immune globulin in tetanus neonatorum. *Lancet* 1971; 1:1146–1149.
18. Mease PJ, Ochs HD, Wedgwood RJ: Successful treatment of echovirus meningoencephalitis and myositis-fasciitis with intravenous immune globulin therapy in a patient with x-linked agammaglobulinemia. *N Engl J Med* 1981; 304:1278–1280.
19. Modlin JF: Fatal echovirus 11 disease in premature neonates. *Pediatrics* 1980; 66:775–780.
20. Nagington J, Wreghitt TG, Gandy G, et al: Fatal echovirus 11 in outbreak in special-care baby unit. *Lancet* 1978; 2:725.
21. Prorenzano WR, Wetterlow LJ, Sullivan CL: Immunization and antibody response in the newborn infant: I. Pertussis inoculation within 24 hours of birth. *N Engl J Med* 1965; 273:959–965.
22. Rager-Zisman B, Allison AC: The role of antibody and host cells in the resistance of mice against infection by coxsackie B3 virus. *J Gen Virol* 1973; 19:329.
23. Report of the Committee on Infectious Diseases, 21 ed. Elk Grove Village, Ill, American Academy of Pediatrics, 1989, pp 5–60.
24. Sidiropoulous D, Boehme U, Muralt GV, et al: Immunoglobulin supplementation in prevention or treatment of neonatal sepsis. *Pediatr Infect Dis* 1986; 5:S193–S194.
25. Stabile A, Pesaresi MA, Miceli Sopo S, et al: Effective high-dose intravenous gammaglobulin therapy for passive immune thrombocytopenia in the neonate. *Eur J Pediatr* 1987; 146:90–91.
26. Stabile A, Sopo SM, Romanelli V, et al: Intravenous immunoglobulin for prophylaxis of neonatal sepsis in premature infants. *Arch Dis Child* 1988; 63:441–443.

17

Hypoglycemia and Hyperglycemia

Lawrence D. Lilien, M.D.

Gopal Srinivasan, M.D.

Tsu F. Yeh, M.D.

Rosita S. Pildes, M.D.

HYPOGLYCEMIA DEFINED

Hypoglycemia should be defined as the state of potentially damaging cellular glucose insufficiency of the central nervous system; however, except for relying on nonspecific symptoms attributed to low glucose levels, there is no way to determine when an infant has cellular glucose insufficiency. Because determining clinical glucose insufficiency at the cellular level is beyond our present ability, definitions have been based on statistical data: two standard deviations below the mean glucose level for a given infant population constitutes hypoglycemia. Of course, the particular infant population used to generate the statistical distribution will affect the definition. Since the original data for 1953 to 1967[6–8] were published, there have been many changes in perinatal practices, for example, more frequent use of maternal intravenous infusions and tocolytic agents and earlier routine infant feeding. Therefore our arbitrary definition is in a constant state of flux. Recent data (Fig 17–1)[19] on healthy full-term neonates born to healthy mothers and fed formula from 3 to 4 hours after birth led to the following definition of neonatal hypoglycemia:

For neonates weighing 2.5 kg or more:

0–3 hours postnatal age: plasma glucose <35 mg/dL

4–24 hours postnatal age: plasma glucose <40 mg/dL

1–7 days postnatal age: plasma glucose <45 mg/dL

Studies in neonates weighing less than 2.5 kg are difficult to perform because parenteral fluids are used frequently. Therefore the definition used

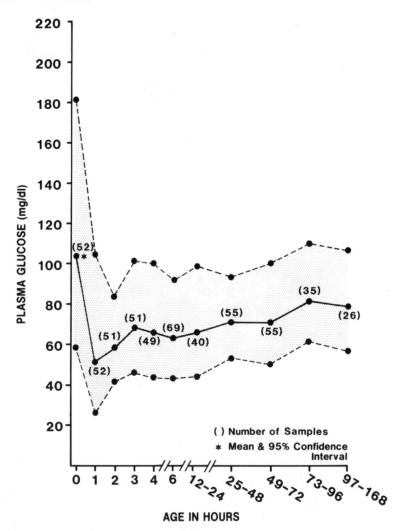

FIG 17–1.
Plasma glucose levels in healthy neonates delivered vaginally with birth weight 2.5 to 4.0 kg. (From Srinivasan G, et al: *J Pediatr* 1986; 109:114–117. Used by permission.)

is similar to that originally recommended by Cornblath and Reisner[6] and modified for plasma:

For neonates weighing less than 2.5 kg:

    0–72 hours postnatal age: plasma glucose <25 mg/dL

    4–7 days postnatal age: plasma glucose <45 mg/dL

Though most discussions of hypoglycemia state that two glucose levels in the hypoglycemic range are necessary to diagnose clinical hypoglycemia, one glucose level in the hypoglycemic range in a symptomatic infant and two glucose levels 30 to 60 minutes apart in an asymptomatic infant should suffice to initiate intravenous therapy. Many infants recover spontaneously; hence a second glucose level is drawn at the time glucose is infused.

Symptomatic vs. Asymptomatic Hypoglycemia

It is important to determine whether an infant is symptomatic for hypoglycemia, because it has been shown that symptomatic infants are more likely to suffer CNS morbidity;[17] thus these infants demand more rapid therapy. Clinical manifestations of hypoglycemia are nonspecific and include tremors or jitteriness, irritability, exaggerated Moro reflex, apneic spells, cyanotic spells, convulsions, limpness, lethargy, hypothermia, high-pitched cry, vomiting, cardiac failure, cardiac arrest, and sweating. Clinical signs are usually alleviated immediately with concomitant correction of the glucose level; however, some symptoms may persist despite what was thought to have been rapid, corrective therapy. According to some authors these infants would not be classified as having symptoms, because the "presumed symptom" was not alleviated by therapy.[8]

MEASUREMENT OF GLUCOSE

The type of sample obtained and the method of analysis are critical in interpreting glucose concentration. Plasma glucose values are on average 15% higher than whole blood glucose values. Whole blood includes red blood cells, which have a lower water content and therefore a lower glucose concentration. Similarly, whole blood with a higher hematocrit value has a lower glucose level than whole blood with a lower hematocrit value. Because the rate of in vitro glycolysis is high in neonatal red blood cells, blood samples should be stored on ice or the cells should be separated immediately from the plasma. If a whole blood sample stands at room temperature the blood glucose level may drop 15 to 20 mg/dL/hr.

In many nurseries rapid assessment of whole blood glucose concentrations is accomplished by a glucose oxidase-peroxidase chromagen test-strip method, either alone or with a reflectance colorimeter (e.g., Chemstrip bG/Accu-Chek II, Glucostix/Glucometer II). These methods are neither precise nor accurate, and 95% confidence intervals are wide. These methods are also hematocrit dependent.[1] For these reasons abnormal or borderline values (<40 mg/dL) should be checked by a standard laboratory method. Therefore, the main use of test strips is for screening purposes and for trending.

DIFFERENTIAL DIAGNOSIS

The differential diagnosis of neonatal hypoglycemia has four main categories[18]:

I. Asymptomatic (transient)
II. Symptomatic (transient, idiopathic)
III. Specific etiology (persistent)
   A. Hyperinsulinism
      1. Maternal diabetes
      2. Erythroblastosis
      3. Beckwith-Wiedemann syndrome
      4. Beta cell nesidioblastosis-adenoma spectrum
      5. Leucine sensitivity
      6. Maternal drugs (tolbutamide, chlorpropamide, benzothiadiazide, β-sympathomimetic tocolytic agents)
   B. Endocrine disorders
      1. Panhypopituitarism
      2. Isolated growth hormone deficiency
      3. Cortisol deficiency
         a. Corticotropin unresponsiveness
         b. Isolated glucocorticoid deficiency
         c. Maternal steroid therapy
         d. Adrenal hemorrhage
         e. Adrenogenital syndrome
      4. Hypothyroidism
      5. Glucagon deficiency
   C. Hereditary defects in metabolism
      1. Carbohydrate metabolism
         a. Galactosemia
         b. Glycogen storage disease type 1
      2. Amino acid metabolism
         a. Maple syrup urine disease
         b. Propionic acidemia
         c. Methylmalonic acidemia
         d. Hereditary tyrosinemia
IV. Associated with other neonatal problems
   A. Iatrogenic
      1. Excessive dextrose fluids in intrapartum period
      2. Maternal starvation before delivery
      3. Following abrupt cessation of intravenous fluids
      4. Following exchange transfusion
      5. Hypothermia
      6. Malpositioned umbilical artery catheter
   B. Miscellaneous
      1. Neonatal infection
      2. Cardiac malformation
      3. Hypothermia
      4. Hyperviscosity
      5. Chronic diarrhea

6. Anti-insulin antibodies
7. CNS abnormalities
8. Intravenous indomethacin

Asymptomatic Transient Hypoglycemia

More than 95% of all neonatal hypoglycemia falls in the category of asymptomatic transient hypoglycemia and frequently is seen before the onset of the first feeding. It may therefore represent the normal physiologic drop caused by the withdrawal of substrate supplied by the mother. The true incidence is impossible to ascertain, as its presence frequently is discovered by chance sampling. Routine glucose sampling in healthy term infants has shown that approximately 10% have glucose levels in the first 4 hours that are by definition hypoglycemic.[19] More than half of these glucose levels correct themselves by the time the repeat glucose test is done. The significance of asymptomatic transient hypoglycemia with respect to potential morbidity is unknown.

Symptomatic Transient, Idiopathic Hypoglycemia

The incidence of transient, idiopathic hypoglycemia varies between 1.3 and 3 per 1,000 live births. These infants have one or more of the symptoms of hypoglycemia. The majority of these infants are of low birth weight, and 75% of them are small for gestational age (SGA). The pathogenesis of symptomatic transient idiopathic hypoglycemia is[18]:

I. Inadequate production of glucose
    A. Decreased glycogen and fat stores
    B. Defective gluconeogenesis
    C. Decreased glucose-sparing substrates
        1. Ketones
        2. Glycerol
    D. Delayed induction of phosphoenolpyruvate carboxykinase (PEPCK)
II. Excessive utilization of glucose
    A. Increased peripheral glucose disappearance in some infants
    B. Inadequate counterinsulin hormones
    C. Increased needs
        1. Increased oxygen consumption in SGA infants
        2. Anoxia
        3. Large brain-liver ratio
    D. Hyperinsulinism

As is expected from the proposed pathogenesis, the hypoglycemia is usually self-limited; however, recurrences are common during the first few days as intravenous fluids infiltrate or are too rapidly discontinued before oral feedings are well tolerated.

Persistent Hypoglycemia: Specific Cause

If we exclude hyperinsulinism secondary to maternal diabetes, the incidence of the sum total of all these entities in the third category is significantly less than 1 per 1,000 live births. These disease states represent hormone excess or deficiency or enzyme deficiency and are not primary substrate problems. Of these, the hyperinsulin diseases predominate. Most of the diseases associated with hyperinsulinism, with the exception of beta cell nesidioblastosis-adenoma spectrum and leucine sensitivity, are self-limited, and recurrences tend to be infrequent within a few days. The remaining hormone and enzyme deficiencies need specific hormone replacement or dietary restriction to control the hypoglycemia. Thus their control is somewhat dependent on how rapid the diagnosis is made.

Diagnostic Evaluation

A maternal history and physical examination of the infant are mandatory for the diagnosis. Important maternal history includes history of diabetes, toxemia, hypertension, blood group incompatibility, familial history of hypoglycemia, and unexplained stillbirth or infant death. Physical examination of the infant will determine if the infant is small or large for gestational age, is postmature, has erythroblastosis, or is an infant of a prediabetic or diabetic mother. If the hypoglycemia is persistent, however, it is imperative that the workup be escalated to find the cause and allow for fine tuning of therapy. At this time one searches for more specific physical findings, observes the clinical course of hypoglycemia, and initiates a blood workup. For example, macrosomia, abnormal umbilicus, vertical ear lobe grooves, and large tongue are diagnostic of Beckwith-Wiedemann syndrome. Small genitalia in a male with widely spaced nipples, cleft lip or palate, or other facial anomalies may point to pituitary deficiency. Cataracts, jaundice, vomiting, hepatomegaly, and reducing substances in the urine suggest galactosemia. The presence of chubby, doll-like facies and hepatomegaly without a history of maternal diabetes may suggest glycogen storage disease. Because neonatal hypoglycemia usually is associated with a fasting state, a history of symptoms immediately after milk intake suggests leucine sensitivity or galactosemia. In an infant who is appropriate for gestational age (AGA) and lacks any positive physical findings, has a noncontributory maternal history, and has severe persistent hypoglycemia resistant to conventional medical management, beta cell nesidioblastosis-adenoma spectrum is highly suggested. Initial laboratory determinations, preferably at the time of hypoglycemia, should show glucose, insulin, human growth hormone, and cortisol levels. Because human growth hormone levels are normally very high in cord blood, a cord blood sample for human growth hormone may be used instead of a sample at the time of hypoglycemia. Thyroid function should also be checked. If glycogen storage disease is suspected, determinations of pH and lactate, pyruvate, and ketone levels are added to the workup. If any of the disorders of amino acid metabolism are suspected, then amino acid levels in urine, blood, or both should be determined.

TREATMENT

The management of neonatal hypoglycemia includes the identification of infants at risk for hypoglycemia, the initiation of oral feedings within 3 to 4 hours after birth, and the minimization of caloric usage by decreasing environmental stress. Management also entails monitoring for clinical symptoms of hypoglycemia and glucose level determinations. In asymptomatic high-risk infants, glucose levels should be checked before the first feeding and randomly before subsequent feedings. If glucose screening is done by such methods as Dextrostix or Chemstrip bG, abnormal or borderline levels should be checked in the laboratory.

In general, the type of treatment is determined by whether the hypoglycemia is transient or persistent, is symptomatic or asymptomatic, and has a specific cause. For treatment purposes, both one hypoglycemic level with concomitant symptoms or two hypoglycemic levels without symptoms are treated with intravenous glucose infusion. Oral glucose is not therapy for these infants. For example, if the infant is an asymptomatic healthy infant who has had a routine Chemstrip bG or glucose level determination in the hypoglycemic range, oral feedings may be given while a repeat glucose level determination is performed. Usually the short interval between the screening and the repeat test is sufficient time for the hypoglycemia to self-correct. Because approximately 10% of healthy term AGA infants have transient asymptomatic hypoglycemia, it would be impractical to start routine intravenous glucose infusions in all of these infants. If, however, the infant remains hypoglycemic, then intravenous glucose must be given.

Symptomatic or questionably symptomatic hypoglycemia should be treated immediately with intravenous glucose, although a preinfusion glucose level is repeated to confirm the diagnosis. Moreover, any second hypoglycemic episode with or without symptoms that cannot be attributed to an infiltrated intravenous infusion or a premature drop in intravenous infusion rate merits further workup (i.e., determining concentrations of glucose, insulin, cortisol, human growth hormone, and thyroxine) and escalation of therapy, as outlined in the following section.

Intravenous Glucose

Infants with asymptomatic hypoglycemia respond within 10 to 20 minutes to 10% glucose solution infused at a rate of 8 mg/kg/min (4.8 mL 10% dextrose in water (D/W)/kg/hr).[12] Infants with symptomatic or persistent hypoglycemia who require immediate correction respond to a minibolus of 200 mg/kg (2 mL 10% D/W per kilogram) injected over 1 minute followed by continuous glucose infusion of 8 mg/kg/min (Fig 17–2).[13] Glucose levels should be determined hourly until they become stable, and the infusion rate should be decreased by 2 mg/kg/min decrements as glucose values stabilize. In infants with two or more hypoglycemic episodes, glucose should be administered through two peripheral intravenous sites to ensure uninterrupted glucose infusion in case of infiltration. Infants with persistent hypoglycemia who are being fed formula should be given feedings by continuous nasogastric drip, not by bolus feeding. With continuous nasogastric drip feeding and continuous intravenous glucose infusion, glucose levels are more likely to reach a steady state and should not have the peak and trough levels that are expected with bolus carbohydrate intake. Therefore, glucose levels can be checked at any time and without concern whether the sample was drawn at peak or trough times. Glucose infusions may be increased up to 12 to 14 mg/kg/min. Further increases may produce fluid overload, venous thrombosis, or slough at the intravenous site; thus hydrocortisone is added to the regimen.

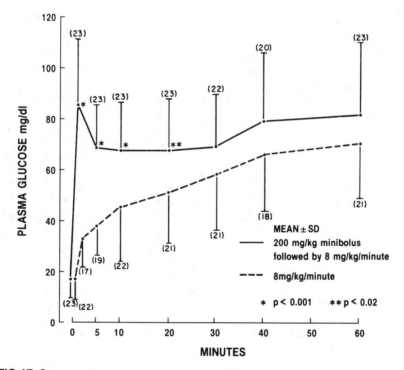

FIG 17–2.
Treatment in 23 hypoglycemic neonates with 200 mg/kg glucose minibolus followed by 8 mg/kg/min constant glucose infusion, compared with treatment in 22 hypoglycemic neonates with 8 mg/kg/min constant glucose infusion. (From Lilien LD, et al: *J Pediatr* 1980; 97:295–298. Used by permission.)

Hydrocortisone

If plasma glucose values are not above 40 mg/dL shortly after intravenous glucose therapy is begun or if hypoglycemia recurs, then hydrocortisone 10 mg/kg/day is given in two doses intravenously, intramuscularly, or orally. Hydrocortisone has been shown to (1) reduce peripheral glucose utilization, (2) increase the effects of exogenous glucagon, and (3) enhance gluconeogenesis. As the net effect of raising glucose levels takes approximately 6 to 8 hours, increased glucose infusion rates may be necessary until the hydrocortisone exerts its effect. When normoglycemia has been maintained for several days, intravenous fluids are tapered first and hydrocortisone is continued until the infant is stable for approximately 3 days after intravenous fluids have been discontinued. Hydrocortisone usually is given for a total of 5 to 7 days. Infants not responding to hydrocortisone may need additional or alternative therapy, depending on the cause of hypoglycemia.

Epinephrine

If hypoglycemia does not respond to intravenous glucose plus hydrocortisone, then a trial dose of epinephrine 1:1,000 (0.01 mL/kg) is administered subcutaneously. If this trial dose is successful, then a maintenance dose of epinephrine 1:200 in 25% glycerine solution (Sus-Phrine; 0.005 to 0.01 mL/kg every 6 hours) is administered subcutaneously or ephedrine sulfate (0.05 mg/kg/3 hr) is given orally. Epinephrine mobilizes stored fuels from the liver by glycogenolysis, stimulates gluconeogenesis, stimulates lipolysis in adipose tissue, augments glucagon secretion, and suppresses insulin secretion. Because of the latter effect, epinephrine has been recommended in infants with hyperinsulinism and has been used particularly in infants of diabetic mothers. On the other hand, epinephrine may cause adverse effects by raising blood lactate levels.

Diazoxide

Diazoxide (10 to 15 mg/kg/day in three to four divided doses), a nondiuretic thiazide given intravenously or orally, inhibits pancreatic insulin release and therefore is often effective in persistent hypoglycemia caused by hyperinsulinism. Failure to respond to diazoxide, however, does not mean that an infant does not have hyperinsulinemia. Failure or transient success frequently is followed by partial pancreatectomy. Side effects of diazoxide include hyperglycemia, hirsutism, ketosis, thrombocytopenia, leukopenia, depressed immunoglobulin levels, sodium retention, and hypotension. Intravenous diazoxide must be given slowly to permit serum protein binding and therefore less hypotensive side effects. Recently, long-term treatment with diazoxide for up to 8 years in infants with persistent neonatal hyperinsulinemic hypoglycemia has been reported.[22]

Glucagon

Glucagon is a single chain of 29 amino acids and has a mass of approximately 3,500 daltons. It contains no cysteine and therefore has no disulfide linkages. Glucagon (0.3 mg/kg intravenously or intramuscularly) has no place in the treatment of neonatal hypoglycemia except as specific therapy for glucagon deficiency. For maintenance therapy in glucagon deficiency, zinc protamine glucagon, 0.1 to 0.5 mg/kg every 12 hours intramuscularly[11] or in combination with somatostatin in beta cell nesidioblastosis-adenoma spectrum is used.[4] In some term neonates insulin-glucagon molar ratios may be more important than the absolute concentration of insulin.[15] Low hepatic production in infants with transient glucagon deficiency and normal absolute insulin levels may be corrected by boluses of glucagon. Because glucagon raises blood glucose through glycogenolysis and gluconeogenesis, it is usually ineffective in SGA neonates with depletion of glycogen stores or defective gluconeogenesis. However, continuous glucagon infusion (0.5 g/day) has been used in SGA infants with elevated glucose levels in the majority of infants examined within 3 hours.[5] Because glucagon may stimulate insulin release and concomitant rebound hypoglycemia, glucagon should be followed by continuous glucose infusion.

Human Growth Hormone

Human growth hormone is a single chain of 191 amino acids, has a molecular weight of approximately 22,000, and has two disulfide bonds. Natural sequence growth hormone (Eli Lilly, Indianapolis) or methionyl growth hormone (Genentech Inc., San Francisco), 50 to 60 μg/kg intramuscularly or subcutaneously three times per week, is effective in infants with hypoglycemia secondary to growth hormone deficiency.[14]

Somatostatin

Somatostatin (somatotropin release inhibiting hormone) is a single chain of 14 amino acids, has a molecular weight of approximately 1,800, and has one disulfide bond. Somatostatin (3.5 to 45 μg/kg/hr by continuous intravenous infusion) suppresses insulin as well as glucagon secretion. It has been useful for preoperative control in infants with suspected beta cell nesidioblastosis-adenoma spectrum.[10] In a newborn with nesidioblastosis, use of long-acting somatostatin analog, SMS 201-995, at a dosage gradually increasing from 2 to 50 μg/24 hr resulted in a dramatic fall in insulin levels.[3] No rebound was observed during short-term interruptions of SMS 201-995 infusion. In two other reports subtotal pancreatectomy for nesidioblastosis failed to prevent recurrent postoperative hypoglycemia; therefore, subcutaneous SMS 201-995 was used for long periods without causing significant side effects.[9, 2]

Pancreatectomy

In persistent cases of beta cell nesidioblastosis-adenoma spectrum in which all other measures have failed, early central venous catheter placement along with near-total (95%) pancreatectomy is recommended.[23] In general, taking into account a workup and various attempts of medical management, surgery should be performed within 2 to 3 weeks of the onset of hypoglycemia. In most infants near-total pancreatectomy is curative; however, if hypoglycemia recurs or persists and cannot be controlled medically, total pancreatectomy has been effective.

HYPERGLYCEMIA DEFINED

Hyperglycemia has been defined as plasma glucose values greater than 150 mg/dL. The incidence of hyperglycemia varies depending on the birth weight of the infant, the degree of stress, and the rate of dextrose infusion. The incidence also depends on how frequently blood and urine are monitored for glucose. In our nursery, monitoring blood Chemstrip bG levels and urine glucose every 8 hours and adjusting amounts of dextrose infused has curtailed dramatically the incidence of significant hyperglycemia.

Clinical Significance

Hyperglycemia in premature infants is a more frequent problem than hypoglycemia. Hyperglycemia has been associated with increased mortality, increased incidence of intraventricular hemorrhage, and increased incidence of major handicaps in very low-birth-weight infants. However, no studies to date have included a sufficient number of infants to make definitive conclusions. It is even more difficult to predict the absolute levels of hyperglycemia at which untoward CNS effects may be detected. Hyperglycemia may cause cerebral hemorrhage by increasing serum osmolarity to greater than 300 mOsm/L. Glucose values of greater than 400 mg/dL would increase serum osmolarity to greater than 300 mOsm/L. Hyperosmolarity greater than 300 mOsm/L causes water to move from the intracellular to the extracellular compartment. The resulting contraction of the intracellular volume in the brain of very low-birth-weight infants may result in cerebral hemorrhage.

Etiologic Factors

There is no true differential diagnosis for hyperglycemia that lists specific disease states, as there is for hypoglycemia. Therefore the most common etiologic factors associated with hyperglycemia are:

1. Stress
   a. Asphyxia
   b. Respiratory distress
   c. Intraventricular hemorrhage
   d. Infection
   e. Surgical procedures
2. Parenteral infusions
   a. Glucose
   b. Lipids
3. Drugs (theophylline, caffeine, dexamethasone)
4. Transient or permanent diabetes mellitus

TREATMENT

Primary therapeutic goals in treatment of hyperglycemia are prevention and early detection to avoid the need for more complex intervention. Infants at risk (i.e., premature infants with some of the above associated factors) need determination of glucose levels before dextrose infusion, approximately 3 hours following infusion, and every 8 hours until stable. It is also important to monitor urine glucose, daily weights, and daily intake and outputs to help quantitate any degree of diuresis. All intravenous fluids must be delivered by volumetric pumps capable of providing very small amounts at a steady rate. Following the administration of lipid infusions or the initiation of methylxanthine therapy, glucose levels should also be monitored.

Initial therapy is determined by whether hyperglycemia is transient or persistent. In general, transient glucose values greater than 200 mg/dL do not require aggressive intervention unless they result in significant osmotic diuresis and weight loss. Decreasing parenteral glucose by decreasing rate or concentration of glucose infusion usually corrects hyperglycemia. If glucose levels are greater than 300 mg/dL non-glucose–containing solutions may be used for short periods. Solutions containing less than 2.5% dextrose should be avoided since they may have changes in pH when prepared. In addition, such hypotonic solutions could cause hemolysis with resulting hyperkalemia.

With proper choice of initial glucose infusion rates, blood and urine glucose monitoring, and early adjustment of glucose infusion rates if glucose levels increase, insulin is rarely required. However, if glucose levels exceed 300 mg/dL despite lowering the amount of glucose infused, then insulin may be administered.

Several methods of administering insulin have been tried. We have had success using a single dose of subcutaneous or intravenous crystalline insulin, 0.1 to 0.2 U/kg, to lower glucose level, and then maintain normal glucose level by lowering the glucose infusion rate. Repeat doses every 6 to 12 hours are rarely necessary. Continuous insulin infusions have been used in very low-birth-weight infants (i.e., less than 1,250 g) to increase caloric intake or control hyperglycemia.[2, 16, 20] No consistent dose of insulin was used in these studies. In two of the studies albumin (approximately 0.3 g/dL) was used to minimize insulin loss by absorption to glass and plastic surfaces. A starting dose of 0.10 U/kg/hr, increased as necessary, is infused by separate syringe pump "piggyback" into the infusion set as close as possible to the patient, between the patient and the in-line filter. Albumin is not needed, because the amount of tubing used is minimal.

REFERENCES

1. Bekefi D, et al: Reflectometric blood glucose determination in the neonatological intensive care: Haematocrit dependence. *Exp Clin Endocrinol* 1984; 83:178–183.
2. Binder ND, et al: Insulin infusion with parenteral nutrition in extremely low birth weight infants with hyperglycemia. *J Pediatr* 1989; 114:273–280.
3. Bruining GJ, et al: Normalization of glucose homeostasis by long-acting somatostatin analog SMS 201-995 in a newborn with nesidioblastosis. *Acta Endocrinol Suppl* 1986; 279:334–339.
4. Bloomgarden ZT, et al: Treatment of intractable neonatal hypoglycemia with somatostatin plus glucagon. *J Pediatr* 1980; 96:148–151.
5. Carter PE, Lloyd DJ, Duffy P: Glucagon for hypoglycemia in infants small for gestational age. *Arch Dis Child* 1988; 63:1264–1266.
6. Cornblath M, Reisner SH: Blood glucose in the neonate, clinical significance. *N Engl J Med* 1965; 273:378–381.
7. Cornblath M, Pildes RS, Schwartz R: Hypoglycemia in infancy and childhood. *J Pediatr* 1973; 83:692–693.
8. Cornblath M, Schwartz R: *Carbohydrate Metabolism in the Neonate,* ed 2. Philadelphia, WB Saunders Co, 1976.
9. Jackson JA, et al: Long-term treatment of refractory neonatal hypoglycemia with long-acting somatostatin analog. *J Pediatr* 1987; 111:548–551.
10. Kitson HF, et al: Somatostatin treatment of insulin excess due to B-cell adenoma in a neonate. *J Pediatr* 1980; 96:145–148.
11. Kollee LA, et al: Persistent neonatal hypoglycemia due to glucagon deficiency. *Arch Dis Child* 1978; 53:422–424.
12. Lilien LD, Grajwer LA, Pildes RS: Treatment of neonatal hypoglycemia with continuous intravenous glucose infusions. *J Pediatr* 1977; 91:779–782.
13. Lilien LD, et al: Treatment of neonatal hypoglycemia with minibolus and intravenous glucose infusion. *J Pediatr* 1980; 97:295–298.
14. Lovinger RD, Kaplan SL, Grumbach MM: Congenital hypopituitarism associated with neonatal hypoglycemia and microphallus: Four cases secondary to hypothalamic hormone deficiencies. *J Pediatr* 1975; 87:1171–1181.
15. Mehta A, et al: Effect of diazoxide or glucagon on hepatic glucose production rate during extreme neonatal hypoglycaemia. *Arch Dis Child* 1987; 62:924–930.
16. Ostertag SG, et al: Insulin pump therapy in the very low birth weight infant. *Pediatrics* 1986; 78:625–630.
17. Pildes RS, et al: A prospective controlled study of neonatal hypoglycemia. *Pediatrics* 1974; 54:5–14.

18. Pildes RS, Lilien LD: Carbohydrate metabolism in the fetus and neonate, in Fanaroff AA, Martin RJ (eds): *Behrman's Neonatal-Perinatal Medicine, Diseases of the Fetus and Infant.* St Louis, CV Mosby Co, 1987, pp 1049–1077.
19. Srinivasan G, et al: Plasma glucose values in normal neonates: A new look. *J Pediatr* 1986; 109:114–117.
20. Vaucher YE, Walson PD, Morrow G: Continuous insulin infusion in hyperglycemic, very low birth weight infants. *J Pediatr Gastroenterol Nutr* 1982; 1:211–217.
21. Wilson DC, Carson DJ, Quinn RJ: Long-term use of somatostatin analogue SMS 201-995 in the treatment of hypoglycaemia due to nesidioblastosis. *Acta Paediatr Scand* 1988; 77:467–470.
22. Wuthrich C, Schubiger G, Zuppinger K: Persistent neonatal hyperinsulinemic hypoglycemia in two siblings successfully treated with diazoxide. *Helv Paediatr Acta* 1986; 41:455–459.
23. Warden MJ, German JC, Buckingham BA: The surgical management of hyperinsulinism in infancy due to nesidioblastosis. *J Pediatr Surg* 1988; 23:462–465.

18

Disorders of Calcium and Magnesium Homeostasis

Maria Lourdes Cruz, M.D.

Reginald C. Tsang, M.B.B.S.

NORMAL PHYSIOLOGY

Calcium

Calcium (Ca) is the most abundant mineral in the human body. The skeleton contains 99% of body Ca, and the remaining 1% is distributed in intravascular, interstitial, and intracellular fluids. Two forms of Ca are present in serum: (1) an undissociated form either bound to protein (30% to 55%) or complexed to different anions (5% to 15%), and (2) an ionized form (50%). Only the ionized form is considered physiologically active. Ionized and protein-bound Ca are in equilibrium, and the acid-base status partly controls the distribution. Acidosis increases the flux of Ca from bone to extracellular space and decreases the proportion of protein-bound Ca, thereby increasing the serum concentration of physiologically active Ca.[17, 28] Alkalosis reverses these effects.

In utero, Ca is actively transported across the placenta from mother to fetus; it is derived largely from the maternal skeleton.[32] During the last trimester, daily maternal-fetal fluxes may reach 150 mg/kg fetal body weight, whereas postnatal Ca retention from milk feedings ranges from 15 mg/kg body weight on day 1 of life to 45 mg/kg body weight on day 3. Therefore the Ca supply is abruptly and drastically reduced in the first few days of life when compared with the amount the fetus received in utero.[32] Serum concentrations of Ca in cord blood are at the highest level for any stage of life (and are higher than maternal levels), and thereafter there is a transient decline at 24 to 48 hours followed by a return to normal values.[17] The daily enteric requirement is approximately 60 elemental Ca mg/kg/day for term infants. The requirements may be higher for preterm infants, up to maximum values of 200 mg/kg/day.[7]

Once milk feedings are started, Ca absorption occurs primarily in the duodenum. Factors that increase Ca absorption include the presence of lactose and medium-chain triglycerides. The percentage of Ca absorbed is higher with human milk feedings than with cow milk–derived formulas, but the absolute quantity absorbed is lower because the Ca content of human milk is lower than cow milk formula. Loss of Ca occurs primarily through the fecal route, although increased urinary losses can occur secondary to increased sodium and protein intake, increased extracellular fluid, decreased phosphate, glucose loading, metabolic acidosis, and furosemide.

An important determinant of serum Ca concentrations is parathyroid hormone (PTH). In brief, PTH increases serum Ca concentrations by mobilization of Ca from bone, increased renal tubular reabsorption of Ca, and stimulation of 1,25-dihydroxyvitamin D_3 [1,25-$(OH)_2$]D production, which mediates intestinal Ca absorption. Calcitonin (CT) lowers serum Ca concentrations by inhibiting bone resorption and possibly by increasing renal Ca clearance. Both hormones are subject to a feedback regulation by Ca: low serum Ca concentrations stimulate PTH secretion, whereas high serum Ca concentrations stimulate CT secretion.

Phosphorus

Phosphorus (P) along with Ca is essential for bone mineralization, with 85% to 90% of total body P being located in the skeleton. As with Ca, in utero P is actively transported from mother to fetus. Endogenous P stores are released postnatally during breakdown of tissue glycogen. This factor, together with a decreased renal excretion (secondary to the normally decreased glomerular filtration rate and increased tubular P reabsorption in newborns), leads to an increased P load for the infant. Intestinal P absorption is very high in infancy, apparently occurring throughout the small intestine. The daily enteric requirement is approximately 40 mg/kg/day in term infants and 100 to 120 mg/kg/day in preterm infants.[7]

Changes in serum P concentrations directly affect serum Ca concentrations. Hyperphosphatemia has a hypocalcemic effect through physiochemical effects by blunting end organ (bone) response to PTH and 1,25-$(OH)_2$D. In contrast, in hypophosphatemia, calcium entry into bone is reduced, and active demineralization of bone may take place in order to raise serum phosphate concentrations,[12] leading to hypercalcemia. Thus the dietary Ca:P ratio can be an important determinant of mineral homeostasis, especially in infancy. A Ca:P ratio of roughly 2:1 in the diet appears to be optimal for term infants. This ratio is found in human milk, but most proprietary infant formulas have a lower Ca:P ratio.

Magnesium

Magnesium (Mg) is the second most common intracellular cation. Fifty percent of body Mg is in bone, the rest being distributed between muscle and soft tissue. Mg is an important component of the adenylate cyclase system and of the enzymes involved in the synthesis of ribosomal proteins. Fifty-five percent to 60% of Mg is in the ionized and presumably active form. As with Ca, acidosis tends to increase serum Mg concentrations whereas alkalosis decreases extracellular Mg concentrations.[22]

In utero, increasing amounts of Mg are transported (presumably by active transport) against a concentration gradient from mother to fetus after the fifth month of gestation. In contrast to Ca and iron transfer, where fetal mineral status is protected at the expense of the mother, fetuses of Mg-deprived rat mothers are Mg deficient.[26] Postnatally, fractional enteric Mg absorption is high compared with that of adults and is further increased by dietary protein, medium-chain triglycerides, and phosphate supplements to full-term breast-fed infants. Mg loss occurs mainly through the kidneys.[27] The daily requirement for Mg is approximately 6 to 8 mg/kg for an infant.

The effects of PTH on Mg are similar to the effects of PTH on Ca: PTH increases serum Mg concentrations by mobilizing bone Mg, possibly indirectly increasing intestinal Mg absorption [by production of $1,25\text{-}(OH)_2D$] and decreasing renal Mg excretion. Calcitonin tends to decrease serum Mg concentrations, presumably by blocking the effects of PTH on bone. Both hormones in turn are sensitive to feedback regulation by Mg in a manner similar to that for Ca. Mg and Ca also interact in a variety of ways. In the intestinal lumen Mg decreases Ca absorption, and Ca excretion is increased at the renal tubular level in the presence of high levels of filtered Mg.[28] Likewise, acute hypermagnesemia may lead to hypocalcemia by inhibition of PTH secretion and stimulation of CT secretion,[22] whereas acute hypomagnesemia theoretically may increase serum Ca concentrations by increasing PTH concentrations. Paradoxically, however, and the major exception to this relationship, is the hypocalcemic effect of chronic hypomagnesemia. This has been attributed to hypoparathyroidism secondary to Mg deficiency, PTH end organ unresponsiveness, and inhibition of the heteroionic bone exchange of Mg for Ca.[31] Finally, serum Mg concentrations may also be affected by P. Hyperphosphatemia tends to increase Mg deposition into bone, thereby depressing serum Mg concentrations.

The complex interactions of Ca, P, and Mg are summarized in Figure 18–1. Note that these relationships are those of acute excesses of each mineral and that the relationships of these minerals at depressed levels cannot be extrapolated from the diagram.

Parathyroid Hormone

PTH is an important regulator of serum Ca concentrations. It acts on bone, intestine, and kidney to increase serum Ca and Mg concentrations while decreasing serum P concentrations. In turn, Ca and Mg exert an acute negative feedback effect on PTH; however, chronic hypomagnesemia decreases PTH

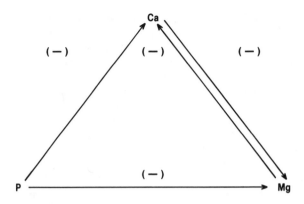

FIG 18–1.
Interactions of Calcium *(Ca)*, phosphorus *(P)*, and magnesium *(Mg)*.

secretion, presumably by inhibition of the adenylate cyclase system necessary for PTH secretion. PTH is degraded primarily in the kidney.

The fetal parathyroid gland is functionally active by the twelfth week of gestation, but since its activity appears to be affected by existing serum Ca concentrations and the fetus is normally hypercalcemic, parathyroid gland function is thought to be suppressed in utero. After birth, however, serum PTH concentration increases in healthy full-term infants, presumably in response to the transient hypocalcemia that occurs normally in the first few days of life.[21]

Calcitonin

CT lowers serum Ca and P through inhibition of bone resorption and possibly increased renal clearance of Ca and P. Calcitonin production is increased when serum Ca concentrations are elevated.[4] Fetal CT function appears to be autonomous of the mother, and CT probably does not cross the placenta. Serum CT concentrations are relatively high at birth, with further increases in the postnatal period.[31] High serum CT concentrations in the neonate possibly protect the skeleton from excessive bone resorption and protect against acute hypercalcemia during milk feedings,[32, 33] but may also aggravate the tendency toward hypocalcemia at this age.

Vitamin D

Vitamin D is ingested as ergocalciferol (vitamin D_2) or cholecalciferol (vitamin D_3) or is produced endogenously in the skin as vitamin D_3. Conversion of vitamin D to 25-(OH)D occurs in the liver; subsequent conversion of 25-(OH)D to 1,25-(OH)$_2$D occurs in the kidney. The 1,25-(OH)$_2$D form is the active metabolite of vitamin D. Its production is stimulated by PTH and hypophosphatemia, and it increases the absorption of Ca from the intestine, facilitates PTH-induced mobilization of Ca and P from bone, and increases Ca and P reabsorption in the kidney tubules. Although 1,25-$(OH)_2D$ appears to cross the placenta, its concentration in cord blood of the newborn may appear to be decreased when compared with maternal levels. The fetoplacental unit appears to synthesize 1,25-$(OH)_2D$,[19] although the functional significance of this synthesis is unclear. Concentrations of 1,25-$(OH)_2D$ in an infant reach normal adult levels by 24 hours of age.[23] The increased postnatal serum concentrations of 1,25-$(OH)_2D$ could be related to the postnatal fall in serum Ca and the resultant increase in PTH secretion. Normal daily requirements for vitamin D are considered to be 400 IU in infants. This amount is available with normal intake of standard vitamin D–fortified infant formulas but not human milk.

A summary of these different perinatal events and the effects of the various hormones on Ca, P, and Mg is shown in Table 18–1.

HYPOCALCEMIA

Classification

Neonatal hypocalcemia is defined as total serum Ca less than 7.8 mg/dL in term infants and less than 7 mg/dL in preterm infants or serum ionized Ca level less than 4.4 mg/dL[11, 29] as determined by newer, ion-selective electrodes. Neonatal hypocalcemia can be divided into early or late hypocalcemia. Early hypocalcemia occurs within the first 3 days of life, with the lowest serum Ca occurring at 24 to 48 hours of life,[40] whereas late hypocalcemia occurs generally after the first week of life. The time of onset of hypocalcemia depends primarily on the underlying mechanism; that is, early neonatal hypocalcemia is a result of perinatal or intrauterine events, whereas late hypocalcemia is either the result of dietary alteration or a manifestation of a congenital defect[14, 34–37] (Table 18–2). In some cases the distinction between the two classes may not be clear. It is important to know that with proper treatment, most cases of early hypocalcemia resolve within the first week of life. Prolonged hypocalcemia should prompt the physician to investigate such conditions as congenital hypoparathyroidism or DiGeorge syndrome.

Diagnosis

The hypocalcemic infant may exhibit signs of neuromuscular hyperactivity (muscle twitching, tremors, seizures, laryngospasm), or lethargy, or may be totally asymptomatic. Chvostek's sign (twitching of upper lip or mouth after stimulation of the facial nerve at the level of the external auditory meatus) or Trousseau's phenomenon (carpopedal spasm after application of a blood

TABLE 18–1.
Perinatal Events and Effects of Various Hormones on Calcium (Ca), Magnesium (Mg), and Phosphorus (P)

	Perinatal Events			Site of Action			
	Placental Transfer	Serum Concentration in Cord Blood	Postnatal Serum Concentration	Intestine	Bone	Kidney	Net Effect on Blood Concentration
Parathyroid hormone	No	Low	Increase	—	↑ Ca,P,Mg release	↑ Ca,Mg reabsorption ↓ P reabsorption ↑ 1,25-OH₂D production	↑ Ca, ↓ P, ↑ Mg
Calcitonin	No	High	Increase	—	↓ Ca,P release	↑ Ca,P,Mg excretion	↓ Ca,P,Mg
1,25-(OH)₂D	(Yes)	Low	Increase	↑ Ca,P absorption	↑ Ca,P release	↑ Ca,P reabsorption	↑ Ca,P

pressure cuff inflated above systolic blood pressure for 3 minutes) may be observed in a term infant; preterm infants are usually asymptomatic.

Confirmation of the diagnosis of hypocalcemia is made from the determination of serum Ca concentrations. It is important to note, however, that decreases in the active, ionized Ca fraction may occur without a decrease in total Ca concentrations, as in alkalosis, binding of Ca in "exchange" transfusions with citrated blood, and raised free fatty acids from lipid infusions. Hypoalbuminemia may cause an artifactual decrease in total Ca concentration without an actual decrease in ionized Ca. Hypomagnesemia and hyperphosphatemia may be present with hypocalcemia, depending on the cause of the disease. Prolonged QT intervals (QT_c greater than 0.4 second, or Q_oT_c greater than 0.2 seconds, both corrected for heart rate) may also be present. The QT interval may be helpful in following clinical progress with treatment but is a poor predictor of ionized Ca concentration.[33] Assays of PTH, CT, and vitamin D metabolites are recommended for the diagnosis of prolonged, refractory, or recurrent hypocalcemia.

Treatment

Symptomatic hypocalcemia should be treated. Calcium gluconate 10%, containing 9.4 mg elemental Ca/mL (102 mg Ca gluconate/mL), given intravenously at 2 mL/kg (equivalent to 18 mg elemental Ca/kg or 200 mg Ca gluconate/kg) over 10 minutes with heart rate monitoring is usually effective. This dose should be followed by intravenous Ca supplementation with elemental Ca, 75 mg/kg/day (approximately 700 to 800 mg Ca gluconate/kg/day), until normocalcemia is achieved. Thereafter the elemental dose should be decreased to 37 mg/kg/day for 1 day, then 18 mg/kg for another day, and then totally withdrawn, provided daily serum Ca determinations during replacement therapy are normal. An alternative regimen consists of 75 mg elemental Ca/kg/day for 2 days and then abrupt withdrawal of Ca, provided serum Ca concentrations are normal. These regimens have been formulated to help prevent iatrogenic hypercalcemia and also prevent potential parathyroid gland suppression and rebound hypocalcemia. If serum Ca concentrations do not revert to normal, one may delay the sequential dose reduction until normocalcemia is achieved.

Several precautions must be taken during Ca infusion. First, rapid infusions may cause bradycardia or cardiac arrest. Therefore, heart rate monitoring is necessary at all times, and tubing with Ca solutions must be labeled to prevent accidental "flushing" of lines with the Ca-enriched solution. Continuous infusion is also preferred over bolus therapy (unless the infant has active seizures) because the increase in serum Ca concentration after bolus therapy is short-lived, decreasing to 50% of the increase after 30 minutes. Second, Ca should not be given intra-arterially, because of potential vascular complications such as intestinal bleeding and skin necrosis, depending on the site of the intra-arterial catheter. Intramuscular administration may cause tissue necrosis. Ca must not be given through umbilical venous catheters

TABLE 18–2.
Classification of Neonatal Hypocalcemia

Etiology	Frequency of Hypocalcemia	Proposed Pathogenetic Mechanisms	Comment
Early			
Prematurity	1/3	Functional hypoparathyroidism* Hypercalcitonemia Decreased oral feeds 1,25-$(OH)_2$ D resistance in very low-birth-weight infants	Gestational age more important than weight[36]; higher incidence with increased prematurity[39]
Asphyxia	1/3	Hypercalcitonemia End organ resistance to PTH Alkalosis from bicarbonate therapy or hyperventilation Hyperphosphatemia (from tissue catabolism)	Concomitant prematurity aggravates hypocalcemia[40]
Infant of insulin-dependent mother	1/2	Functional hypoparathyroidism–maternal hypomagnesemia (from urinary losses), leads to chronic fetal hypomagnesemia, ↓ PTH secretion Hypercalcitonemia Decreased oral feeds from respiratory distress	Severity of hypocalcemia proportional to severity of maternal diabetes; usually with hypomagnesemia Infants of mothers with gestational diabetes are probably less prone to develop hypocalcemia than infants of insulin-dependent diabetics
Infant of hyperparathyroid mother	Rare	Maternal hypercalcemia leads to fetal hypercalcemia and fetal parathyroid gland suppression	Transient
Maternal anticonvulsant therapy	Rare	Increased hepatic metabolism of vitamin D	Maternal vitamin D therapy may be helpful

Late			
Iatrogenic			
"Exchange" transfusion	Variable	Citrate in acid-citrate dextrose blood binds Ca	Transient; may not need prophylactic Ca
Alkalosis (metabolic or respiratory)		Lowers ionic fraction of Ca	
Lipid infusion		Formation of free fatty acid–Ca soaps	In vitro
Phototherapy		(?)Decreased melatonin secretion; increased bone Ca uptake in rats	
Congenital hypoparathyroidism	Always	Agenesis/dysgenesis/hypoplasia of parathyroid gland: X-linked/autosomal dominant/sporadic	Rare; lifelong vitamin D treatment
		DiGeorge syndrome	Thymic aplasia, T cell and immune defect
			Heart/aortic arch defects, hypoplastic mandible, ear defects
			Compensatory hyperparathyroidism may relieve hypocalcemia but may aggravate rickets
Disorders of vitamin D metabolism	Frequent		
Vitamin D deficiency Diet		↓ Intestinal absorption of Ca and P	
Liver/kidney disease		↓ Conversion of vitamin D to 25-(OH)D or 1,25-(OH)$_2$D	
1,25-(OH)$_2$ vitamin D unresponsiveness		Receptor defect; ↓ intestinal absorption of Ca and P	
Neonatal systemic lupus erythematosus	Rare	Antiparathyroid gland antibodies(?)	Seizures at 7 weeks[13]
Maternal hypovitaminosis D	Occasional	Fetal and neonatal hypovitaminosis D leads to ↓ intestinal absorption of Ca and P after birth	Maternal therapy indicated if detected during pregnancy

(Continued)

TABLE 18–2 (cont.).

Nutritional High P feeds	Frequent	Increased Ca-P complex deposition Blunted end organ response to PTH	Present formulas in U.S. have lower P than in cow milk P high in evaporated cow milk and some cereals
Chronic hypomagnesemia	Frequent	Decreased adenylate cyclase—stimulated PTH release; decreased bone Mg-Ca exchange; end organ unresponsiveness to PTH	

*The concept of functional hypoparathyroidism is controversial. Some workers[35,36,40] have found delayed or inadequate response to hypocalcemia; others[4] have found an appropriate response.

situated near the heart or within the liver. If the infant is already receiving oral feeds, then oral Ca supplementation at the same doses, given at 4- to 6-hour intervals, is preferred over intravenous therapy. Preparations such as Ca glubionate (Neo-Calglucon) are hypertonic and can provoke diarrhea; theoretically, they may also predispose to necrotizing enterocolitis. Thus 10% IV Ca gluconate solution is the preparation of choice for enteric administration. Third, intravenous sites must be checked regularly for proper placement, because Ca in soft tissue causes skin sloughing. Fourth, Ca is incompatible with bicarbonate and must be given in separate intravenous lines. Last, calcium chloride usually is avoided in infants because it can cause metabolic acidosis.

Treatment of asymptomatic hypocalcemia is controversial. In theory, infants with Ca concentrations in the hypocalcemic range are at risk for potential adverse cardiovascular and CNS effects. Treatment with Ca may cause some risk. In clinical practice, many neonatologists arbitrarily decide to treat only when severe hypocalcemia occurs, that is, when total serum Ca is less than 6 mg/dL in preterm infants and less than 7 mg/dL in term infants or ionized Ca is less than 3.4 mg/dL in all infants. In all cases, treatment of underlying causes must be instituted as well.

More recently, vitamin D metabolites ($1,25\text{-}(OH)_2D$) have been used in the prevention and treatment of neonatal hypocalcemia. However, since this approach is still experimental, its use is not routinely recommended at this time. Furthermore, there appears to be resistance to $1,25\text{-}(OH)_2D$ in very low-birth-weight infants, and the supraphysiologic doses required have not been proved safe.[9, 39]

Prevention

Another area of controversy in Ca therapy is prophylactic Ca supplementation. In general, premature or birth-asphyxiated infants may benefit from prophylactic Ca supplementation from day 1 of life at approximately 35 mg/kg/day elemental Ca (300 to 400 mg/kg/day Ca salt) without detrimental effects on P, Mg, and PTH concentrations.[1, 13, 18] The infant can then be weaned from supplements after 3 days, provided serum Ca concentrations are normal, since the infant's hormonal regulatory mechanisms should be functional at this time. Iatrogenic causes of hypocalcemia (discussed earlier) should be avoided or minimized, and mothers taking anticonvulsants may benefit from vitamin D supplementation.

Prognosis

In a study by Cockburn et al.[3] of 75 newborns with seizures secondary to (late neonatal) hypocalcemia, there was associated hypomagnesemia and hyperphosphatemia; 65% of these infants were healthy, and 11% were developmentally delayed at 1 year of age. There were single instances of ataxia, dystonia, and spasticity. Electroencephalographic abnormalities may persist

TABLE 18–3.
Classification of Neonatal Hypercalcemia

Cause	Pathogenetic Mechanism	Manifestations	Treatment
Parathyroid disorders			
Primary hyperparathyroidism		Usually autosomal recessive, with hypophosphatemia, hyperphosphaturia, hypercalciuria nephrocalcinosis, demineralization	Surgical removal of parathyroid gland; otherwise, prognosis is poor
Secondary hyperparathyroidism	Maternal hypoparathyroidism and hypocalcemia lead to fetal parathyroid gland hyperplasia	As in primary hyperparathyroidism, but transient biochemical features	Supportive
Benign familial hypocalciuric hypercalcemia	May or may not include neonatal hyperparathyroidism	Usually autosomal dominant; hypotonia, constipation, feeding problems	Supportive
Idiopathic infantile hypercalcemia	?: Vitamin D hyperresponsivity, abnormal calcitonin secretion	May be associated with Williams syndrome (elfin facies, mental retardation, supravalvular aortic stenosis, failure to thrive); usually detected after neonatal period	Low Ca/low vitamin D diet Avoid sunlight
Nutritional			
Hypophosphatemia	Mobilization of Ca from bone	Usually in low-birth-weight infants fed human milk; can lead to rickets	Need P and Ca supplement
Vitamin D intoxication	Increased intestinal absorption of Ca	Infants of food faddists	
Vitamin A intoxication	Increased bone resorption of Ca		
Subcutaneous fat necrosis	Abnormal fat metabolism; Ca release from tissue	Usually in asphyxiated, hypothermic babies or large infants with trau-	Low Ca/vitamin D diet, hydration/furosemide

Disorder	Mechanism	Clinical features	Treatment
	(?) Abnormal vitamin D sensitivity	matic delivery	
	Macrophage release of 1,25-$(OH)_2$D(?)	Painless, sharply demarcated plaques over bony prominences/buttocks/cheeks; skin lesions appear shortly after birth; hypercalcemia later	
Thyroid disorders			
Hypothyroidism	Increased intestinal Ca absorption(?)	—	Treatment of primary thyroid disorder
Hyperthyroidism	Increased bone resorption of Ca	—	
Iatrogenic			
Overtreatment of hypocalcemia		—	Avoidance or cessation of causative agent
Excess Ca prophylaxis in "exchange" blood transfusion		—	
Thiazide treatment	Decreased Ca excretion	—	

for several months.[6] The ability to respond to social stimuli was affected in asymptomatic hypocalcemic newborns evaluated at birth by Chan et al.,[2] but 3- and 6-month Gesell developmental examinations were normal. Tooth enamel hypoplasia has also been reported.[15, 25]

HYPERCALCEMIA

Etiology

Hypercalcemia is defined as total serum Ca concentration of greater than 10.8 mg/dL or ionized Ca greater than 5.6 mg/dL.[24] Elevated serum total Ca concentrations are usually associated with elevated ionized Ca, unless there is concomitant hyperproteinemia, which may lead to falsely elevated total Ca. Hypercalcemia occurs rarely in the neonate, and when identified, the most probable cause is iatrogenic (overtreatment of hypocalcemia or excessive Ca prophylaxis in "exchange" blood transfusions). Recently the use of thiazide diuretics in the neonatal intensive care unit has been associated with hypercalcemia. Human milk feeding in preterm infants may also lead to hypophosphatemia because of the low P content of human milk, and this in turn may cause secondary hypercalcemia. Otherwise, the differential diagnosis for neonatal hypercalcemia consists of a group of uncommon disorders (Table 18–3).

Treatment

Aside from treatment of underlying causes (iatrogenic or nutritional), supportive therapy in the form of fluid replacement in cases of dehydration control may be necessary. Otherwise, with total serum Ca concentrations of less than 12.5 mg/dL, treatment may not be necessary unless the patient has symptoms. Furosemide at 1 mg/kg/dose is effective over the short term as a calciuretic agent when given every 2 to 4 hours for 1 or 2 days, but fluid support may be necessary. Glucocorticoids at 1 mg/kg/day for 3 to 4 days decrease intestinal absorption but are usually slow acting. Other modes of therapy, including phosphates, prostaglandin synthetase inhibitors, and CT are rarely used.

HYPOMAGNESEMIA

Classification

Hypomagnesemia is defined as serum concentration less than 1.6 mg/dL.[30] Most cases of hypomagnesemia are transient, with the exception of those secondary to intestinal and renal transport defects, both of which require lifetime replacement. Clinical signs and symptoms, usually evident at serum concentrations of 1.2 mg/dL, include apnea, bradycardia, neuromuscular excitability, weakness, and Trousseau's and Chvostek's signs. Laboratory findings include hypocalcemia, hyperphosphatemia, and T wave inversion (Table 18–4).

Treatment

Mild asymptomatic hypomagnesemia needs no treatment provided the cause of hypomagnesemia can be eliminated and the patient has adequate dietary Mg intake. One should also determine if there is concomitant hypocalcemia, as hypocalcemia often will not resolve if there is underlying hypomagnesemia. Short-term therapy consists of 0.1 to 0.2 mL/kg of 50% $MgSO_4 \cdot 7H_2O$ USP (contains 49.3 mg of elemental Mg per milliliter or 500 mg of $MgSO_4$ per milliliter; the dose is therefore about 5 to 10 mg/kg of elemental Mg or 50 to 100 mg/kg of $MgSO_4$) by the intramuscular route, or by slow intravenous infusion over 60 minutes. If enteric treatment is undertaken, the same dose should be diluted to a 5% or 10% solution and can be given every 8 to 12 hours. Serum Mg concentration should be monitored every 2 hours, and cardiac monitoring should be used to detect complications such as prolongation of atrioventricular conduction time, atrioventricular block, and sinoatrial block. Other clinical symptoms of Mg toxicity include CNS or respiratory depression, hypotension, intestinal ileus, and urinary retention.

When tolerated, maintenance therapy can be given orally as 50% $MgSO_4 \cdot 7H_2O$ USP at 0.4 to 0.8 mL/kg/day (20 to 40 mg elemental Mg/kg/day or 200 to 400 mg $MgSO_4$/kg/day) diluted to a 10% solution and given in four equal doses. This higher dose is necessary because of the normally low intestinal absorption of Mg, and may be cautiously given up to 100 to 120 mg/kg/day if definite Mg malabsorption is documented. Large doses, however, may cause diarrhea.

Prognosis

Three children receiving chronic Mg supplementation for specific Mg malabsorption showed normal physical and mental development on follow-up examination. It is assumed that early recognition and treatment of hypomagnesemia results in good outcome.

HYPERMAGNESEMIA

Hypermagnesemia is defined as serum Mg concentrations greater than 2.5 mg/dL. In neonates, the most common cause of hypermagnesemia is maternal Mg therapy for preeclampsia or premature labor. Prematurity and perinatal asphyxia may aggravate the problem because of decreased urinary excretion. Mg-containing antacids, which are on rare occasions administered

TABLE 18–4.
Classification of Neonatal Hypomagnesemia

Cause	Pathogenetic Mechanism	Comments
Decreased supply		
Infant of diabetic mother (IDM)	Maternal urinary Mg losses	Occurs in 38% of IDMs Degree of hypomagnesemia directly proportional to severity of maternal diabetes
Infant of alcoholic mother	Poor maternal diet Increased urinary losses of Mg (in rats)	Seen in experimental rats Concomitant growth retardation and zinc deficiency
Small for gestational age	Decreased maternal supply or poor placental transfer	Especially in infants of primiparous mothers with toxemia
Intestinal Mg malabsorption		
Primary	Intestinal receptor defect onset 2 to 4 wks; Ca deficiency also	Rare; usually male
Acquired	Surgical resection: decreased absorptive surface Ileostomy/obstruction: change in bacterial flora	
Prematurity Inadequate parenteral supplementation	Decreased stores	
Increased loss		
"Exchange" transfusion	Mg-citrate complex formation	
Biliary atresia/hepatitis	Secondary to hypoalbuminemia and hypoaldosteronism; increased urinary losses	
Thiazides/furosemide	Urinary losses; aggravated by increased Na/Ca in renal tubular lumen	
Renal tubular defect	Tubular receptor defect	
Disorders of homeostasis:		
Hypoparathyroidism	Decreased bone Mg mobilization Decreased renal Mg reabsorption Hyperphosphatemia; increased Mg deposition in bone	Duration of hypomagnesemia dependent on cause and duration of hypoparathyroidism

to infants, may cause hypermagnesemia.[8] Clinical manifestations include respiratory and neuromuscular depression. The duration of weakness is directly proportional to the duration of maternal therapy but may not correspond to the degree of maternal hypermagnesemia.[10] Clinical symptoms improve in 24 to 48 hours. Offspring of mothers given Mg may demonstrate hypocalcemia,[20] increased serum calcium concentration,[5] or normocalcemia.[16] The hypocalcemia may be attributed to suppression of PTH secretion by the high Mg concentrations, whereas the increase in serum calcium is thought to be secondary to increased heteroionic bone Mg exchange for Ca. The factors that control this varied Ca response are unknown.

Treatment of hypermagnesemia is mainly expectant and includes discontinuation of medications containing Mg, and cardiorespiratory support. Urinary Mg excretion may be enhanced by furosemide, 1 mg/kg/dose every 2 to 4 hours, but this must be supported by fluid replacement. If the infant shows signs of neuromuscular toxicity, 10% CA gluconate, 0.1 to 0.3 mL/kg/dose (approximately 1 to 3 mg elemental Ca/kg/dose) by slow intravenous infusion, may result in reversal of toxicity. Exchange blood transfusion or dialysis may be needed in extreme cases.

REFERENCES

1. Brown DR, Tsang RC, Chen I: Oral calcium supplementation in premature and asphyxiated neonates. *J Pediatr* 1976; 89:973–977.
2. Chan GM, et al: Neurologic development of prematures treated for neonatal hypocalcemia (abstract). *Pediatr Res* 1977; 11:561.
3. Cockburn F, et al: Neonatal convulsions associated with primary disturbance of calcium, phosphorus, and magnesium metabolism. *Arch Dis Child* 1973; 48:99–108.
4. David L, Salle BL, Putet G, et al: Serum immunoreactive calcitonin in low birth weight infants; effects of intravenous calcium infusion; relationships with early changes in serum calcium, phosphorus, magnesium, parathyroid hormone, and gastric levels. *Pediatr Res* 1981; 15:803–808.
5. Donovan EF, Tsang RC, Steichen JJ, et al: Neonatal hypermagnesemia: Effect on parathyroid hormone and calcium homeostasis. *J Pediatr* 1980; 96:305–310.
6. Eriksson M, Zetlerstrom R: Neonatal convulsions. *Acta Paediatr Scand* 1979; 68:807–811.
7. Greer FR, Tsang RC: Calcium, phosphorus, magnesium and vitamin D requirements for the preterm infant, in Tsang RC (ed): *Vitamin and Mineral Requirements in Preterm Infants.* New York, Marcel Dekker, 1985, pp 99–136.
8. Humphrey M, Kennon S, Pramanik AK: Hypermagnesemia from antacid administration in a newborn infant. *J Pediatr* 1981; 98:313–314.
9. Koo WWK, Tsang RC, Poser JW, et al: Elevated serum calcium and osteocalcin levels from calcitriol in preterm infants. A prospective randomized study. *Am J Dis Child* 1986; 140:1152–1158.
10. Lipsitz PJ: The clinical and biochemical effects of excess magnesium in the newborn. *Pediatrics* 1971; 47:501.

11. Loughead JL, Mimouni F, Tsang RC: Serum ionized calcium concentration in normal neonates. *Am J Dis Child* 1988; 142:516–518.

12. Lyon AJ, McIntosh N: Calcium and phosphorus balance in extremely low birth weight infants in the first six weeks of life. *Arch Dis Child* 1984; 59:1145–1150.

13. Moudgil A, Kishore K, Srivastava RN: Neonatal lupus erythematosus, late onset hypocalcemia, and recurrent seizures. *Arch Dis Child* 1987; 62:736–739.

14. Nervez CT, et al: Prophylaxis against hypocalcemia in low birth weight infants requiring bicarbonate infusion. *J Pediatr* 1975; 87:439–442.

15. Purvis RJ, Barrie WJ, Mackay GS, et al: Enamel hypoplasia of the teeth associated with neonatal tetany: Manifestation of maternal vitamin D deficiency. *Lancet* 1973; 2:811–814.

16. Rasch DK, Huber PA, Richardson CJ, et al: Neurobehavioral effects of neonatal hypermagnesemia. *J Pediatr* 1982; 100:272–276.

17. Root AW, Harrison HE: Recent advances in calcium metabolism. *J Pediatr* 1976; 88:1–18, 177–199.

18. Salle BL, et al: Prevention of early neonatal hypocalcemia in low birth weight infants with continuous calcium infusion. *Pediatr Res* 1977; 11:1180–1185.

19. Salle BL, Senterre J, Glorieux PH, et al: Vitamin D metabolism in preterm infants. *Biol Neonate* 1987; 52(suppl 1):119–130.

20. Savory J, Monif GR: Serum calcium levels in cord sera of the progeny of mothers treated with magnesium sulfate for toxemia of pregnancy. *Am J Obstet Gynecol* 1971; 110:556–559.

21. Schedewie HK, et al: Parahormone and perinatal calcium homeostasis. *Pediatr Res* 1979; 13:1–6.

22. Schedewie HK, Fisher DA: Perinatal mineral homeostasis, in Tulchinsky D, Ryan KJ (eds): *Maternal Fetal Endocrinology.* Philadelphia, WB Saunders Co, 1980, pp 355–386.

23. Specker BL, Lichtenstein P, Mimouni F, et al: Calcium-regulating hormone and mineral from birth to 18 months of age: A cross-sectional study. II. Effects of sex, race, age, season and diet in serum minerals, parathyroid hormone, and calcitonin. *Pediatrics* 1986; 77:891–896.

24. Steichen JJ, et al: Perinatal vitamin D homeostasis: 1,25(OH) D in maternal, cord and neonatal blood (abstract). *Clin Res* 1977; 25:567.

25. Stimmler L, Snodgrass GJAL, Jaffe E: Dental defects associated with neonatal symptomatic hypocalcemia. *Arch Dis Child* 1973; 48:217–220.

25a. Stromme JH, Nesbakken R, Norman T, et al: Familial hypomagnesemia: A follow-up examination of three patients after 9 to 12 years of treatment. *Pediatr Res* 1981; 15:1134–1139.

26. Suh SU, Firek AF: Magnesium and zinc deficiency and growth retardation in offspring of alcoholic rats. *J Am Coll Nutr* 1982; 1:192–198.

27. Tsang RC: Neonatal magnesium disturbances. *Am J Dis Child* 1972; 124:282–293.

28. Tsang RC, Donovan EF, Steichen JJ: Calcium physiology and pathology in the neonate. *Pediatr Clin North Am* 1976; 23:611–626.

29. Tsang RC, Oh W: Neonatal hypocalcemia in low birth weight infants. *Pediatrics* 1970; 45:773–781.

30. Tsang RC, Oh W: Serum magnesium levels in low birth weight infants. *Am J Dis Child* 1070; 120:44–47.

31. Tsang RC, Steichen JJ: Calcium and magnesium homeostasis in the newborn, in Avery GB (ed): *Neonatology: Pathophysiology and Management of the Newborn.* Philadelphia, JB Lippincott Co, 1981, pp 600–611.

32. Tsang RC, Steichen JJ, Brown DR: Perinatal calcium homeostasis: Neonatal hypocalcemia and bone demineralization. *Clin Perinatol* 1977; 4:385–409.
33. Tsang RC, Steichen JJ, Chan GM: Neonatal hypocalcemia: Mechanism of occurrence and management. *Crit Care Med* 1977; 5:56–61.
34. Tsang RC, et al: Hyocalcemia in infants of diabetic mothers. *J Pediatr* 1972; 80:384–395.
35. Tsang RC, et al: Possible pathogenetic factors in neonatal hypocalcemia of prematurity. *J Pediatr* 1973; 82:423–429.
36. Tsang RC, et al: Neonatal parathyroid function: Role of gestational age and postnatal age. *J Pediatr* 1973; 83:728–738.
37. Tsang RC, et al: Neonatal hypocalcemia in infants with birth asphyxia. *J Pediatr* 1974; 84:428–433.
38. Tsang RC, et al: Hypomagnesemia in infants of diabetic mothers: Perinatal studies. *J Pediatr* 1976; 89:115–119.
39. Venkataraman PS, Tsang RC, Steichen JJ, et al: Early neonatal hypocalcemia in extremely preterm infants. High incidence, early onset, and refractoriness to supraphysiologic doses of calcitriol. *Am J Dis Child* 1986; 140:1004–1008.
40. Venkataraman PS, Tsang RC, Chen IW, et al: Pathogenesis of early neonatal hypocalcemia: Studies of serum calcitonin, gastrin, and plasma glucagon. *J Pediatr* 1987; 110:599–603.

19

Renal Failure

Eunice G. John, M.D.
Tsu F. Yeh, M.D.

Acute renal failure (ARF) may be defined as a sudden impairment of glomerular and tubular function that results in oliguria, anuria or polyuria, water and electrolyte imbalance, acid-base disturbances, and accumulation of nitrogenous wastes such as urea and creatinine. Causative factors usually are categorized as prerenal, renal, or postrenal:

1. Prerenal causes
   a. Hypovolemia: hemorrhage, dehydration, sepsis, phototherapy, hyperosmotic intravenous fluid
   b. Hypoperfusion: hypoxia, hypotension, respiratory distress syndrome (RDS), cardiac failure, medication-induced hypotension, tolazoline therapy, postcardiac surgery, positive pressure ventilation
2. Renal causes
   a. Congenital: bilateral renal dysplasia, agenesis, multicystic or polycystic kidneys, congenital nephritis or nephrotic syndrome
   b. Acquired: intravascular coagulation, renal vein thrombosis, cortical or medullary necrosis
   c. Ischemic: shock, dehydration, hypotension, hypoxia, RDS
   d. Nephrotoxic: aminoglycosides and methicillin therapy, hemoglobin, myoglobin, bilirubin, contrast material and indomethacin administration
   e. Miscellaneous: acidosis, hyperuricemia of the newborn, polycythemia; tolazoline, papaverine, and catecholamine administration; urinary tract infection (viral or bacterial)
3. Postrenal causes
   a. Congenital obstructive uropathy: posterior urethral valve, uterocele, pelvic ureteral obstruction, urethral diverticulum, urethral strictures, neurogenic bladder, megacystis-megaureter syndrome, and tumor

CLINICAL FEATURES AND LABORATORY TESTS

Clinical findings are determined mainly by the disease or disorder that produces ARF. Oliguria is the most important sign of ARF. However, there may be normal or increased urine output if ARF is secondary to aminoglycoside antibiotic therapy, nephrogenic diabetes insipidus, or partial urinary obstruction. Edema is usually secondary to fluid overload. Abdominal distention or flank masses may be present depending on the cause. Neonates with bilateral renal agenesis or severe dysplasia have features of Potter facies and usually a history of oligohydramnios. Seizures may be observed as a result of associated hypoxia, intracranial hemorrhage, cerebral edema, hypoglycemia, hyponatremia, hypocalcemia, hypertension, uremia, or infection.

Hypotension may occur early in the course of ARF. Hypertension is often due to fluid overload or excessive secretion of renin and aldosterone. If the blood pressure is increased considerably, the possibility of renal cortical necrosis and renal artery thrombosis or embolism should be considered. Most neonates with intrinsic ARF have microscopic or gross hematuria or proteinuria.

Impairment of renal function may be confirmed by blood and urine tests (Table 19–1). Glomerular filtration rate (GFR) is the best parameter to follow changes in renal function.[5, 24] In premature and newborn infants, accurate calculation of GFR with serum creatinine levels and body length without urine collection awaits further clarification (Table 19–2).[17, 21, 39, 40]

PATHOPHYSIOLOGY

Much controversy surrounds the pathogenetic mechanisms (Fig 19–1) involved in the development and sustenance of ARF following hemorrhage, dehydration, or sepsis. Maintenance of ARF long after the removal of the insult has been attributed to tubular obstruction from cell debris and back-diffusion of filtrate through the damaged tubular walls. Recently the emphasis has shifted toward reduced cortical blood flow and diminished glomerular filtration as the principal function abnormalities in ARF. Several studies have shown that catecholamine release, increased sympathetic tone, and activation of the renin-angiotensin system may account for the reduction of renal cortical blood flow.[8, 20] The decrease in cortical blood flow leads to tubular damage and loss of sodium, which in turn stimulates the macula densa and release of more renin. This occurrence initiates the afferent arteriolar and glomerular mesangial contraction and decreases GFR. It is possible that a vicious circle be created: afferent arteriolar vasoconstriction would induce further renin release and thus maintain the oliguric state long after cessation of the initial insult. In the presence of damage to the macula densa, however, lack of renin production will result in continued loss of salt and water secondary to tubular damage, which accounts for high-output renal failure in some patients.

TABLE 19–1.
Diagnostic Indices in Neonatal Acute Renal Failure

Findings	Prerenal Oliguria Without Renal Failure	Prerenal and Intrinsic Renal Failure
Serum		
Sodium	Normal or elevated	Low normal or elevated
Potassium	Normal or elevated	Normal or elevated
Blood urea nitrogen	Normal or elevated	Elevated
Creatinine	Normal or elevated	Elevated
Calcium	Normal	Low
Phosphorus	Normal	Normal or elevated
Urine		
Red blood cells, protein, casts, and tubular cell casts	Usually absent	Present
Specific gravity	Increased	Low
Urine volume	Low	Low in 60%–80% (<1 mL/kg/hr); normal or high in 40% (>2.4 mL/kg/hr)
Urine osmolarity (mOsm/ kg water)	Increased >300–400	Decreased <300
Urine Na (mEq/L)	<30 mEq/L (preterm infant) <20 mEq/L (term infant)	>30 mEq/L
Creatinine clearance	Normal or decreased	Decreased
U/P creatinine	>20:1	<10:1
U/P urea	>20:1	<10:1
U/P osmolarity	>1.5:1	<1.5:1
$FE_{Na}\%$*	<1% (term infant) <3% (preterm infant)	>2% (term infant) >3% (preterm infant)
RFI†	<3%	>3%

*FE_{Na} = excreted fraction of filtered sodium = $\dfrac{UNa}{Ucr} \times \dfrac{Pcr}{PNa} \times 100$, where UNa = urinary sodium, Ucr = urinary creatinine, Pcr = plasma creatinine, and PNa = plasma sodium.

†RFI = renal failure index = $\dfrac{UNa}{Ucr} \times Pcr$.

TABLE 19–2.
Estimates of Glomerular Filtration Rate Derived from Body Length and Surface Area

Patients	Calculation*		Reference
VLBW infants*	0.27 × Lcm/Pcr	[mL/min/1.73 m²]	Fornell and John [17]
Premature infants	0.35 × Lcm/Pcr	[mL/min/1.73 m²]	Schwartz et al.[40]
Full-term infants	0.45 × Lcm/Pcr	[mL/min/1.73 m²]	Schwartz et al.[40]
Children 1 to 16 years	0.55 × Lcm/Pcr	[mL/min/1.73 m²]	Schwartz et al.[39]

*Lcm = body length, in centimeters; Pcr = plasma creatinine [mg%].
†VLBW = very low birth weight infants.

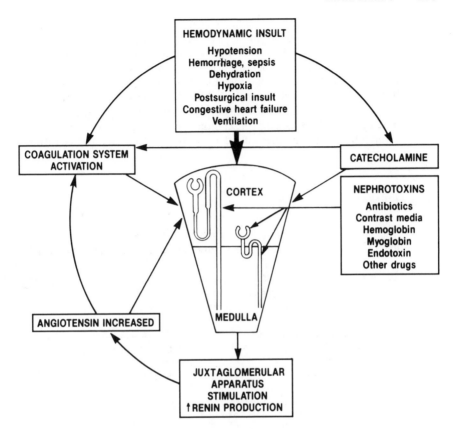

FIG 19–1.
Pathophysiology of acute renal failure (ARF) is multifactorial. Pathogenesis of ARF may begin with an ischemic or toxic event that activates the renin-angiotensin system; increase in angiotensin activity then constricts afferent arterioles and reduces glomerular filtration rate, and produces further tubular damage. Initial vascular event also can directly stimulate catecholamine release, activate coagulation system, and thus cause renal damage. (From Hostetter TH, Wilkes BM, Brenner BM: Mechanisms of impaired glomerular filtration in acute renal failure, in Brenner BM, Stein JH (eds): *Contemporary Issues in Nephrology,* vol 6, *Acute Renal Failure.* New York, Churchill Livingstone, 1980. Used by permission.)

Increased fibrin degradation products are found frequently in the serum and urine in patients with ARF. Temporary obstruction of peritubular capillary or capillary vessels is an important factor in initiating the changes in tubular necrosis.

In summary, the pathophysiology of ARF ranges from vascular and glomerular events to deranged tubular function, and probably reflects interaction between all three components (Fig 19–2).

In recent years, pathophysiologic changes at the cellular level have been studied in ARF of multiple origin. These changes include perturbations in mitochondrial respiration and intracellular calcium homeostasis, cellular lipid metabolism, free radical production, adenosine metabolism, and derangement of subcellular structures. In experimental models, treatment with adenosine triphosphate (ATP), calcium channel blockers, phospholipid inhibitors, and maneuvers designed either to detoxify oxygen free radicals or to prevent production significantly enhance postischemic functional recovery.[12, 41] Whether such therapeutic measures are effective in ARF in humans awaits further investigations.

MANAGEMENT

Prompt and adequate restoration of plasma volume; treatment of shock, left ventricular dysfunction, and sepsis; and cessation of administration of

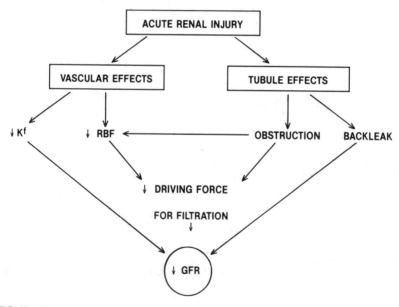

FIG 19–2.
Schematic representation of mechanisms generally considered to initiate and maintain the defect in glomerular filtration rate (GFR) in acute renal failure. It should be noted that tubule backleak reduces measured GFR. K_f = measure of renal function compared with normal; RBF = renal blood flow. (From Hostetter TH, Wilkes BM, Brenner BM: Mechanisms of impaired glomerular filtration in acute renal failure, in Brenner BM, Stein JH (eds): *Contemporary Issues in Nephrology* vol 6, *Acute Renal Failure*. New York, Churchill Livingstone, 1980. Used by permission.)

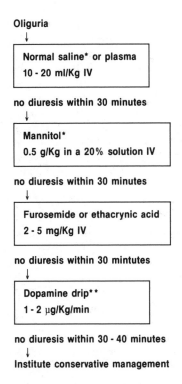

Oliguria
↓

| Normal saline* or plasma |
| 10 - 20 ml/Kg IV |

no diuresis within 30 minutes
↓

| Mannitol* |
| 0.5 g/Kg in a 20% solution IV |

no diuresis within 30 minutes
↓

| Furosemide or ethacrynic acid |
| 2 - 5 mg/Kg IV |

no diuresis within 30 mintutes
↓

| Dopamine drip** |
| 1 - 2 μg/Kg/min |

no diuresis within 30 - 40 minutes
↓
Institute conservative management

* In congestive heart failure should be used with caution.

**In addition to dopamine, (26, 45,48) theophylline in micro-
molar concentration (0.5 mg/Kg/dose) can be tried. (19)

FIG 19–3.
Guidelines for management of acute renal failure and oliguria. (From Hostetter TH, Wilkes BM, Brenner BM: Mechanisms of impaired glomerular filtration in acute renal failure, in Brenner BM, Stein JH (eds): *Contemporary Issues in Nephrology*, vol 6, *Acute Renal Failure*. New York, Churchill Livingstone, 1980. Used by permission.)

toxic substance and vasodilator medications may reduce the number of patients in whom renal failure progresses from prerenal oliguria or functional renal failure to true renal failure (Fig 19–3).

Diuretic Therapy

Mannitol given intravenously is an osmotic diuretic neither metabolized nor reabsorbed by the renal tubules. There are several plausible mechanisms by which mannitol and furosemide diuretics might exert a beneficial effect:

1. They may act by increasing the filtrate and thereby minimizing obstruction of the tubule by cell debris.

2. Mannitol and loop diuretics are vasodilators, which might directly reverse the arteriolar vasoconstriction now thought to be one of the principal factors in the pathophysiology of acute tubular necrosis.
3. Mannitol may overcome the backdiffusion phenomenon by shrinking swollen capillary endothelium.
4. Mannitol may decrease renin secretion by the ischemic kidney.
5. Mannitol may improve renal function nonspecifically by extracellular fluid expansion and reduction of viscosity.
6. Loop diuretics also may improve renal function nonspecifically by reducing volume overload and thereby improving left ventricular function in patients with congestive heart failure and prerenal oliguria.

It also has been demonstrated that furosemide can convert oliguric to nonoliguric ARF, which is easier to manage and may carry a better prognosis than oliguric ARF.[7, 33] In the presence of initial response, continuous infusion of intravenous furosemide may be more effective than intermittent bolus therapy in sustaining polyuria.

Dopamine

The third endogenous catecholamine, dopamine, increases myocardial contractility and heart rate by direct action on beta adrenergic receptors. It also releases norepinephrine from myocardial catecholamine storage sites. Dopamine differs from other sympathomimetic amines in exerting unusual vasodilation in the renal, mesenteric, coronary, and intracerebral arterial vascular beds and is mediated by dopaminergic receptors[13, 14, 18] (see also Chapters 8 and 12).

Other Therapeutic Measures

Thromboxane Synthetase Inhibitor
Renal generation of thromboxane is increased in certain types of experimental ARF. Thromboxane is a potent vasoconstrictor formed in platelets and in various organs, including the kidney. In systemic sepsis the plasma concentration of thromboxane is increased, which has been linked to renal dysfunction. Cummings et al.[10] demonstrated the protective effect of thromboxane synthetase inhibitor on renal function in systemic sepsis.

Atrial Natriuretic Peptide
Atrial natriuretic peptide (ANP) used at a high dose in the isolated kidney significantly improves renal functional recovery. It is more protective in the isolated kidney perfusion than verapamil. With its ability to increase single nephron filtration as well as distal delivery of solutes and fluid, ANP probably exerts protective effect similar to mannitol and furosemide. Studies with ^{31}P

also demonstrated acceleration of cellular ATP regeneration as well as trends toward more rapid reduction of intracellular inorganic phosphate concentrations and correction of intracellular acidosis in rats with ARF treated with ANP.[31]

Theophylline
Adenosine mediates renal hemodynamic changes in various models of ARF. The combination of high angiotensin II and adenosine renal contents is encountered in pathophysiologic conditions such as renal ischemia or hypoxemia, both conditions associated with sustained preglomerular vasoconstriction. A beneficial effect of theophylline (adenosine antagonist) has been demonstrated in ARF induced by hypercapnea, endotoxin, radiocontrast products, and amphotericin B as well as in myoglobinuric ARF.[19]

Thyroxine
Animals treated postischemically with thyroxine (T_4) showed accelerated and sustained recovery from ARF. The beneficial effect appears to be related to cellular ATP mechanisms (recovery of ATP), essential for the restoration of sublethally injured cells.[44]

Fluid and Electrolyte Requirement
Water requirement is limited to insensible loss and replacement of urinary output and other abnormal losses. The figure for insensible water loss is approximately 20 mL/kg/day (300 mL/m²/day). Careful weighing of patients once or twice a day is the only effective means of monitoring fluid balance. Normally a loss of 1% to 2% of body weight per day is expected.

Sodium
Newborn infants with complete anuria require no sodium intake. In infants with urine output, sodium losses in the urine and other drainage fluid should be replaced with a solution containing the lost amount of sodium.[15] In the presence of acidosis, sodium bicarbonate should be administered instead of sodium chloride solution to replace sodium loss. Hyponatremia in ARF is due to dilution of the sodium content of the extracellular water. It can be slowly corrected by restriction of fluid until the extracellular content is normal. Symptomatic hyponatremia must be corrected promptly. Sodium should be infused to bring serum concentration to 124 mEq/L, which yields an amount equal to the result of multiplying the concentration deficit (measured serum sodium to desired serum sodium) by 0.7 (distribution space for total body water) and by body weight (kilograms). The sodium should be infused over 60 to 120 minutes. In the presence of congestive heart failure or severe fluid overload, peritoneal dialysis should be instituted. Certain drugs have a high sodium content and may provide metabolic load: for example, carbenicillin (4.7 mEq/g), penicillin G (1.7 mEq/million units), ampicillin (3 mEq/g), cephalothin (2.5 mEq/g), sodium polystyrene sulfonate (65 mEq/g), Fleet Phospho-Soda (24 mEq/5 mL).

Potassium

The single major consequence of hyperkalemia is its effect on cardiac conduction, which may lead to asystole and death. The prevention and treatment of hyperkalemia include (1) elimination of all sources of potassium intake, (2) provision of adequate caloric intake, (3) prompt treatment of infection, (4) surgical debridement of devitalized tissues, and (5) elimination of accumulated blood and use of fresh blood for transfusion. Frequent ECGs and serum potassium determination should be obtained.

ECG changes secondary to hyperkalemia include, in order of severity, tall peaked T waves, heart block with widening QRS complex, arrhythmia, and cardiac arrest. Mild hyperkalemia may be treated with ion-exchange resins, for example, sodium polystyrene sulfonate (Kayexalate), 1 g/kg, repeated as necessary. Rectal administration is the preferred route, because the greatest rate of sodium-potassium exchange occurs in the colon.[3] Oral administration is also effective, but onset of action is somewhat delayed. Simultaneous administration of 20 mL/g 70% sorbitol or 4 mL/g 10% dextrose per dose will hasten the onset of action because each acts as an osmotic cathartic; the ensuing diarrhea helps in potassium and water elimination. The resin removes potassium from the body at a rate of approximately 1 mEq/g resin,[3] but adds an equal amount of sodium. This amount may be dangerous in a patient who already has volume overload. Sodium polystyrene sulfonate administration may not be advisable in premature or hypotensive infants. It can produce rectal bleeding and is contraindicated in patients with diarrhea, gastrointestinal bleeding, necrotizing enterocolitis, and abdominal surgery.

Moderate hyperkalemia (6.5 to 7.5 mEq/L) without changes in the ECG should be treated with intravenous sodium bicarbonate, 10% glucose with or without insulin, and sodium polystyrene sulfonate enema.

Severe hyperkalemia (7.5 mEq/L) with ECG changes is a medical emergency and should be treated with an infusion of 0.5 mL/kg to 1 mL/kg 10% calcium gluconate solution given over 10 minutes while monitoring the ECG. This solution does not affect the serum potassium levels per se, but diminishes the toxic effect on the heart. Onset of action is within 1 to 5 minutes, and the effects last for more than 2 hours. Hypernatremia and congestive heart failure may preclude the use of sodium bicarbonate in ARF. In addition, infusion of 1 mL/kg of a solution of 25% glucose containing insulin 0.3 to 0.5 U/mL accelerates intake of potassium ions (K^+) into cells. Because 3% sodium bicarbonate and 25% glucose solutions are hypertonic, they should be used with caution in premature infants with or without cerebral bleeding. The high incidence of hypoglycemia in premature infants and infants with cardiogenic shock after cardiac surgery precludes the use of insulin.[27] The beneficial effect does not occur until 2 to 3 hours after the administration of insulin and glucose, and may last for 6 to 24 hours. If a patient with high serum K^+ does not respond to sodium polystyrene sulfonate therapy, peritoneal dialysis should be used to remove excess potassium.

Acidosis

Metabolic acidosis is an inevitable consequence of ARF. Acidosis should be treated if serum bicarbonate is less than 15 mEq/L. The correction of acidosis in ARF is complicated by the need to restrict sodium. The amount of base given is determined from the product of base deficit concentration multiplied by 0.3 and by body weight (in kilograms) and is infused over 3 to 12 hours. In infants with severe acidosis (causing myocardial dysfunction or hypotension resistant to sympathomimetic medications), rapid intravenous administration of sodium bicarbonate may be required. Carbenicillin, paraldehyde, and acetazolamide may promote acidosis during therapy.

Hypocalcemia and Hyperphosphatemia

The treatment of hyperphosphatemia and hypocalcemia is aimed initially at lowering the serum phosphate level. This measure alone sometimes leads to elevated serum calcium levels. Supplying additional calcium in a patient with hyperphosphatemia is ineffective and dangerous because it can cause metabolic calcification. Phosphorus accumulation can be prevented to some extent by reducing the catabolic rate, by restricting protein intake, and by orally administering aluminum hydroxide (60 mg/kg), which reduces the absorption by binding phosphorus in the intestine.

Aluminum hydroxide can produce constipation and fecal impaction. Once serum phosphorus levels are normal or near normal (5 to 6 mg/dL), a calcium supplement may be given in the form of calcium gluconate or calcium carbonate. Calcium carbonate has the advantage of correcting acidosis as well. Symptomatic hypocalcemia should be treated with intravenous calcium, given as 10% calcium gluconate, 0.5 to 1 mL/kg, administered slowly over 4 to 10 minutes with ECG monitoring; rapid infusion of calcium can precipitate cardiac arrest. Repeated doses are often needed to control hypocalcemia. If hypocalcemia is persistent, synthetic vitamin D preparations such as dihydrotachysterol (0.1 to 0.4 mg/day) are used to improve intestinal absorption of calcium. Oral calcium should be started if the gastrointestinal system allows oral intake.

Anemia

Mild to severe anemia is a complication of ARF. Patients with ARF may be extremely sensitive to the volume expansion caused by transfusion, and hypertension and congestive heart failure may develop. Other complications of blood transfusion in patients with ARF are hyperkalemia, azotemia, and pyrexia. Therefore, fresh packed cells, 5 to 10 mL/kg, should be used for transfusion, preferably in combination with an exchange transfusion or dialysis.

Hypertension

Hypertension is not a prominent feature of ARF in the newborn except when associated with renal vascular lesions. When it develops, however, it is secondary to fluid overload in the majority of patients or to renin-angiotensin catecholamine disturbance. If the patient does not respond to salt and fluid restriction, dialysis is indicated. Treatment also includes the use of antihypertensive drugs. Captopril is effective in treating intractable hypertension (see also Chapter 9).

Infection

Newborns and small infants with ARF are prone to infection as a result of several factors, including the presence of indwelling catheters, malnutrition, and postsurgical wounds. They should be treated vigorously with antibiotics, because resistance to infection is low in ARF. Because many antibiotics are excreted primarily by the kidneys, their dosage must be adjusted according to the patient's renal function to avoid potentially serious complications.

ADJUSTMENT OF MEDICATION IN RENAL FAILURE

General Considerations

Prescription of drugs for patients with renal failure should incorporate adjustment of dosage regimens to avoid accumulation and its adverse effects. Medications can be classified on the basis of need for dosage adjustment in renal failure:

1. *No modification required:* isoxazolyl penicillins (oxacillin, cloxacillin, dicloxacillin, nafcillin), clindamycin, erythromycin, doxycycline, rifampin, ethionamide.
2. *Moderate modification required:* chloramphenicol succinate, lincomycin, pentamidine, isoniazid, amphotericin B, caffeine, theophylline, paraldehyde.
3. *Major modification required:* penicillin G, methicillin, ampicillin, amoxicillin, carbenicillin, cephalosporins, vancomycin, aminoglycosides, sulfonamides, ethambutol, paraminosalicyclic acid, viomycin, flucytosine, digoxin, indomethacin, magnesium sulfate, furosemide, mannitol.

In recent years it has been widely recognized that the altered physiology of renal failure may involve other organs vital to drug elimination (e.g., liver and plasma protein).[46] Further complicating factors involved in renal failure are (1) changes in volume of distribution, (2) changes in binding of drug to plasma proteins, (3) irregular gastrointestinal absorption, and (4) dialysis treatment. If a drug is excreted to a significant extent in an unchanged form by the kidney, the amount of drug administered must be reduced in the presence of renal failure,[47] in one of two ways: (1) the normal dose of the drug can be maintained but the interval between successive doses increased; (2) the dose can be reduced and the dosing interval remain unchanged. Sometimes a combination of these approaches is the best formulation of a dosage regimen.

The dosing interval of drugs excreted 100% unchanged by the kidney can be altered according to the formula[4]

$$\text{Normal dosing interval} \times \frac{\text{Normal creatinine clearance}}{\text{Patient's creatinine clearance}}$$

Alternatively, the dose may be altered according to the formula[4]

$$\text{Normal dose} \times \frac{\text{Patient's creatinine clearance}}{\text{Normal creatinine clearance}}$$

Most drugs, however, are not excreted entirely unchanged by the kidney; rather, metabolism plays a significant role in their elimination. In this situation a given reduction in renal function obviously will cause a lesser increase in half-life than a drug that is excreted entirely by the kidney. Calculation of dosing intervals or dose becomes more difficult.

To calculate dosing interval, the following formula may be used[4]:

$$\text{Normal dosing interval} \times \frac{1}{F(K_f - 1) + 1}$$

where F equals the fraction of the absorbed dose normally eliminated unchanged by the kidney and K_f is a measure of renal function compared with normal renal function:

$$K_f = \frac{\text{Patient's creatinine clearance}}{\text{Normal creatinine clearance}}$$

For example, consider a drug that under normal conditions is excreted 60% unchanged by the kidney and is normally administered every 6 hours. Creatinine clearance is 10% of normal:

$$6 \text{ hours} \times \frac{1}{0.6\,(0.1 - 1) + 1} = 13 \text{ hours}$$

To change the dose and maintain the normal dosing interval, the following formula can be used[4]:

$$\text{Normal dose} \times \frac{F\,(K_f - 1) + 1}{1}$$

These formulas provide a general approach for drug dosing in renal failure. Certain limitations and assumptions are made in the use of these formulas. It is assumed that renal clearance of drug is directly related to creatinine clearance; other factors that affect drug handling in the body, such as absorption, distribution, hepatic and cardiac function, and protein binding, are assumed to be unaltered by renal failure. It is also assumed that the metabolism of a given drug does not change in renal failure and that the metabolites are neither active nor toxic. Other methods, using elimination constants, are available,[11] but few drugs can be applied in newborns.

The following list should serve as a guideline in the drug treatment of renal failure:

1. Do not use drugs in renal failure unless definite indications are present.
2. If the dosage regimen of a drug in renal failure has been determined in a well-controlled study, it should be used in preference to the previously discussed formulas.
3. When the drug has not been studied but some information is available, such as the percentage of excretion by the kidney, it is possible, with use of the previously discussed formulas, to make a rough estimate of the proper dose in renal failure.
4. If an assay procedure for the drug is available, periodic measurement of blood levels of drug is advisable for any schedule (e.g., digoxin, aminoglycosides). By obtaining peak and trough drug levels, the half-life and other values can be calculated to individualize the therapy.
5. Careful monitoring for toxicity and pharmacologic effect is mandatory in all cases.

Aminoglycosides

Sirinavin et al.[42] found that in the presence of diminished renal function, half-life and elimination of aminoglycosides correlated significantly with serum creatinine levels. When renal function was unstable and changing daily, however, gentamicin half-life cannot be reliably predicted from the serum creatinine value.

Nephrotoxicity and ototoxicity are more frequent in patients with impaired renal function. Aminoglycoside-induced renal failure is usually reversible and is frequently nonoliguric. Aminoglycosides are dialyzed during hemodialysis and peritoneal dialysis (Table 19–3); thus an additional dose should be administered after hemodialysis and peritoneal dialysis in patients with renal failure.

TABLE 19–3.
Dialyzability of Drugs*

Drug	Peritoneal Dialysis	Hemodialysis
Antimicrobial agents		
Amikacin	Yes	Yes
Amoxicillin	?	Yes
Amphotericin B	No	No
Ampicillin	No	Yes
Carbenicillin	Slight	Yes
Cefamandole	No	No
Cefazolin	No	Yes
Cephalothin	Yes	Yes
Chloramphenicol	No	Yes
Clindamycin	No	No
Cloxacillin	No	No
Colistimethate	Yes	No
Dicloxacillin	No	No
Erythromycin	Yes	No
Flucytosine	Yes	Yes
Gentamicin	Yes	Yes
Isoniazid	Yes	Yes
Kanamycin	Yes	Yes
Lincomycin	No	No
Methicillin	No	No
Nafcillin	No	No
Neomycin	?	Yes
Nitrofurantoin	?	Yes
Oxacillin	No	No
Penicillin G	No	Yes
Pentamidine	No	?
Rifampin	No	No
Streptomycin	Yes	Yes
Trimethoprim-sulfamethoxazole	Yes	Yes
Sulfisoxazole	Yes	Yes
Ticarcillin	No	No
Tobramycin	Yes	Yes
Vancomycin	No	No
Antiarrhythmic agents		
Lidocaine	No	No
Procainamide	Yes	Yes
Propranolol	No	No
Quinidine	Yes	Yes
Anticoagulant agents		
Heparin	No	No
Antihypertensive agents		
Diazoxide	Yes	Yes
Hydralazine	No	No
Methyldopa	Yes	Yes

(Continued)

TABLE 19–3. (cont.).

Antimicrobial agents		
Nitroprusside	Yes	Yes
Reserpine	No	No
Corticosteroids		
Cortisone	No	No
Cardiac glycosides		
Digoxin	No	No
Diuretic agents		
Aminophylline	Yes	Yes
Furosemide	No	No
Anticonvulsant agents		
Phenytoin	Yes	No
Diazepam	No	No
Phenobarbital	Yes	Yes

*? = Insufficient data available; yes = alteration in drug dosage recommended.

Penicillin

Penicillin is secreted by the kidneys.[6] There is a logarithmic relationship between rising penicillin half-life and falling GFR.[36] Risks of excessive penicillin levels include hyperkalemia (1.7 mEq potassium/million units penicillin) and seizures.[35] For penicillin G, methicillin, and ampicillin, dosage modification is needed when creatinine clearance falls below 10 to 15 mL/min.[2] Carbenicillin dosage should be decreased in patients with creatinine clearance below 30 mL/min. Hemodialysis and peritoneal dialysis generally do not remove penicillin and methicillin.

Cloxacillin, dicloxacillin, oxacillin, and nafcillin are excreted essentially unchanged by the liver in the anephric state, and no dose adjustment is required in patients with renal failure.

Cephalosporins

Cephalosporins are eliminated primarily by the kidney. These drugs need to be administered in modified dosage when creatinine clearance falls below 25% of normal levels. For cephalothin and cefazolin, after loading dose, a maintenance dose of one fourth to one half the loading dose should be administered every 8 to 18 hours. For cefazolin, the maintenance dose should be administered every 48 to 72 hours, when GFR is less than 10 mL/min/1.73 m².[24] Ceftriaxone has the longest half-life and thus should be used with caution in the newborn.[32] Cephalosporin antibiotics can be nephrotoxic; therefore, cephalosporin administration should be limited in patients with renal impairment.

Chloramphenicol

Thirty-five percent of chloramphenicol succinate (prodrug) is cleared through the renal route. In newborns the immature function of the liver and the kidneys is responsible for the prolonged half-life and susceptibility to toxic effect. In the newborn there is an inverse correlation between serum creatinine and total body clearance of chloramphenicol succinate.[38] The dosage must be reduced by as much as 25% to 42% to compensate for the increased retention of chloramphenicol succinate. Chloramphenicol may cause gray syndrome, impairment of erythropoiesis, and anemia in renal failure.

Cardiac Glycosides

Serum digoxin half-life is longer in premature infants than in term infants. The total body clearance of digoxin is 1.34 mL/min/kg in the premature infant, significantly less than in the full-term infant, and is related to reduced renal excretion.[23]

Digoxin undergoes little metabolism in the body, and 70% to 90% is excreted by glomerular filtration and tubular secretion.[22] The renal excretion rate of digoxin is directly related to GFR; its clearance also is directly related to postnatal age.[22]

In the newborn and premature infant decreasing the digoxin dosage to the same extent as creatinine clearance usually gives serum levels in the nontoxic range; however, serum levels of digoxin should be closely followed in these patients. Evidence of digitalis toxicity also should be monitored. Neither digoxin nor digitoxin are removed significantly by dialysis.

Caffeine and Theophylline

Caffeine is largely excreted unchanged in the urine in neonates, indicating deficiency in the capacity to metabolize caffeine. Similarly in neonates given theophylline, a considerably high ratio of caffeine to theophylline is found, compared with that in adult patients. Because caffeine is cleared by the kidney, its level should be carefully monitored and dosage should be adjusted (see also Chapters 4 and 5).

Indomethacin, Tolazoline, and Magnesium

Indomethacin and tolazoline have adverse effects on renal blood flow and function and can worsen existing renal damage in azotemic patients (see Chapters 8 and 10).[9, 25, 28, 29, 34]

Magnesium-containing medications should be avoided in patients with renal failure. Accumulation of magnesium occurs in renal failure and can cause hypotension, hypotonia, respiratory arrest, and coma.

PERITONEAL DIALYSIS

In neonates with renal failure, peritoneal dialysis is preferred because of its relative safety and rapid institution. There are no absolute contraindications for dialysis; the indications are severe fluid overload, hyperkalemia, severe electrolyte derangements, and severe CNS depression due to uremia. In many neonates ARF does not require dialysis and can be managed by the previously discussed guidelines for conservative therapy. Dialysis should not be avoided, however, when conservative therapy has failed.

Although description of the technique of peritoneal dialysis[30] is not pertinent to this discussion, a point should be made concerning type of dialysis solution (Table 19–4). Commercial dialysate solutions contain lactate as a substitute for bicarbonate. The net result of the metabolism of lactate is the generation of 1 mol bicarbonate. Thus this solution is satisfactory as long as the oxidation of lactate is possible; however, many neonates with ARF are hypoxic and cannot metabolize lactate. Use of commercial dialysate in these infants results in movement of lactate from the peritoneal cavity to the extracellular fluid and in the loss of bicarbonate from the extracellular fluid into the peritoneal cavity. The result is a progressive metabolic acidosis characterized by a high anion gap due to loss of bicarbonate into peritoneal dialysate, with accumulation of lactate ions in extracellular fluid. If such metabolic acidosis with high anion gap occurs in the infant receiving peritoneal dialysis, a dialysis solution that contains bicarbonate instead of lactate should be made (Table 19–5). Because calcium may precipitate in the solution containing bicarbonate, calcium should be eliminated from the dialysate but administered intravenously. To remove extra fluid rapidly, dialysate containing 2.5% or 4.25% glucose should be used. During initial dialysis in the hyperkalemic patient, potassium should not be added to the dialysate. In patients receiving digitalis, however, addition of potassium (3.5 to 4.0 mEq/L) to the dialysate is desirable to avoid hypokalemia and digitalis toxicity. Many drugs are dialyzable during peritoneal dialysis (see Table 19–3). Thus the appropriate amount of medications should be added to the dialysate fluid to supplement for losses during peritoneal dialysis. Peritonitis, which is a complication of peritoneal dialysis, can be treated by adding antibiotics to the peritoneal fluid.

In recent years continuous arteriovenous hemofiltration (CAVH) or continuous arteriovenous hemofiltration plus dialysis (CAVH-D) has been used in adults and children as well as in newborn infants as alternative treatment in critically ill patients when hemodialysis or peritoneal dialysis is precluded because of the patient's clinical condition or because of technical problems. The known advantages of this treatment are simplicity and rapid and easy application. There is no need for specialized equipment or staff, and there is good clinical tolerance.[37] However, one should be cautious and avoid overheparinization to prevent CNS bleeding in neonates.

TABLE 19–4.
Composition of Dialysis Fluid

Dialysis Fluid (Manufacturer)	Na (mEq/L)	P (mEq/L)	Ca (mEq/L)	Mg (mEq/L)	Chloride (mEq/L)	Lactate (mEq/L)	Glucose (%)	Osmolarity (mOsm/L)
Inpersol (Abbott)	140.5	—	3.5	1.5	101	44.5	1.5	371.5
Dianeal (Baxter)	141.5	—	3.5	1.5	101	45.0	1.5	372.5

TABLE 19–5.
Peritoneal Dialysis Solution Containing Bicarbonate

Component	Volume (mL)	Na⁺ (mEq)	Cl⁻ (mEq)	Mg⁺⁺ (mEq)	SO₄⁼ (mEq)	HCO₃⁻ (mEq)	Glucose (g)
NaCl (0.45%)	916.0	70	70	—	—	—	—
NaCl (2.5 mEq/mL)	12.0	30	30	—	—	—	—
NaHCO₃ (mEq/mL)	40.0	40	—	—	—	40	—
MgSO₄ (10%)	1.8	—	—	1.5	1.5	—	—
50% Dextrose in water	30.8	—	—	—	—	—	15
Total	999.8	140	100	1.5	1.5	40	15

Nutrition

The importance of dietary management of ARF has been stressed in recent years.[1] At least 1 to 1.5 g/kg/day protein or 80 to 120 mg/day nitrogen[16] and 30 to 40 calories/kg/day should be provided to prevent a negative protein and caloric balance. One interesting approach to the management of ARF consists of providing a mixture of essential L-amino acids along with a full caloric intake using high concentrations of glucose delivered by way of a central venous catheter. Hyperalimentation consists of essential and nonessential amino acids and histidine, a necessary amino acid in patients with uremia. The theoretical basis for this approach is the observation that ammonia, formed from urea by the flora of the gastrointestinal tract, can be used as a source of nonessential nitrogen. With adequate caloric intake and exogenous provision of all essential amino acids, protein synthesis and new cell growth can occur, with attendant uptake of potassium, phosphate, and magnesium from the extracellular fluid. Amino acid treatment increases the synthesis of renal membrane choline-containing phospholipids and decreases the level of renal functional insufficiency.

These patients also require vitamins D, B complex, and C and folic acid supplementation. Plasma levels of vitamin A and retinol-binding protein concentrations are high in uremic patients.[43] Therefore vitamin A supplements should be avoided in patients with renal failure. Formulas low in sodium, potassium, and phosphorus should be used for feeding in infants with ARF. Breast milk or S-M-A and S-29 formulas are more suitable than cow's milk and other formulas with high solute content. The addition of glucose polymers (Polycose) and medium-chain triglycerides to formula helps to increase caloric intake without causing volume overload.

PROGNOSIS

A significant number of children who have apparently recovered from ARF continue to have renal dysfunction.

Despite the general availability of peritoneal dialysis, a recovery rate from neonatal ARF of less than 50% has been reported. The prognosis depends largely on the nature and severity of the initial damage and the skill with which chemical disturbances are managed. Use of continuous ambulatory peritoneal dialysis in the newborn with or without renal anomalies may change in part the prognosis in some patients who do not recover from ARF and subsequently develop chronic renal failure.

REFERENCES

1. Abel RM, et al: Improved survival from acute renal failure after treatment with intravenous essential L-amino-acids and glucose. *N Engl J Med* 1973; 288:695–699.
2. Altman G, et al: Blood levels of ampicillin, kanamycin and gentamicin in the uremic patients. *J Med Sci* 1970; 6:683–690.
3. Anand SK: Acute renal failure in the neonate. *Pediatr Clin North Am* 1982; 29:791–800.
4. Anderson RJ, Gambertoglio JG, Schrier RW: Fate of drugs in renal failure, in Brenner B, Rector FC Jr (eds): *The Kidney,* vol 2. Philadelphia, WB Saunders Co, 1976, pp 1911–1948.
5. Aperia A, et al: Postnatal development of renal function in pre-term and full-term infants. *Acta Paediatr Scand* 1981; 70:183–187.
6. Barnett HL, et al: Renal clearances of sodium penicillin G, procaine penicillin G, and inulin in infants and children. *Pediatrics* 1949; 3:418–422.
7. Cantrovich F, et al: High dose furosemide in established renal failure. *Br Med J* 1973; 4:449–450.
8. Carriere S, Daigneault B: Effect of retransfusion after hemorrhage hypotension in intrarenal distribution of blood flow in dogs. *J Clin Invest* 1970; 49:2205–2217.
9. Catterton Z, Sellers B, Gray G: Inulin clearance in the premature infant receiving indomethacin. *J Pediatr* 1980; 96:737–739.
10. Cummings AD, McDonald JW, Lindsay RM, et al: The protective effect of thromboxane synthetase inhibition on renal function in systemic sepsis. *Am J Kid Dis* 1989; 13:114–119.
11. Dettli L: Individualization of drug dosage in patients with renal failure. *Med Clin North Am* 1974; 58:977–985.
12. Dickman KG, Jacob WR, Mandel LJ: Renal metabolism and acute renal failure. *Pediatr Nephrol* 1987; 1:359–366.
13. Driscoll DJ, Gillette PC, McNamara DG: The use of dopamine in children. *J Pediatr* 1978; 92:309–314.
14. Durairaj SK, Haywood LJ: Hemodynamic effects of dopamine patients with resistant congestive heart failure. *Clin Pharmacol Ther* 1978; 24:175–185.
15. Engle WD: Evaluation of renal function and acute renal failure in the neonate. *Pediatr Clin North Am* 1986; 33:129–151.
16. Fildes RD, Springale JE, Feld LG: Acute renal failure: II. Management of suspected and established disease. *J Pediatr* 1986; 109:567–571.
17. Fornell L, John EG: Glomerular filtration rate in infants. *J Pediatr* 1985; 106:346–347.

18. Goldberg LI: Drug therapy dopamine, clinical uses of an endogenous catecholamine. *N Engl J Med* 1974; 291:707–710.
19. Gouyon JB, Guignard JP: Functional renal insufficiency: Role of adenosine. *Perinatol Nephrol Biol Neonate* 1988; 53:237–242.
20. Grand-Champ A, et al: Relationship between renin and intrarenal hemodynamics in hemorrhagic hypotension. *J Clin Invest* 1971; 50:970–978.
21. Guignard JP, John EG: Renal function in the tiny, premature infant. *Clinics Perinatol* 1986; 13:377–401.
22. Halkin H, et al: Steady state serum digoxin concentration in relation to digitalis toxicity in neonates and infants. *Pediatrics* 1978; 61:184–188.
23. Hastreiter AR, et al: Digoxin pharmacokinetics in premature infants. *Pediatr Pharmacol* 1982; 2:23–31.
24. Hines LB, et al: Cefazolin in children with renal insufficiency. *J Pediatr* 1980; 96:335–339.
25. John EG, Assadi FK, Samuel S, et al: The effect of dopamine on renal functions in newborn puppies. *Int J Pediatr Nephrol* 1984; 8:28.
26. John EG, Bhat R, Assadi FK, et al: Effect of tolazoline on renal function in newborn puppies. *Dev Pharmacol Ther* 1986; 9:402–411.
27. John E, Bhat R, Vasan U, et al: Effect of intravenous indomethacin on renal function of premature infants. *Pediatr Res* 1980; 14:601.
28. John EG, Bhat R, Vidyasagar D: Renal response to tolazoline in normal and hypoxemic newborn puppies. *Pediatr Res* 1979; 14:514.
29. John EG, Levitsky S, Hastreiter AR: Management of acute renal failure complicating cardiac surgery in infants and children. *Crit Care Med* 1980; 8:562–569.
30. Kanarek K, Root E, Sidebottom EA, et al: Successful peritoneal dialysis in an infant weighing less than 800 grams. *Clin Pediatr* 1981; 21:166–169.
31. Masahiko N, Joseph L, Shapiro P, et al: In vitro and in vivo protective effect of atriopeptin III on ischemic acute renal failure. *J Clin Invest* 1987; 80:698–705.
32. Melvin IM: Ceftriaxone and more to come. *J Pediatr* 1983; 103:70–72.
33. Mielth RG: Furosemide in acute renal failure, in Friedman EA, Eliator ME (eds): *Conference on Acute Renal Failure,* (NIH) 74–608, 974. Brooklyn, N.Y., U.S. Department of Health, Education and Welfare, 1975, pp 263–264.
34. Naujoks S, Guignard JP: Renal effects of tolazoline in rabbits. *Lancet* 1979; 2:1075–1076.
35. Oldstone MBA, Nelson E: Central nervous system manifestations of penicillin toxicity in man. *Neurology* 1966; 16:693–700.
36. Plaut ME, et al: Penicillin handling in normal and azotemic patients. *J Lab Clin Med* 1969; 174:12–18.
37. Ronco C, Brendolan A, Bragantine L, et al: Treatment of acute renal failure in newborn by continuous arteriovenous hemofiltration. *Kidney Int* 1986; 19:908–915.
38. Sack CM, et al: Chloramphenicol succinate kinetics. *Pediatr Pharmacol* 1982; 2:93–103.
39. Schwartz GJ, et al: A simple estimate of glomerular filtration rate in children derived from body length and plasma creatinine. *Pediatrics* 1976; 58:259–263.
40. Schwartz GJ, et al: A simple estimate of GFR in children. *J Pediatr* 1984; 104:849–854.
41. Shapiro JLC, Cheung C, Itabashi A, et al: The effect of verapamil on renal function after warm and cold ischemia in the isolated perfused rat kidney. *Transplantation* 1985; 40:496–600.

42. Sirinavin S, McCracken GH, Nelson JD: Determining gentamicin dosage in infants and children with renal failure. *J Pediatr* 1980; 96:331–334.

43. Smith FR, Goodman DWS: The effects of disease of the liver, thyroid and kidneys on the transport of vitamin A in human plasma. *J Clin Invest* 1971; 50:2426–2436.

44. Sutter PM, Thulin G, Stromski M, et al: Beneficial effect of thyroxine in the treatment of ischemic acute renal failure. *Pediatr Nephrol* 1988; 2:1–7.

45. Tulassay T, Seri I, Mackay T, et al: Effects of dopamine on renal function in premature neonates with respiratory distress syndrome. *Int J Pediatr Nephrol* 1983; 4:19.

46. Whelton A: Antibiotic pharmacokinetics and clinical application in renal insufficiency. *Med Clin North Am* 1982; 267–280.

47. Yaffe SJ, Chudzik GM: Drugs and the kidney, in Edelman CM (ed): *Pediatric Kidney Disease,* vol 1. Boston, Little, Brown & Co, 1978; pp 809–832.

48. Yeh TF, Cuevas D, John E, et al: Effect of dopamine during first 3 days of life in preterm newborns. *Clin Res* 1985; 33:897.

20

Fluid and Electrolyte Therapy in the Neonate

Paul Y. K. Wu, M.D.

Fluid therapy is one of the most important adjuncts in the management of neonates, particularly the low-birth-weight (LBW) infant. The fetus undergoes constant changes in body water concomitant with changes in body composition.[11, 13] Total body water (TBW) and extracellular water (ECW), as percentages of body weight, gradually decrease with advancing gestational age, whereas intracellular water increases with gestational age.[11–13] These dynamic changes in body water assume practical importance because the distribution factor of drugs or electrolytes will vary with the maturity of the infant. For example, the formula used for correction of plasma sodium concentration is:

$$(C_d - C_i) \times D_f \times \text{Wt in kg} = \text{mEq required}$$

where C_d = plasma concentration desired (mEq/L), C_i = present plasma concentration (mEq/L), and D_f = distribution factor as a fraction of body weight.

Postnatally, fluid therapy should take into account (1) changes in body composition, (2) changes in nutrition, (3) changes in renal development and function, (4) changes imposed by external environment, and (5) water required for growth. It has been postulated that the fetus has "fluid overload" and therefore needs to undergo some contraction in body water during the early postnatal period.[17] However, the extent to which this contraction should occur is controversial. With moderate fluid intake, the contraction ranges from 10% to 15% TBW in infants less than 1,000 g body weight to 2% to 4% TBW in term infants, with maximum contraction occurring within the first 3 postnatal days. Except for very low-birth-weight (VLBW) infants, most infants regain their water loss by 7 to 10 days of life.

Changes in nutritional components such as water, caloric density, and electrolytes have a major effect on water balance. Higher caloric density formulas will increase the so-called hidden intake. Normally about 12 mL water is derived from the oxidation of 100 kcal nutrients (proteins, fats, or carbohydrates). While this addition of water may not have a significant impact on healthy term infants, it needs to be taken into consideration in smaller preterm infants.

CHANGES IN RENAL DEVELOPMENT AND FUNCTION

The primary function of the kidney is to regulate water and electrolyte homeostasis within the body. The glomerular filtration rate (GFR) in term neonates is only about 25% that in adults. Nevertheless, there is a rapid rise in GFR after delivery, particularly in infants of 34 weeks or more gestation.[2, 19] This has been attributed to a decrease in vascular resistance and a rise in systemic blood pressure.[14] Preterm infants have even lower GFR. During the first 2 days after birth the GFR in a neonate tends to be lower than on subsequent days. While anatomic and functional development continues to mature long after birth, the neonate, even the VLBW infant, is capable of excreting the loads of sodium, water, and acid that are normally presented to it, and can maintain water and electrolyte balance. In the neonate, the volume of urine excreted is dependent on (1) fluid intake, (2) the amount of solute (i.e., urea, electrolytes, glucose) for excretion, and (3) the limits of concentrating and diluting abilities of the developing kidney. The amounts of solute for urinary excretion vary from about 10 to 30 mOsm per 100 calories metabolized,[16] depending on whether the neonate is fed low solute and protein milk (i.e., breast milk or special low solute formulas) or high solute and protein formulas. The diluting capacity of the kidney is 30 to 50 mOsm/L, and its concentrating capacity is 700 mOsm/L. Thus if 30 mOsm is to be excreted and the limit of concentrating ability is 700 mOsm/L, the minimal volume of urine would be 43 mL and the maximum volume 600 mL if the diluting capacity is 50 mOsm/L. The amount of fluid supplied for urine water should be such that it will not tax the diluting or concentrating capacity of the kidney. In most infants, if 80 mL of water is provided per 100 calories metabolized, urine osmolality will be in the region of 100 to 300 mOsm/L.

CHANGES IMPOSED BY THE EXTERNAL ENVIRONMENT

Insensible Water Loss

Insensible water loss (IWL) constitutes one of the principal components of output in water balance. This is defined as nonvisible loss of water through evaporation from the skin and respiratory tract.

Insensible water loss from the skin depends on:

TABLE 20–1.
Insensible Water Loss (IWL) in Infants
Inside a Single-Wall Incubator in a
Neutral Thermal Environment*

Body Weight (g)	IWL (mL/kg/day)
≥1,000	64 ± 4
1,001–1,250	56 ± 7
1,251–1,500	38 ± 7
1,501–1,750	22 ± 6
1,751–2,000	17 ± 3

*From Wu PYK, Hodgman JE: *Pediatrics*
1974; 54:704–712. Used by permission.

1. *Effective surface area for evaporation.* Compared with older children and adults, the preterm infant is at a special disadvantage. Immaturity of the cornified layer of the skin and a larger body surface area relative to body mass result in passive evaporation of large amounts of body water.[4,6,22,23] In addition, hypotonic preterm infants generally lie in an extended abducted position, thus exposing more surface area for IWL.

2. *Velocity of air movement over body surface.* This is dependent on the air flow in the nurseries and inside the incubators. The higher the air flow, the greater the evaporative loss.

3. *Pressure of water vapor on the skin.* This will vary according to climate, air temperature, dimensions of the space in which the infant is placed, and provision of humidified air around the infant.

Insensible water loss from the respiratory tract depends on:

1. Absolute humidity of the inspired and expired air.
2. Respiratory minute volume.

Recognition of the importance of thermoregulation in the reduction of morbidity and mortality in neonates has led to the introduction of a large variety of warming devices, all of which have a role in affecting IWL and thus determining the amount of fluid therapy for the infant. Several investigators have reported the IWL in neonates nursed under various types of devices.[4,6,22,23] In general, the more immature an infant the greater the IWL (Table 20–1). Radiant warmers with open bed platforms impose greater IWL on infants than incubators do (Table 20–2). Shielding of infants under radiant warmers with transparent plastic sheets, or heat shields and double-wall incubators will reduce the IWL by 30% to 50%.

Increased Insensible Water Loss

The following factors are associated with increased IWL:

1. Prematurity/IWL (100% to 300%) is inversely correlated with advancing gestational age. Thus an infant with a gestational age of 24 weeks may have IWL of 3 mL/kg/hr, while one of 36 weeks will have IWL of 0.7 mL/kg/hr when nursed in a conventional single-wall incubator.
2. Radiant warmer with open bed (50% to 100%).
3. Forced convection (30% to 50%).
4. Phototherapy (10% to 50%). Earlier studies reported that phototherapy increases IWL. With proper temperature control and newer types of phototherapy lamps (e.g., equipped with exhaust fan to cool ballast), the amount of IWL due to phototherapy can be reduced.
5. Hyperthermia (30% to 50%). For each 1° C rise in body temperature IWL can be increased by 30%.
6. Tachypnea (20% to 30%).
7. Activity and feeding.
8. Decrease ambient humidity.

Decreased Insensible Water Loss

Factors associated with decreased IWL are:

1. Endotracheal intubation on assisted ventilation (30%).
2. Nasal continuous positive airway pressure (30%).
3. Humidified hood (20% to 30%).
4. Decreased activity.
5. Additional or high humidity in incubator/environment.
6. Decreased heat loss (e.g., thermal blankets, heat shields, double-walled incubators) (30% to 50%).

TABLE 20–2.
Insensible Water Loss (IWL) in Infants Under Radiant Warmers

Reference	Body Weight (kg)	IWL (mL/kg/hr)
Wu and Hodgman[23]	<1.5	2.45 ± 0.40
Williams and Oh[23]	3.24 ± 0.97	1.49 ± 0.40
Bell et al.[6]	0.79–1.31	2.43 ± 0.24
Baumgart et al.[4]	1.01–1.5	2.66 ± 0.20
	1.51–m 2.00	0.52 ± 0.01

TABLE 20–3.
Factors in Neonatal Water Balance

Intake	Output
Parenteral fluids	Insensible water loss
Medications and infusions:	Urinary output
Sodium bicarbonate	Stool (generally <10% of total output)
Albumin, plasmanate	Gastrointestinal tract loss (gastric aspirate,
Plasma	third spacing)
Blood (over blood replacements)	Sweat (negligible)
Other blood products	Blood for chemistry studies, accidental blood
Other intravenous medications	loss
Oral intake	
Hidden intake (12 mL/100 kcal)	

FLUID THERAPY

In theory, water balance can be achieved if intake is equal to output. However, various factors need to be taken into account in the balance, and these are shown in Table 20–3.

In the neonate the aim of fluid therapy is not to maintain an absolute balance, in which intake is equal to output, but to endeavor to allow for extrauterine adaptation and contraction of body water, change in metabolic rate, nutrition, environmental conditions, and kidney functions, as well as postnatal growth. In addition, any underlying pathologic condition will impose other considerations on fluid requirements. Careful documentation of intake and output is essential. In general, fluid therapy for the neonate in a thermal-neutral environment can be estimated to be equal to IWL plus urinary output with addition of 10% for losses in the stool and 10% to 15% more for growth.

Because urinary output is lower in the early postnatal period (first 2 days) and because of the need for postnatal body water contraction, the fluid therapy advocated for the first day is 60 to 75 mL/kg/24 hr, with subsequent increment as urinary output increases.

The addition of electrolytes to fluids will depend on urinary output and plasma concentrations of electrolytes. In general, sodium and potassium can be added to intravenous fluids between 24 and 48 hours after birth. The maintenance doses are 2 to 3 mEq/kg/24 hr.

Evaluation of Water Balance

The following parameters are useful as a guide to monitoring water balance:

1. *Changes in Body Weight.* During the first few days postnatally any

change in weight represents change in body water (e.g., wt = 1 mL water). However, when the infant is taking adequate calories, a gain in weight represents gain in body tissue and body water. The percentage of the weight due to water will vary with the maturity of infant.

2. *Hematocrit.* Hemaconcentration may be a reflection of increased loss of ECW, whereas a decrease in hematocrit without other signs of blood loss may represent overhydration.

3. *Serum osmolarity, electrolytes and proteins.* As with hematocrit, changes in concentration may represent underhydration or overhydration.

4. *Urinary flow rate, osmolarity, specific gravity, urinary electrolytes, blood urea nitrogen, and creatine.* The normal urinary flow rate in a neonate is 2.5 to 4 mL/kg/hr. A decrease, in the absence of renal disease, represents underhydration. A single urinary specific gravity should not be used as an index of the degree of hydration. Neonates, especially the VLBW infants or infants with perinatal asphyxia, may lose large amounts of salt in the urine and thereby show higher specific gravity. However, once the diagnosis is made, sequential changes in osmolarity or specific gravity may be helpful in evaluation of the success of therapy.

5. *Clinical signs of dehydration or overhydration.* Mild dehydration (5%) may be associated with dry skin and mucous membrane and slightly sunken fontanelles. Moderate (10%) dehydration is associated with accentuation of the signs found in mild dehydration, with loose abdominal skin turgor, sunken fontanelles and eyeballs, and oliguria with signs of circulatory insufficiency (tachycardia, tachypnea, poor capillary filling, poor skin perfusion, mottled skin). With more severe dehydration clinical signs of shock will become apparent.

6. *Central venous pressure.* While central venous pressure may not be helpful initially in the evaluation of hydration, serial determinations are invaluable in situations requiring rapid intravascular expansion. Continuous or sequential changes in central venous pressure may reflect the adequacy of fluid or volume expanders such as colloids. During the early part of replacement therapy, pressure changes are minimal initially; however, as expansion nears completion, central venous pressure rises.

7. *Water balance studies.* For a more precise assessment of fluid therapy, water balance studies may be performed. The steps for the study are:

1. Choose duration of study period (e.g., 8, 12, or 24 hours).
2. Start period after passage of urine.
3. Weigh infant (wt_i).
4. Record all "intake" during period.

5. Collect urine in previously weighed urine collection bags (or previously weighed diapers).
6. Collect stools in previously weighed diapers.
7. At end of period, weigh infant (wt_f), urine bag, and diapers.
8. Differences in wt_f − (wt_i + weight of intake) will give change in weight for that period.
9. Differences in initial and final weights of urine bags (diapers) will give the weight of urine (g). (For quantity, weight of urine ÷ specific gravity of urine = mL of urine).
10. Differences in initial and final weight of diapers with stool will give weight of stool.

In summary:

$$\text{Balance} = \text{Intake} - (\text{IWL} + \text{urine} + 10\% \text{ stool wt})$$

where IWL = Δwt − (urine and 10% stool wt).

Changes in Serum Sodium Concentration: Dilution vs. Urinary Excretion

In instances when a neonate has been overhydrated or has excessive sodium excretion, it is necessary to know how much of the resultant drop in serum sodium concentration is a result of dilution and how much is due to excretion. Apart from monitoring the serum and urinary sodium levels and urinary output, the following examples of calculation of water distribution with water load may be helpful.

With water load, the excess of water is distributed uniformly in the ICW and ECW compartments, leading to a drop in osmolal concentrations. For example:

1. If infant birth weight = 4 kg, then TBW (4 × 0.75) = 3 L, ICW = 1.75 L, and ECW = 1.25 L.

If infant gains 300 g (300 mL H_2O) and initial serum osmolality (Osm) = 300 mOsm/L, then expected

$$\text{Serum Osm} = \frac{300 \times 0.3}{(3 + 0.3)} = 270 \text{ mOsm/L}$$

and gain in H_2O is

$$\text{ECW} = \frac{1.75 \times 0.3}{3.0} = 0.175 \text{ L (175 mL)}$$
$$\text{ICW} = \frac{1.25 \times 0.3}{3.0} = 0.125 \text{ L (125 mL)}$$

2. If infant birth weight = 1 kg, then TBW = $(1 \times 0.85) = 850$ mL.

If weight gain = 100 g = 100 mL H_2O, then resultant TBW = $(850 + 100) = 950$ mL.

If initial serum Na = 140 mEq/L, then expected

$$\text{Serum Na concentration} = \frac{0.85}{0.95} \times 140 = 125 \text{ mEq/L}$$

SPECIAL CONSIDERATIONS

Very Low-Birth-Weight Infants

This group of infants, particularly those who weigh less than 1000 g, pose a major challenge to fluid therapy. The immaturity of the regulatory mechanisms and environmental factors impose a very narrow margin of safety between the adequacy of fluid therapy and overhydration or underhydration on these infants. During the first week of life they are specially at risk for developing a syndrome associated with hypernatremia, hyperglycemia, oliguria, and hyperkalemia.[3, 5]

Conversely, because of the high fractional excretion of sodium,[9] these infants may be dehydrated and become hyponatremic during the diuretic phase in the first 2 postnatal weeks. Great care must be taken to prevent the infant from getting too much fluids, with concomitant increase in glucose intake. Excessive fluid may compound the problems of hyperglycemia and hyponatremia. The concentration of glucose in intravenous fluids should be adjusted to maintain glucose administration to 4 to 5 mg/kg/min. Excessive glucose, which is osmotically active and easily diffuses from intravascular into extracellular fluid, causes a shift of water from the intracellular to the extracellular compartment, resulting in a fall in sodium concentration.

Care needs to be taken to prevent excessive evaporative loss by the use of double-wall incubators, heat shields, and even increased humidity. At the same time, we advocate a more conservative fluid intake. We have usually prescribed fluids as follows: 60 mL/kg/24 hr for the first 24 to 48 hours; then, depending on urinary output, fluid intake may be increased to 60 to 80 mL/kg/24 hr at 48 to 96 hours, and 90 to 120 mL/kg/24 hr at 96 to 144 hours. For most infants the subsequent fluid intake may be between 130 and 160 mL/kg/24 hr when they are nursed in an incubator.

Perinatal Asphyxia, Respiratory Distress Syndrome, and Acute Renal Failure

The effects of perinatal asphyxia on kidney functions have been a subject of considerable interest. Data available indicate that asphyxia may be associated with the elevation of certain hormones that are related to kidney functions, such as antidiuretic hormone (ADH), and the renin-angiotensin-aldosterone system. In addition asphyxia can cause decrease in renal blood flow, leading to acute renal failure or acute tubular necrosis. Frequently it is difficult to separate the symptoms ascribed to inappropriate ADH (SIADH; syndrome of inappropriate ADH secretion) from those of the diuretic phase of renal failure. Asphyxiated neonates have an increase in urine flow and sodium excretion after the initial oliguric phase.[1, 8, 10, 18, 20, 21] These infants are also prone to cerebral edema. Great care must therefore be exercised in prescribing fluids in order to prevent overexpansion of ECW or dehydration. Careful monitoring of body weight, urinary output, and serum and urinary electrolyte levels will assist in modifying fluid and electrolyte therapy. Attention must be paid initially to correcting prerenal factors that may decrease renal blood flow and GFR, for example, impaired myocardial contractility, decreased intravascular volume, oncotic pressure, blood pressure, hypoventilation, and hypoxia. Adjuncts to fluid therapy may therefore include cardiotonic drugs, volume expanders including colloids, and assisted ventilation. Once prerenal problems are corrected, the treatment of SIADH or the oliguric phase of renal failure is water restriction initially. When hyponatremia is severe (serum concentration less than 130 mEq/L), seizures can occur in the infant who is already prone to seizures as a result of hypoxic-ischemic insult. Correction of hyponatremia with hypertonic saline solution may be necessary to raise the serum sodium concentration to about 130 mEq/L in order to reduce the risk of seizures. This may be followed by administration of a diuretic (e.g., furosemide). This combination will cause a rise in serum sodium concentration with concurrent diuresis. Generally, most infants respond to this therapy within 48 to 72 hours by decreasing sodium excretion and increasing urinary excretion. During the polyuric phase of acute tubular necrosis, in which the infant may lose large amounts of water and sodium, great care must be taken to prevent dehydration by providing extra fluids, but not to the extent of matching urinary output. This fine tuning involves careful evaluation of water balance.

Bronchopulmonary Dysplasia

Infants with bronchopulmonary dysplasia have special problems. Because of abnormal lymphatic drainage or accompanying right-sided heart failure or left ventricular function, they are particularly susceptible to pulmonary edema. The need for fluid restriction must be balanced against the need to provide adequate calories in a volume of fluid that will meet their growth requirements as well as the physiologic demand of the kidneys. Lacking data for a more rational basis for fluid requirements, we have generally prescribed a more conservative fluid intake, 120 to 140 mL/kg/24 hr, with a moderately high caloric density type of formula, 24 kcal/30 mL. When clinical signs of increased pulmonary fluid develop, diuretics are used. With roentgenographic, electrocardiographic, and echocardiographic evidence of cor pulmonale, digitalis is used as an adjunct to therapy.

Infants With Congenital Heart Disease

Several factors require attention in prescribing fluid for infants with congenital heart disease. Drugs used for the management of these infants may cause changes in urinary output and sodium excretion (e.g., digitalis and diuretics). In addition, hypokalemia can also result from the use of hydrochlorothiazide. Judicious selection of diuretics may minimize potassium loss, such as the use of spironolactone (Aldactone) which increases sodium and water excretion while retaining potassium.

Second, there is a need to replace IWL and urinary water losses as well as electrolytes to maintain normal fluid tonicity. Thus fluid restriction should not be as aggressive as in older children. In general, 80 to 120 mL/kg/24 hr of fluid can be provided together with the nutrients, electrolytes, and trace metals to maintain the nutritional needs and fluid requirements of the neonate.

Frequent monitoring of body weight, presence of pulmonary and systemic edema, and serum electrolyte concentrations will be necessary, particularly in the early phase of management. Care needs to be taken to provide the infant's fluid and electrolyte needs by evenly distributing them throughout the 24 hours to avoid sudden changes in circulatory blood volume.

Patent Ductus Arteriosus

An increased incidence of PDA with congestive cardiac failure in infants receiving higher fluid intake during the early postnatal days was reported by Bell et al.[7] Current practice recommends partial replacement of urine volume and IWL with a modest amount of fluid intake (90 to 120 mL/kg/24 hr). Urinary output must be monitored carefully, particularly in infants given indomethacin, because kidney functions may be compromised with this drug,[15] and further fluid restrictions are necessary to prevent overexpansion of ECW and development of edema.

Fluid Therapy After Cardiopulmonary Bypass

Cardiopulmonary bypass may be associated with retention of water and sodium from the pump prime. Hyponatremia is also a common result of disproportionate water retention. Greater restriction of fluid is therefore necessary in the immediate postoperative period (60 mL/kg/24 hr). When serum sodium concentration falls to low levels (less than 125 mEq/L), the risk of seizure is increased. Conversely, hyponatremia may be seen in infants given large amounts of sodium bicarbonate. In these instances, sodium restriction with more liberalization of fluids will be necessary.

Hypokalemia is often associated with cardiac surgery and potentiates the pharmacologic effects of digitalis. It can be treated by administration of potassium at 0.3 mEq/kg/hr until normal serum concentration (4 to 4.5 mEq/L) is attained.

Gastrointestinal Fluid Loss

Gastrointestinal fluid loss is a major complication associated with intestinal infection and with anatomic and enzymatic defects. The goals of fluid therapy are (1) to correct preexisting deficits, (2) to estimate and replace ongoing abnormal losses, and (3) to provide for normal maintenance fluid intake.

The causes of fluid loss need to be taken into account, since the type of fluid and electrolyte replacements will vary according to the underlying condition of the infant. In the neonate, losses due to diarrhea are isotonic, so that replacement can be made with isotonic saline solution. With concurrent metabolic acidosis, a portion of the chloride can be replaced by bicarbonate to achieve a concentration of 24 mEq/L.

All weight loss in the neonate can be assumed to be water with accompanying electrolytes. Thus total weight loss in grams is equivalent to milliliters of fluid to be replaced as isotonic solution. Generally, half of the estimated loss can be replaced over the first 12 hours with a sodium-containing solution, an additional fourth over the next 12 hours, followed by another fourth of fluid containing both sodium and potassium if urinary output has been reestablished. Potassium should be withheld from the initial hydrating solution. Once urinary function is reestablished (urinary flow rate greater than 2 mL/kg/hr), 1 mEq/kg/24 hr may be added to the infusion in addition to the usual maintenance allotment of 2mEq potassium/kg/24 hr. Regain of weight to preillness level and elimination of signs of dehydration, along with improvement in urinary function with fall in serum blood urea nitrogen and creatinine concentration, are indicators of successful therapy.

Obstructive surgical conditions of the gastrointestinal tract may be associated with vomiting as a major symptom. With obstructive lesions of the upper gastrointestinal tract (pyloric stenosis), there is loss of acidic gastric fluid with resultant hypochloremic metabolic alkalosis and contraction of extracellular fluid space. This change in ECW stimulates aldosterone production, which promotes maximal sodium and chloride reabsorption while promoting hydrogen and potassium ion excretion. This may result in severe hypokalemia. Therapy is aimed initially at reexpansion of ECW with isotonic sodium chloride. Once reexpansion is accomplished and urinary flow rate increases, aldosterone is suppressed and sodium and bicarbonate are excreted in the urine. Supplemental potassium should be added. For severe hypochloremia, arginine hydrochloride (2 to 4 mmol/kg given intravenously over 6 to 12 hours) may be used to correct acid-base balance.

Obstructive lesions of the lower gastrointestinal tract are accompanied by loss of alkaline or neutral fluid. Rehydration can be achieved as with losses in the upper tract; in addition, the volume of nasogastric drainage should be

TABLE 20–4.
Estimate of Daily Fluid Requirement

	mL/kg/day	mL/100 kcal
Insensible water loss	25–50	30–40
Urine	60–95	50–80
	(2.5–4 kg/hr)	
Stool	10–15	10
Growth	10–15	12
Hidden intake (oxidation)	15	12
Total	100–160	80–140

replaced with an equal volume of intravenous fluid containing sodium and potassium content similar to the nasogastric drainage as analyzed by the clinical laboratory.

In addition to deficit correction, the neonate undergoing surgery will require intraoperative fluid therapy to compensate for blood loss and third space losses (translocated fluid that is sequestered in the tissue spaces as a result of surgical trauma). The amount of fluid loss will depend on the underlying disease and type of surgery. These amounts are difficult to judge with accuracy. For major abdominal surgery, 10 to 15 mL/kg/hr may be empirically used. Supplemental serum albumin (5% solution), 10 to 15 mL/kg, may be added if fluid requirement exceeds 25 to 30 mL/kg/hr or serum total solids are less than 3.5 to 4 g/dL.

SUMMARY

In summary, fluid and electrolyte therapy for the neonate must take into account the dynamic changes in body water as a result of changes with maturity, nutrition, development of the kidney, losses as a result of environmental influences, and underlying disease. In general, the fluid requirement for the neonate will depend on IWL, urinary excretion, stool water, and water for growth (Table 20–4).

Sequential monitoring and assessment of clinical, biophysical, and biochemical changes are necessary to maintain fluid and electrolyte homeostasis.

REFERENCES

1. Alward CT, Hook JB, Helmrath TA, et al: Effects of asphyxia on renal function in the newborn piglet. *Pediatr Res* 1978; 12:225–228.
2. Apnea A, Broberger O, Elinda G, et al: Postnatal development of renal function in pre-term and full-term infants. *Acta Paediatr Scand* 1981; 70:183–187.
3. Baumgart S: Radiant energy and insensible water loss in premature newborn infant under a radiant warmer. *Clin Perinatol* 1982; 8:483–504.

4. Baumgart S, Engle WD, Fox WW, et al: Radiant warmer power and body size as determinants of insensible water loss in the critically ill neonate. *Pediatr Res* 1981; 15:1495–1499.
5. Baumgart S, Langman CB, Sosulski R, et al: Fluid, electrolyte, and glucose maintenance in the very low birthweight infant. *Clin Pediatr* 1982; 21:199–206.
6. Bell EF, Neidich GA, Cashore WJ, et al: Combined effect of radiant warmer and phototherapy in insensible water loss in low-birthweight infants. *J Pediatr* 1979; 94:810–813.
7. Bell EF, Warburton D, Stonestreet BS, et al: Effect of fluid administration on the development of symptomatic patent ductus arteriosus and congestive heart failure in premature infant. *N Engl J Med* 1980; 302:598.
8. Daniel SS, Hussain MK, Milliez J, et al: Renal response of the fetal lamb to complete occlusion of the umbilical cord. *Am J Obstet Gynecol* 1978; 131:514–519.
9. Engelke SC, Shah BC, Vasan U, et al: Sodium balance in very low birth weight infants. *J Pediatr* 1978; 93:837–841.
10. Feldman W, Drummolnd KW, Klein M: Hyponatremia following asphyxia neonatorum. *Acta Pediatr Scand* 1970; 59:52–57.
11. Friis-Hansen B: Changes in body water compartments during growth. *Acta Paediatr Scand [Suppl]* 1957; 110:1–68.
12. Friis-Hansen B: Body composition during growth. In vivo measurements and biochemical data correlated to differential anatomical growth. *Pediatrics* 1971; 47:264–274.
13. Friis-Hansen B: Water distribution in the foetus and newborn infant. *Acta Paediatr Scand [Suppl]* 1983; 305:7–11.
14. Gruskin AB, Edelman CM, Jr, Yuan S: Maturational changes in renal blood flow in piglets. *Pediatr Res* 1970; 4:7–13.
15. Halliday HL, Hirata T, Brady JP: Indomethacin therapy for large patent ductus arteriosus in the very low birth weight infant: Results and complications. *Pediatrics* 1979; 64:154–159.
16. Holliday MA, Segar WE: The maintenance need for water in parenteral fluid therapy. *Pediatrics* 1957; 19:823–832.
17. Kagan BM, Stanincora V, Felix NS, et al: Body composition of premature infants: Relation to nutrition. *Am J Clin Nutr* 1972; 25:1153–1164.
18. Lagercrantz H, Bislo HP: Catecholamine release in the newborn infant at birth. *Pediatr Res* 1977; 11:889–893.
19. Leake RD, Trygstad CW: Glomerular filtration rate during the period of adaptation to extrauterine life. *Pediatr Res* 1977; 11:959–962.
20. Paxson CL Jr, Stoerner JW, Durson SE, et al: Syndrome of inappropriate antidiuretic hormone secretion in neonates with pneumothorax or atelectasis. *J Pediatr* 1977; 91:459–463.
21. Weinberg JA, Weitzman RE, Zahauddin S, et al: Inappropriate secretion of antidiuretic hormone in a premature infant. *J Pediatr* 1977; 90:111–114.
22. Williams PR, Oh W: Effects of radiant warmers on insensible water loss in newborn infants. *Am J Dis Child* 1974; 128:511–514.
23. Wu PYK, Hodgman JE: Insensible water loss in preterm infants: Changes with postnatal development and non-ionizing radiant energy. *Pediatrics* 1974; 54:704–712.

21

Diuretic Therapy

William Oh, M.D.

Diuretics are pharmacologic agents used for the removal of pathologically accumulated excess body fluid through the kidney. Diuretics are commonly used in the newborn; indications include generalized edema, fluid overload, congestive heart failure, pulmonary edema, and hypertension. Several diuretic agents are available commercially; however, only a few are used commonly in the newborn. In this chapter we discuss the pharmacology, indications, dosage, administration, and possible complications of these agents when used in the newborn period.

As shown in Table 21–1, at least five types of diuretic agents are available for therapeutic usage. The most commonly used agent in the newborn is furosemide. Furosemide is used intravenously because of its rapid onset of action for short-term therapy; it is also available in an oral form so that maintenance therapy can be given infants who can tolerate oral intake. Another frequently used diuretic agent is spironolactone; its use is desirable when prolonged diuretic therapy is indicated, as in hypertension. More recently diuretics have been used as an adjunct therapeutic agent in the management of low-birth-weight (LBW) infants with chronic lung disease. We discuss its therapeutic efficacy and potential complications.

PHARMACOLOGY

When given intravenously, diuretics such as furosemide exert a diuretic action within 15 to 30 minutes of administration, and the action will last for approximately 2 to 4 hours.[14] Although furosemide does not alter the glomerular filtration rate, it does inhibit chloride reabsorption along the proximal tubule (ascending limb of Henle's loop), which results in increased excretion of sodium, chloride, and potassium, with significant osmotic diuresis. In addition, furosemide enhances excretion of calcium.[15] Although the

TABLE 21–1.
Diuretic Agents

Drug (Trade Name)	Mechanism of Action	Route of Administration*	Onset of Action	Dose
Furosemide (Lasix)	Loop diuretics; inhibits sodium and chloride reabsorption in proximal tubule	IV, IM PO	15–30 min 30–60 min	1 mg/kg/dose 1–3 mg/kg/dose
Chlorothiazide (Diuril)	Inhibits sodium and chloride reabsorption along the distal tubules	PO	1–2 hr	20–40 mg/kg/24 hr
Hydrochlorothiazide (HydroDIURIL)	Similar to chlorothiazide	PO	1–2 hr	2–4 mg/kg/24 hr
Spironolactone (Aldactone)	Competitive antagonist of aldosterone	PO	3–5 days	1.5–3.0 mg/kg/day
Ethacrynic acid (Edecrin)	Similar to furosemide	IV PO	10–20 min 1 hr	1 mg/kg/dose 1–3 mg/kg/day

half-life of furosemide is relatively longer in newborns,[2] particularly in LBW infants, the duration of pharmacologic action of the drug is relatively short, lasting approximately 2 to 4 hours after a 1 mg/kg intravenous dose.

Spironolactone is also often used in newborns, particularly if prolonged diuretic therapy is desirable, such as in treatment of hypertension and congestive heart failure. This drug is a competitive antagonist for aldosterone, a hormone that decreases excretion of sodium and chloride.[8] It takes much longer for spironolactone to begin acting after oral administration, but the duration of action is also much longer and sustained.

The precise mechanism of chlorothiazide and hydrochlorothiazide in the newborn and pediatric patient is still unclear, although the consensus is that these drugs inhibit sodium and chloride reabsorption along the distal tubules of the kidney.[4] Both drugs are given orally, and onset of action is approximately 1 to 2 hours after administration, with duration of action approximately 6 to 12 hours.

INDICATIONS FOR DIURETIC THERAPY

Fluid Overload

Fluid overload is particularly common in LBW infants; fluid and electrolyte therapy can be very challenging in these neonates and often results in either overhydration or dehydration.[13] In fluid overload significant clinical problems can result that necessitate acute and rapid removal of the excess body fluid by use of diuretics. The diuretic (e.g., furosemide) should be given as a single dose. Subsequent requirement for diuretics should be judged on the basis of clinical and fluid and electrolyte status. Furthermore, judicious management of fluid and electrolyte balance should be a high priority to avoid the need for diuretics to treat fluid overload (see Chapter 20).

Pulmonary Edema

Pulmonary edema is a common and clinically significant problem in LBW infants. Because of the limited ability of the kidney to excrete excess fluid, LBW infants are more prone to fluid retention when an inappropriate amount of excess fluid is given.[11] When the excess fluid is given intravenously over a short period, pulmonary edema is a frequent complication and requires immediate attention. In addition to appropriate adjustment of fluid dose, diuretics given systematically can provide immediate relief of adverse clinical manifestations resulting from fluid overload. The diuretic most frequently used under these circumstances is furosemide, at a dose of 1 mg/kg intravenously. The drug can be repeated at the same dose at 12- to 24-hour intervals if signs of pulmonary edema persist.

In LBW infants with patent ductus arteriosus and significant left-to-right shunt, pulmonary edema is also common.[3] The definitive management of this clinical condition is closure of the ductus arteriosus, either with intravenous indomethacin or by surgical ligation. Prior to definitive management, a 1 mg/kg dose of furosemide given intravenously is also indicated to provide immediate relief of the clinical symptoms secondary to pulmonary edema.

Congestive Heart Failure

As in older children, diuretics are part of the therapeutic regimen in the treatment of congestive heart failure in the newborn. Diuretic therapy is particularly useful if congestive heart failure is accompanied by significant peripheral edema and hepatosplenomegaly, indicative of right-sided heart failure.

Hypertension

Most cases of hypertension in the newborn are secondary to acute renal artery thrombosis, particularly in association with prolonged use of an indwelling umbilical artery catheter.[1] Hypertension also may be a sequela of acute renal failure following asphyxia-induced acute tubular necrosis. Diuretics are useful in conjunction with other antihypertensive agents. Spironolactone is often used because of its sustained and prolonged diuretic effect and because the agent can be given orally.

Recent reports have suggested that diuretics such as furosemide can be useful as an adjunct to therapy in such clinical conditions as respiratory distress syndrome (RDS)[6] and bronchopulmonary dysplasia (BPD).[9, 10] The rationale for usage is based on the assumption that RDS and BPD are associated with significant pulmonary edema. Because lack of surfactant is now considered the major cause of RDS, the use of diuretics in this condition is not advisable. The edema in the interstitial tissue found in BPD is only part of the more extensive pathologic findings in this condition. Airway necrosis and fibrotic changes in the pulmonary parenchyma are the major pathologic features; long-term treatment of pulmonary edema with diuretics yields only modest beneficial effects.[10]

DOSAGE AND ADMINISTRATION

The choice of diuretic agent may depend in part on whether the infant can tolerate oral feeding. In situations where oral feeding is not possible, diuretics that can be administered by parenteral routes may be used (e.g., furosemide). Orally administered diuretics are readily absorbed through the intestinal tract, and their duration of action is similar to that of diuretics administered parenterally. The dose, route, and frequency of administration are shown in Table 21–1.

POSSIBLE COMPLICATIONS

There are several potential complications of diuretic therapy in the newborn. Judicious short-term use of diuretics is relatively free of complication, particularly if attention is paid to fluid and electrolyte balance during the course of therapy. However, long-term use of such diuretics as furosemide has been associated with several complications as a result of the effect of furosemide on electrolyte, acid-base, and calcium and phosphate balance, particularly in the VLBW infants.

Furosemide is frequently used as an adjunct to therapy in the management of BPD in LBW infants. Since its usage is associated with increased renal excretion of sodium, potassium, chloride, hydrogen ions, and calcium, these infants are at risk for development of metabolic complications, including hyponatremia, metabolic alkalosis, and calcium deficiency. Calcium deficiency can lead to osteopenia of prematurity, with multiple fractures as a result of deficient calcium storage in the bone.[12, 16] Increased excretion of calcium may also lead to nephrocalcinosis.[7]

Others have recommended the use of diuretics such as chlorothiazide or spironolactone, which do not have as much calciuric effect as furosemide. However, these diuretics may not have as much beneficial effect on the pulmonary function as furosemide.[5] Until more data are available in regard to the therapeutic efficacy of diuretics other than furosemide, the latter should probably be used as an adjunct to therapy of BPD.

REFERENCES

1. Adelman RD: Neonatal hypertension. *Pediatr Clin North Am* 1978; 25:99–110.
2. Aranda JV, et al: Pharmaco-kinetic dispositions and protein binding of furosemide in newborn infants. *J Pediatr* 1978; 93:507–511.
3. Bell EF, Warburton D, Stonestreet BS, et al: Effect of fluid administration of the development of symptomatic patent ductus arteriosus and congestive heart failure in premature infants. *N Engl J Med* 1980; 302:598–604.
4. Beyer KH: The mechanism of action of chlorothiazide. *Ann NY Acad Sci* 1958; 71:363–379.
5. Engelhardt B, Blalock WA, DonLevy S, et al: Effect of spironolactone-hydrochlorothiazide on lung function in infants with chronic bronchopulmonary dysplasia. *J Pediatr* 1989; 114:619–624.
6. Green TP, et al: Furosemide use in premature infants and appearance of patent ductus arteriosus. *Am J Dis Child* 1981; 135:239.
7. Hufnagle KG, Khan SN, Penn D, et al: Renal calcification: A complication of long-term furosemide therapy in premature infants. *Pediatrics* 1982; 70:360–363.
8. Kahuawa CM, Sturtebant FM, VanArman CP: Pharmacology of a new steroid that blocks salt activity of Aldactone and desoxycorticosterone. *J Pharmacol Exp Ther* 1959; 126:123–130.

9. Kao LC, Warburton D, Cheng MH, et al: Effects of oral diuretics on pulmonary mechanics in infants with chronic bronchopulmonary dysplasia: Results of a double blind crossover sequential trial. *Pediatrics* 1984; 74:37–44.
10. Kao LC, et al: Furosemide acutely decreases airways resistance in chronic bronchopulmonary dysplasia. *J Pediatr* 1983; 103:624–629.
11. Leake RD, Zakauddin S, Trygstad CW, et al: The effects of large volume intravenous fluid infusion on neonatal renal function. *J Pediatr* 1976; 89:968–972.
12. O'Brodovich HM, Mellins RB: Bronchopulmonary dysplasia: Unresolved neonatal lung injury. *Am Rev Respir Dis* 1985; 132:694–709.
13. Oh W: Fluid and electrolyte management, in Avery GB (ed): *Neonatology.* Philadelphia, JB Lippincott Co, 1981, pp 643–657.
14. Ross BS, Pollak A, Oh W: The pharmacologic effects of furosemide therapy in low birth weight infant. *J Pediatr* 1978; 92:149–152.
15. Taft H, Roin J: Effect of furosemide administration on calcium excretion. *Br Med J* 1971; 1:437–438.
16. Venkataraman PS, et al: Secondary hyperparathyroidism and bone disease in infants receiving long-term furosemide therapy. *Am J Dis Child* 1983; 137:1157–1161.

22

Seizures

Hilda Goldbarg, M.D.

Tsu F. Yeh, M.D.

Neonatal seizures are a frequent and difficult problem encountered by neo-natologists and pediatric neurologists. Estimates of incidence vary from 1.5 to 3.5 per 1,000 live births. In nurseries and neonatal intensive care units the frequency of seizures has been estimated at 0.8% to 20.1%, respectively. Mortality has been reported, as high as 40% to 60% in earlier reports and as low as 16% in more recent studies.[15]

Neonatal seizures should be considered a symptom of an insult affecting the central nervous system. The seriousness of seizures is manifested by the fact that permanent neurologic deficits may be left as sequelae. Moreover, experimental evidence suggests that seizures themselves may result in cerebral injury. Thus, rapid determination of their cause and subsequent treatment are essential.

ETIOLOGY

Comparing studies before and after 1968,[13-15, 20] it is clear that there have been significant changes in the prevalence of etiologic factors in seizures.

Lombroso[16] showed that seizures secondary to birth trauma and late hypocalcemia have decreased consistently, whereas seizures caused by asphyxia and intracranial hemorrhage have increased. Other etiologic factors have remained unchanged.

Hypoxic Ischemic Encephalopathy

Hypoxic ischemic encephalopathy is a common manifestation of asphyxia in neonates and accounts for 50% to 70% of neonatal seizures. The seizures usually occur in the first 24 hours after birth. They can be multifocal and clonic; subtle seizures can be seen alone or in combination.

The seizures are usually associated with apathy, hypotonia or hypertonia, and absent or depressed infantile reflexes.

Intracranial Hemorrhage

Intracranial hemorrhages were found in 14% to 15% of affected newborns in one large series.[12, 16]

Four major types of intracranial hemorrhages have been described[23]: subdural, primary subarachnoid, periventricular, and intracerebral.

Periventricular and intracerebral hemorrhages are characterized by bleeding into the cerebral white matter, particularly in the centrum semiovale and caudate nucleus. Periventricular and intracerebral hemorrhages are extremely common in premature babies, occurring in 50% to 70%.[10] They are usually associated with a hypoxic event, severe respiratory distress, or both. Seizures develop during the first 24 to 48 hours of life and are subtle, tonic, or multifocal clonic.

Primary subarachnoid hemorrhage occurs primarily in the subarachnoid space and is not an extension of intraventricular or subdural hemorrhage. When it occurs in premature infants, it is usually associated with trauma or hypoxia. In full-term babies with subarachnoid hemorrhage, seizures occur during the second day of life and are characteristically associated with no other clinical abnormalities.

Subdural hemorrhage may be secondary to laceration of the tentorium with rupture of the falx cerebri sinus, vein of Galen, or lateral sinus. When tears occur in the tentorium, the hemorrhage is more frequently infratentorial. Subdural hemorrhage almost always is secondary to traumatic lesions during the delivery period. The seizure usually is due to concomitant cerebral concussion, and may occur in the first 48 hours of life. The frequency of subdural hemorrhage has decreased considerably as a result of improvements in obstetric practice.

Infections

Infections involving the CNS accounted for approximately 17% of cases in the series reviewed.[5, 17] Of the bacterial infections, meningitis secondary to group B hemolytic streptococci[6] and *Escherichia coli* is the most common cause of seizures.

Nonbacterial causes of neonatal seizures include infections with cytomegalovirus, *Toxoplasma,* herpes simplex and rubella viruses, and fungus, such as *Candida albicans.*

Hypoglycemia

Infants of diabetic mothers and infants small for gestational age (SGA) are at higher risk for hypoglycemia. The most frequent symptoms of hypoglycemia are tremors, apnea, poor suck, hypotonia, and convulsions of a subtle or clonic type (for details see Chapter 17).

Hypocalcemia

Hypocalcemia can occur early or late in the neonatal period. Early hypocalcemia is seen at 2 to 3 days of life and is commonly found in babies with perinatal asphyxia or obstetric trauma. Therefore, hypocalcemia usually is accompanied by hypoglycemia, acidosis, or intracranial bleeding. Clinically the neonates show hypotonia, poor suck, depressed infantile reflexes, and subtle or multifocal clonic seizures. Late hypocalcemia occurs at the end of the first week of life. Affected infants are usually full term and large for gestational age. Hypocalcemia is induced by the consumption of a milk preparation with suboptimal ratios of phosphorus to calcium and of phosphorus to magnesium. Hyperphosphatemia and hypomagnesemia are frequent concomitant findings. Clinically the infants show jitteriness, hyperactivity, increased deep tendon reflexes, and seizures (for details see Chapter 18).

Pyridoxine

Pyridoxine dependency is a relatively rare congenital metabolic disturbance that produces neonatal seizures unresponsive to anticonvulsant medication. Pyridoxine is transformed in the body to pyridoxal phosphate, which is an important coenzyme involved in the synthesis of the inhibitory neurotransmitter γ-aminobutyric acid (GABA). Intrauterine convulsions may mark the beginning of the disease.

Developmental Defects

Developmental defects associated with neonatal seizures (i.e., schizencephaly, pachygyria, and polymicrogyria) are related to disturbances of neuronal migration that occur during the third to fifth months of gestation. Clinically, in addition to seizures that appear during the first 2 to 3 days of life the newborns show hypotonia, lethargy, and poor suck.

Drug Withdrawal

Neonatal seizures secondary to maternal narcotic use is a well-recognized syndrome. In one study the incidence of seizures from drug withdrawal in infants exposed to methadone was 7.8%, and to heroin 1.2%. The principal seizure manifestations described were generalized motor or myoclonic[11] (see also Chapter 3).

Familial Seizures

Familial neonatal seizures constitute a separate entity. Convulsions usually start during the second or third day of life, and are focal or multifocal clonic. During interictal periods the infant appears normal. As a rule, the seizures do not respond to anticonvulsant medication. The seizures disappear within days or weeks, and motor and mental development in the infant usually is normal. The condition is inherited as an autosomal dominant trait, and the cause is unknown.

CLINICAL MANIFESTATIONS

In the newborn the clinical manifestations of seizures are varied, and any unusual transient event could well be a seizure. At least four main types are recognized: focal clonic, multifocal clonic, myoclonic, and tonic.

Focal Clonic Seizures

Focal clonic seizures are characterized by clonic movements of one or more of the extremities, involving one limb or segment of the limb or part of the face. The clonic movements usually remain localized. Hemiclonic seizures are not uncommon at this age. These seizures are a common manifestation of focal cerebral injury produced by an infarct or focal intracranial bleed.

Multifocal Clonic Seizures

In this type of seizure the clonic movements shift fairly rapidly from one part of the body to another in a disorderly pattern. Sometimes the movements shift so rapidly that they may simulate generalized clonic seizures.

Myoclonic Seizures

Myoclonic seizures are rather uncommon during the neonatal period. They are characterized by single or repeated jerks that can be focal, multifocal, or generalized (infantile spasms).

Tonic Seizures

Tonic seizures are manifested by tonic extension of limbs and extremities. Eye movements and apnea can accompany the seizures. Tonic posturing is often not a manifestation of true seizures but a release phenomena of brain stem origin caused by functional decortication and disinhibition of normal tonic brain stem facilitory mechanisms.

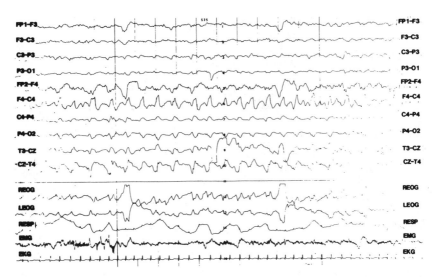

FIG 22–1.
High-voltage sharp waves on right centrotemporal region.

Subtle Seizures

Subtle seizures are characterized by motor automatisms and autonomic signs. Motor automatisms consist of one or more of the following: tonic eye deviation, eye jerking, blinking, lip smacking, or other buccolingual repetitive movements, as well as abnormal limb motions such as swimming, bicycling, or rowing. Autonomic manifestations consist of changes in heart rate, apnea, or changes in rate or depth of respirations.

Electroencephalographic Study

An electroencephalographic (EEG) study should be obtained during the ictal and interictal periods. The ictal tracing can determine the cortical origin of the seizure episodes; the interictal tracing can be of value in estimating prognosis if a sequence of recordings is obtained. A 16-channel machine should be used for the recording of EEG activity in addition to the recording of extraocular movement (EOM), electromyogram, EKG, and respiratory activity. The tracing should be long enough to record awake, quiet, and active sleep periods. Rose and Lombroso[20] classified the ictal EEG abnormality as follows:

1. Focal or unifocal: tracing of sharp waves originating focally, usually associated with peripheral focal clonic seizures (Fig 22–1).
2. Focal pseudo-beta-alpha-theta-delta ictal pattern; usually focal with repetitive waves at frequencies between 0.5 and 12 Hz. Clinically they manifest as subtle, tonic, or myoclonic seizures (Fig 22–2).

3. Multifocal-ictal patterns: usually associated with abnormal interictal activity (low voltage or burst suppression).
4. Low-frequency discharges on low-amplitude background (sharp waves occurring at low frequency, 1 Hz).

The background activity is particularly important in determining outcome and covers a large spectrum. The most severe are: (1) the inactive or isoelectric pattern, with activity below 5MV; and (2) burst suppression or periodic patterns characterized by periods of inactive background (lower than U/O 15 MV) interrupted by bursts of synchronous or asynchronous bursts of activity (Figs 22–3 and 22–4). Intermediate abnormalities consist of low-voltage patterns through all states, interhemispheric amplitude asymmetry, and delayed maturation patterns.

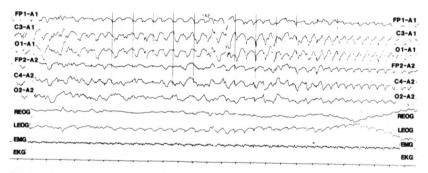

FIG 22–2.
Rhythmic 2 to 3 Hz sharp and slow activity over left hemisphere, spreading to right hemisphere, accompanied by episodes of apnea and rapid horizontal eye movements.

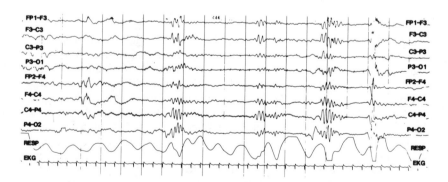

FIG 22–3.
Isoelectric periods interrupted by rhythmic activity at 6 to 7 Hz with sharp waves in right frontal region.

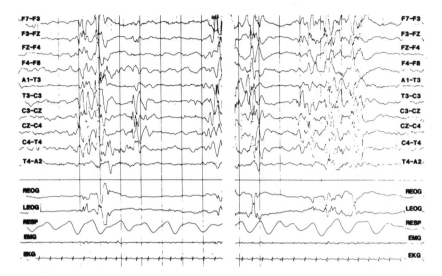

FIG 22–4.
Depression of background activity interrupted by bursts of bilateral spike discharges.

MANAGEMENT OF NEONATAL SEIZURES

General Management

Careful continuous monitoring of respirations and heart rate, proper ventilation, and maintenance of body temperature are essential in neonatal seizures. Electrolyte and pH levels, spinal puncture, and septic workup should be done before institution of specific treatment. In addition, an ultrasound or computed tomographic scan of the head should be obtained to exclude cerebral malformations or intracerebral bleeding. If the cause of seizures remains obscure, investigations should be carried on to exclude the presence of an inborn error of metabolism. The usual battery of tests consists of determination of levels of serum pyruvate and lactate, blood ammonia, urinary organic acids, urinary or blood amino acids, and occasionally, long-chain fatty acids. Chromosomal studies are indicated if dysmorphic features are present in the newborn.

Specific Treatment

If hypoglycemia is present, minibolus and maintenance of intravenous glucose can be given (see Chapter 17). With hypocalcemia an injection of 2.5% to 5% calcium gluconate is administered intravenously with ECG monitoring.

For correction of hypomagnesemia, 2 to 8 mL of a 2% to 3% solution of magnesium sulfate is given intravenously, or 0.2 mL/kg of a 50% solution is given intramuscularly.

Pyridoxine dependency is treated by giving 100 mg pyridoxine intravenously with EEG monitoring. This approach serves the dual purpose of diagnosis and treatment, in that the clinical seizures will stop and the EEG tracing will become normal within minutes after administration.

ANTICONVULSANT THERAPY

When seizures are not secondary to a correctable metabolic abnormality, anticonvulsant medication is indicated. Anticonvulsants used in neonates are shown in Table 22–1.

Phenobarbital

Phenobarbital is the drug of first choice for the treatment of neonatal seizures. Its mechanism of action is still incompletely understood. At therapeutic concentrations it inhibits paroxysmal membrane depolarization shifts that characterize epileptic foci in animals. Phenobarbital is completely absorbed after oral, intramuscular, or intravenous administration. It has a volume of distribution of 0.93 to 0.15 L/g in all neonates at loading doses of 15 to 20 mg/kg.[19] This volume of distribution indicates a predictable plasma level following administration of a loading dose.

TABLE 22–1.
Anticonvulsants in Neonates

Drug	Loading Dose	Mean Serum Half-life	Maintenance Dosage	Serum Therapeutic Range (μg/mL)
Phenobarbital	20–40 mg/kg	100 hr	2–8 mg/kg/day	16–40
Phenytoin	20 mg/kg	6–140 hr	5 mg/kg/day (variable)	10–20
Primidone	15–25 mg/kg	12 hr	12–20 mg/kg/day	6–12
Diazepam	0.3 mg (stat dose) 3–12 mg/day (continuous infusion)	50–400 hr (anticonvulsant activity only) 20 min	10–30 μmol/L	6–12
Lorazepam	0.05 mg/kg	9.4 hr	—	—
Paraldehyde	150 mg/kg/hr for 3 hr	10.2 hr	—	100–250
Lidocaine	4 mg/kg/hr	2.9–3.2 hr	—	0.5–4

Painter et al.[19] found that the neonate binds phenobarbital less well than the older child. Their phenobarbital binding ranged from 6% to 41% (mean ± SD 24.1% ± 8.7%). In older children, mean phenobarbital binding is 41.3% ± 8.4%. Binding seemed to be more impaired in very sick preterm infants. The brain-plasma ratio of phenobarbital is similar in the neonate and older child (0.71 ± 0.2).

The potential toxicity of phenobarbital in the neonate has not been well studied. Svenningen et al.[21] noted a decrease in heart rate below 100 beats/min in the presence of phenobarbital levels of 52 μg/mL. This is important because such relative bradycardia may result in a decrease in cardiac output and compromise cerebral blood flow. Also, Diaz et al.[4] noticed that phenobarbital interferes with brain growth in the experimental rat model. Further studies on the effects of phenobarbital on brain growth and metabolism are warranted.

The half-life of phenobarbital decreases from 100 hours during the first 2 weeks of life to 65 and 45 hours at the end of 2 and 4 weeks of therapy, respectively.[18]

Phenobarbital is administered by an intravenous loading dose of 20 mg/kg; that amount is necessary to obtain blood levels of approximately 20 μg/mL. Clinical effectiveness of phenobarbital is uncommon with serum concentrations below 16 μg/mL. Gal et al.[7] found that 12% of their patients required plasma concentrations above 30 μg/mL to control seizures. They recommend increasing phenobarbital until the seizures stop or a total dose of 40 mg/kg has been administered. Maintenance dose should not exceed 5 mg/kg/day.

Phenytoin

Phenytoin is the second most commonly used anticonvulsant. It is usually given after failure of phenobarbital therapy to control seizures. Its anticonvulsant action differs from that of phenobarbital in that it inhibits post-tetanic potentiation of nerve impulse transmission and limits the spread of epileptiform activity into the surrounding brain. The molecular mechanism of action is unknown.

Phenytoin is insoluble in water at physiologic pH, but is soluble in alkali and propylene glycol, which are used in the parenteral preparation. According to Painter et al.,[19] phenytoin binding ranged from 30% to 91% (mean 70.2% ± 14.0%). The mean brain-plasma ratio was 1.28 ± 0.32.

The metabolism of phenytoin in the neonate is variable. Bourgeois and Dodson[1] reported that the half-life of phenytoin varied between 6 and 140 hours in infants aged 2 to 36 days, after an intravenous loading dose. The effective plasma concentration is 10 to 20 μg/mL, and intravenous loading doses of 20 mg/kg are necessary to obtain concentrations above 15 μg/mL.[19]

The neonate should be carefully monitored during intravenous administration of the drug because of the possible induction of cardiac arrhythmias.

The maintenance dose should not exceed 5 mg/kg/day when the intravenous route is used.

Maintenance administration is also complicated by the nonlinear kinetics of the drug; therefore, blood levels should be carefully monitored.

Diazepam

Diazepam is used commonly when the neonate continues to have seizures after administration of loading doses of phenobarbital and phenytoin, but it also can be used as the initial mode of therapy. Gamstorp and Seden[8] used continuous intravenous infusion of diazepam at rates of 0.7 to 2.75 mg/hr for 6 to 11 days. The medication was slowly tapered when the infant was seizure free for 12 to 24 hours. Thong and Abramson[22] used continuous intravenous infusion of 3 to 12 mg/kg/day, given from 21 hours to 18 days. Plasma concentrations in their series exceeded 35 mol/L in 50% of their population. The volume of distribution of plasma diazepam has been found to vary between 1.3 and 2.6 L/kg, and the half-life varies between 50 and 400 hours. When used as a single dose and not as an infusion, diazepam has a rapid clearance from the brain (20 minutes after intravenous administration); therefore, its effectiveness is limited when used as a single bolus dose. Side effects include hypotension, lethargy, and hypoventilation. There has been some concern regarding the use of diazepam because of the possibility that its vehicle, sodium benzoate, could uncouple bilirubin from albumin and increase the risk of kernicterus. Although kernicterus has not been reported as a complication of diazepam, use of this drug should be considered very carefully in neonates with jaundice.

Lorazepam

Recent literature[3] suggests that lorazepam, a long-acting benzodiazepine, is effective and safe in the management of neonatal seizures. It is given intravenously at a dose of 0.05 mg/kg over 2 to 5 minutes. Human data indicate that the half-life of lorazepam averages 9.4 hours in children and 15.7 hours in adults. Lorazepam rapidly penetrates the CNS and produces minimal cardiovascular and respiratory depression.

Primidone

Primidone can be used as an adjunctive agent in neonates with refractory seizures. It can only be administered by the oral route. The lowest effective dose of 10 to 25 mg/kg is given, followed by a maintenance dose of 10 to 20 mg/kg/day. Toxic effects include somnolence and hypotension.

Paraldehyde

Paraldehyde[9] is also used as an adjunctive agent in the treatment of refractory neonatal seizures. It is given as an intravenous infusion of 150 mg/kg/hr for 3 hours in a form of 5% solution in 5% dextrose. The minimal effective plasma level appears to be 100 μg/mL, and its half-life 10.2 ± 1.0 hours. Toxic effects include hypotension and lipoid pneumonitis.

Lidocaine

Lidocaine can be used for refractory seizures. It is administered at an intravenous dose of 4 mg/kg/hr. Lidocaine appears to be anticonvulsant at serum levels of 0.5 to 4 μg/mL. The half-life of the drug is 2.9 to 3.2 hours. Its toxicity includes seizures, arrhythmias, and hypotension.

Duration of Therapy

If the infant is seizure free after the initial acute episode, anticonvulsants can be discontinued before discharge, even if the neurologic examination shows abnormality. The anticonvulsant therapy is continued after discharge, and the infant should be examined again at 2 to 3 months of age. If no further seizures are reported, the anticonvulsant medication can be tapered and discontinued.

PROGNOSIS

The overall prognosis of neonatal seizures is unknown because large prospective long-term studies in infants with neonatal convulsions are few. Many also believe that the prognosis depends more on the cause of the seizures and the gestational age of the infant than on the seizures themselves.[16, 24] It is also worth mentioning that with the advent of the prolonged EEG, television monitoring of infants is being questioned if many of the so-called subtle seizures represent a true epileptiform phenomena. Until all those factors are taken into consideration a true estimate of the prognosis of neonatal seizures will not be known. The outlook in a newborn with seizures may be evaluated in terms of mortality, morbidity, and long-term findings.[16] A significant decrease in mortality has been noted, from 40% to 60% before 1968 to 15% to 16% between 1968 and 1980. The improvement in mortality seems to be related to better obstetric care and increased sophistication and technology in neonatal intensive care units.

The morbidity, on the other hand, has not changed during the past 20 years, and varies between 70% and 35%. Approximately 35% of neonates do not develop significant neurologic difficulties. Seizures have recurred after the neonatal period in 20% of the infants reported by Dennis.[2]

As part of the U.S. National Collaborative Perinatal Project, Holden et al.[12] found that 277 infants of 5,700 pregnancies developed neonatal seizures; 35% of these neonates died, and 19 of 181 survivors had mental retardation with or without cerebral palsy. Two percent had cerebral palsy alone, and 70% of the survivors had no sequelae.

The incidence of later recurrent seizures varies. Holden et al.[12] report an incidence of 9%, while Rose and Lombroso[20] and Dennis[2] reported recurrence rates of 26% and 20%, respectively. Overall, the worse prognosis is related to the presence of cerebral dysgenesis.

REFERENCES

1. Bourgeois B, Dodson WE: Phenytoin elimination in newborns. *Neurology* 1983; 33:173–178.
2. Dennis JC: Neonatal convulsions: Etiology, late neonatal status, and long-term outcome. *Dev Med Child Neurol* 1978; 20:143–150.
3. Deshmukh A, Witlert W, Schnitzler E, et al: Lorazepam in the treatment of refractory neonatal seizures. *Am J Dis Child* 1986; 140:1042–1044.
4. Diaz J, Schain R, Baileyn BG: Phenobarbital induced brain growth retardation in artificially reared rat pups. *Biol Neonate* 1977; 32:77–82.
5. Feigin R: Bacterial meningitis in the newborn infant, in *Clinics in Perinatology*, vol 4. Philadelphia, WB Saunders Co, 1977, pp 103–116.
6. Franciosi RA, Knostonan JD, Zimmerman RM: Group B streptococcal neonatal and infant infections. *J Pediatr* 1973; 82:707–715.
7. Gal P, et al: Efficacy of phenobarbital monotherapy in the treatment of neonatal seizures, relations to blood levels. *Neurology* (NY) 1982; 32:1401–1404.
8. Gamstorp I, Seden G: Neonatal convulsions treated with continuous diazepam. *Upsala J Med Sci* 1982; 87:143–149.
9. Giacola GP, Gessner PK, Zaleska MM, et al: Pharmacodynamics of paraldehyde disposition in the neonate. *J Pediatr* 1984; 104:291–296.
10. Grunwald P: Subependymal cerebral hemorrhage in premature infants and its relationship to various injurious influences at birth. *Am J Obstet Gynecol* 1951; 61:1285–1292.
11. Herzlinger RA, Krandall SR, Vaughan HG: Neonatal seizure associated with narcotic withdrawal. *J Pediatr* 1977; 91:638–641.
12. Holden KR, Freeman JM, Melitis ED: Outcomes of infants with neonatal seizures, in Wada JA, Penry JK (eds): *Advances in Epileptology: The Xth Epilepsy Internal Symposium.* New York, Raven Press, 1980, pp 155–158.
13. Lombroso CT: Neonatal seizures states, in *Proceedings of the Ninth International Congress of Pediatrics.* Tokyo, University of Tokyo Press, 1965, pp 38–59.
14. Lombroso CT: Seizures in the newborn period, in *Handbook of Clinical Neurology,* vol 15. Amsterdam, North Holland, 1973, pp 189–213.
15. Lombroso CT: Convulsive disorders in newborns, in Thompson RA, Green JR (eds): *Pediatric Neurology and Neurosurgery.* New York, Spectrum, 1978, pp 101–113 and 205–239.

16. Lombroso CT: Status epilepticus, mechanisms of brain damage and treatment, in Escuete AD, et al (eds): *Advances in Neurology*. New York, Raven Press, 1983, pp 101–113.
17. Overall JC Jr: Neonatal bacterial meningitis. *J Pediatr* 1970; 76:499–511.
18. Painter MJ, et al: Phenobarbital and diphenyl hydantoin levels in neonates with seizures. *J Pediatr* 1978; 92:315–319.
19. Painter MJ, Pippenger C, Wasterlain C, et al: Phenobarbital and phenytoin in neonatal seizures: Metabolism and tissue distribution. *Neurology (NY)* 1981; 21:1107–1112.
20. Rose AL, Lombroso CT: Neonatal seizures states: A prospective study in 137 full-term babies. *Pediatrics* 1970; 45:404–425.
21. Svenningen NW, Blennow G, Landroth M, et al: Brain oriented intensive care treatment in severe neonatal asphyxia. *Arch Dis Child* 1982; 57:176–183.
22. Thong YH, Abramson D: Continuous infusion of diazepam in infants with severe recurrent convulsions. *Med Ann DC* 1974; 77–102.
23. Volpe J: Neonatal intracranial hemorrhage, in Volpe J (ed): *Clinics in Perinatology*, vol 4. Philadelphia, WB Saunders Co, 1977, pp 77–102.
24. Volpe JJ (ed): *Neurology of the Newborn*, ed 2. Philadelphia, WB Saunders Co, 1987, p 145.

23

Prevention of Intraventricular Hemorrhage

Tonse N. K. Raju, M.D.

Although the overall incidence of neonatal intraventricular hemorrhage (IVH) has been declining in recent years, severe grades of hemorrhage still occur in 50% to 70% of extremely premature infants of less than 26 weeks gestation and weighing less than 750 g at birth, and somewhat less frequently in those between 27 and 32 weeks' gestation.[13] Thus, although survival rates for premature babies have improved remarkably, because large hemorrhages lead to morbidity in most, IVH continues to be of great concern.

PREVENTION OF INTRAVENTRICULAR HEMORRHAGE

In experimental animals, elevation of systemic blood pressure and volume expansion produce IVH, perhaps because of rupture of the capillary network in the germinal matrix, which lacks sufficient connective tissue. Further, in distressed preterm infants the cerebral blood flow (CBF) could be "pressure passive" because of a loss of CBF autoregulation; in such circumstances sudden changes in blood volume or intravascular pressure could critically alter CBF to the periventricular border zones. Increase in flow could lead to hemorrhage; reduction in flow might cause ischemia, neuronal death, or cystic and periventricular leukomalacia.

Some clinical factors associated with IVH[13] are asphyxia and shock, "fluctuating" CBF velocity, pneumothorax, patent ductus arteriosus (PDA), abnormalities of coagulation and hemostatic mechanisms, and excessive use of heparin. Most of these factors are confounded with prematurity; therefore IVH should be viewed as a multifactorial complication, with prematurity of the developing nervous system and its vascular structures as the most important denominator.

Because alterations in CBF in a structurally susceptible immature nervous

TABLE 23–1.
Prevention of Intraventricular Hemorrhage

	Rationale
Agents affecting CBF	
Phenobarbital	Decreases CBF and $CMRO_2$
	Free radical scavenger
	Stabilizes blood pressure
	Sedative effect
Indomethacin	Cyclooxygenase inhibitor
	Reduces free radical formation
	PDA closure effect
	Capillary endothelial stability
	Reduces CBF
Ethamsylate	Inhibition of capillary bleeding
	Stabilization of capillaries
	Inhibition of prostaglandin synthesis
	PDA closure
	Reduces CBF
Other agents	
Vitamin E	Free radical scavenger
Pancuronium	Stabilization of blood pressure and respiration
	Reduction of "fluctuations" in CBF velocity
Tranexamic acid	Inhibits plasminogen activators
Fresh frozen plasma	Corrects coagulation deficiencies
Vitamin K_1	Corrects coagulation deficiencies

CBF = cerebral blood flow; $CMRO_2$ = cerebral metabolic rate for oxygen; PDA = patent ductus arteriosus.

system seem to be the basis for most IVH, prophylactic trials are directed at preventing excessive CBF and reducing cerebral metabolic rate for oxygen ($CMRO_2$) and toward measures to stabilize cerebral vasculature and endothelium (Table 23–1). It is difficult to derive a unified conclusion from the diverse group of trials, particularly because they vary in patient entry criteria, dose, route, frequency and duration of drug therapy, and study design.

Phenobarbital

Rationale.—The effect of phenobarbital on the cerebral vasculature and CBF has not been studied in human infants; studies in animals, however, indicate that at anticonvulsant doses, phenobarbital lowers the mean arterial blood pressure acutely. It is also possible that phenobarbital widens the upper boundaries of CBF autoregulation and reduces blood pressure swings. Other pharmacologic properties hypothesized to be beneficial are decrease in both the overall and cerebral fraction of oxygen consumption ($CMRO_2$), maintenance of endothelial integrity by antioxidant effect, and decrease in catecholamine release.

Clinical Trials.—Among the clinical trials summarized in Table 23–2, there is much variation in the entry criteria and treatment protocols. Although in 1981 Donn et al.[3] reported a 34% reduction in IVH in the phenobarbital-treated preterm infants, six subsequent trials failed to confirm this observation. Further, two recent trials [5, 11] reported an increased incidence in IVH in the phenobarbital-treated group, although the reason for this discrepant find-

TABLE 23–2.
Prevention Studies: Phenobarbital*

Authors	Total No.	Entry Criteria	Dose (mg/kg)/ Route/ Duration (days)	Conclusions Δ ICH
Postnatal				
Donn et al.	60	<1,500 g	20 mg/kg IV 7 days	Decrease
Hope et al.	35	<33 wk	20 mg/kg PO 5 days	No change
Morgan et al.	60	<1,250 g or <1,500 g, ventilator	20 mg/kg PO 1 day	No change
Whitelaw et al.	60	<1,500 g or <31 wk	20 mg/kg IM/IV 1 day	No change
Bedard et al.	42	<1,500 g, <33 wk or <37 wk, ventilator	20 mg/kg IV 7 days	No change†
Goldstein et al.	129	<1,500 g	20 mg/kg IV 7 days	Decrease
Ruth et al.	52	<1,500 g	20 mg/kg IV 5 days	Decrease
Porter et al.	19	<1,500 g ventilator	20 mg/kg IV 3 days	Increase
Kuban et al.	280	≤1,750 g	20 mg/kg IV 5 days	Increase
Anwar et al.	58	<1,500 g	20 mg/kg IV 7 days	No change
Ruth et al.	101	<1,500 g	30 mg/kg IV 5 days	No change
Antenatal				
Shankaran et al.	46	<35 wk Preterm labor	500 mg IV and 100 mg PO qd	Decrease
Morales et al.	150	<32 wk Imminent delivery	390 mg IV or 720 mg PO	Decrease

*Adapted from Ment LR, Ehraenkranz RA, Duncan LM: *Semin Perinatol* 1988; 12:359–372.
ICH = intracranial hemorrhage.
†Possibly reduced severity.

ing was not clear. The effect of phenobarbital on the severity of IVH has also been controversial.

The two prenatal phenobarbital trials shown in Table 23–2 reported 24% and 26% lower incidence of IVH, along with reduced severe grades of hemorrhages in the treatment groups. In the Shankaran trial,[12] IVH incidence was reduced despite a low serum (cord blood) concentration of the drug. Although the results are promising, the findings of prenatal phenobarbital trials are to be replicated. The effects of confounding variables, such as mode of delivery, antenatal use of dexamethasone, and tocolytic therapy, are to be delineated. Appropriate dose, frequency, and timing of therapy are unclear, as are the magnitude of side effects, such as neonatal depression and acidosis, and the effect on fetal cardiac output. Until these concerns are addressed, *routine* clinical use of antenatal phenobarbital to prevent IVH does not appear to be justified.

Indomethacin

Rationale.—Cerebral prostaglandin cascade is intimately involved in the control of CBF during health and in the pathophysiology of hypoxic ischemic brain injury. A detailed review of pharmacologic properties of indomethacin is beyond the scope of this chapter, but collective evidence strongly suggests that intravenously administered indomethacin prevents prostanoid release into the cerebrospinal fluid and decreases CBF to all regions of the brain.[7] It attenuates the cerebral hyperemia induced by combined severe hypoxia and hypercapnia; in experimental animals subjected to hemorrhagic hypotension, a reduction in both CBF and $CMRO_2$ occurs after administration of indomethacin.[6] Stabilization of blood pressure and microvascular permeability following ischemic insult and early constriction of PDA could all be favorable.

On the other hand, indomethacin treatment could cause far greater reduction in $CMRO_2$ than in CBF. Leffler et al.[6] reported that in 75% of animals given indomethacin after hemorrhagic shock the $CMRO_2$ reduction was so profound as to cause coma.

Clinical Trials.—Five of the nine trials summarized in Table 23–3 reported a statistically significant reduction in the overall incidence of IVH. Only borderline reduction in IVH severity was seen in four of the five studies providing data on IVH grades. However, in a recent study Bada et al.[1] reported a 16% reduction in IVH grades 2 through 4 in indomethacin-treated preterm infants of less than 1,500 g birth weight.

Although no study has reported a higher incidence of major acute complications from indomethacin, long-term follow-up results are not yet available. In view of these concerns, and because there has been only a marginal effect on the overall incidence of IVH (and lack of sufficient data on severe IVH), *routine* early administration of indomethacin for the specific purpose

TABLE 23-3.
Prevention Studies: Indomethacin*

Authors	Total No.	Entry Criteria	Dose/Route/ Duration (days)	Conclusions Δ ICH
Setzer et al.	199	≤1,300	0.4 mg/kg IV 2 days	Decreased
Ment et al.	48	≤1,250	0.1–0.2 mg/kg IV 0.1 mg/kg q 12 hr × 4 days	Decreased
Mahoney et al.	104	700–1,300	0.2 mg/kg IV 0.1 mg/kg at 12 and 36 hr	No change
Rennie et al.	50	<1,750	0.2 mg/kg IV q 24 hr × 2 days	No change
Hanigan et al.	122	501–1,500	0.1 mg/kg IV q 24 hr × 3 days	Variable†
Ment et al.	36	600–1,250	0.1 mg/kg IV q 24 hr × 2 days	Decreased
Bandstra et al.	199	500–1,300	0.2 mg/kg IV 0.1 mg/kg q 12 hr × 2 days	Decreased
Kreuger et al.	87	750–1,500	0.2 mg/kg IV × 1 day	Decreased
Vincer et al.	30	<1,500	0.2 mg/kg IV q 24 hr × 3 days	No change

*Adapted from Ment LR, Ehraenkranz RA, Duncan LM: *Semin Perinatol* 1988; 12:359–372.
ICH = intracranial hemorrhage.
†Lower incidence in 1,000–1,500 g; no change in 501–999 g.

of preventing IVH does not appear to be justified until more studies demonstrate risk-benefit ratios.

Other Agents

Vitamin E

The effect of α-tocopherol on cell membrane protection from oxidative damage caused by free radicals is the primary reason for the use of vitamin E in IVH prevention. In three of four trials listed in Table 23–4, IVH incidence was reduced following administration of vitamin E; one of these trials reported no significant effect on severe grades of IVH. However, Phelps et al.[10] noted an increased incidence of severe IVH in infants weighing less than 1,000 g at birth who were given DL-α-tocopherol in alcohol for prevention of retinopathy of prematurity: 30.9% (14/42) in the treated group vs. 9.3% (4/43) controls.

The side effects of vitamin E are considerable: inhibition of wound healing, fibrinolysis and platelet aggregation, and at high serum concentrations an increased risk of infection and necrotizing enterocolitis. In view of these concerns, and because definitive data on the magnitude of IVH prevention are lacking, we have to conclude that the available literature does not support the *routine* use of vitamin E as prophylaxis against IVH.

Ethamsylate

Ethamsylate is believed to mediate its effect by way of the prostaglandin cascade. Its effects include reduction in capillary bleeding time by reinforce-

TABLE 23–4.
Prevention Studies: Other Agents*

Authors	Total No.	Entry Criteria	Dose/Route/ Duration	Conclusions Δ ICH
Vitamin E				
Chiswick et al.	44	≤32 wk	20 mg/kg/day IM for 3 days	Decreased
Speer et al.	134[†]	<1,500 g, O_2	45 mg/kg IM for 6 days	Decreased[‡]
Phelps et al.	287	<1,500 g or <33 wk	20 mg/kg IV/PO 7 days[§]	No change[‖]
Sinna et al.	231	≤32 wk	20 mg/kg IM 3 days	Decreased
Ethamsylate				
Morgan et al.	70	<1,500 g	12.5 mg/kg IM q 6 hr × 4 days	Decreased
Cooke et al.	91	501–1,500 g, ventilator	12.5 mg/kg IM q 6 hr × 4 days	Decreased
Benson et al.	330	<1,500 g	12.5 mg/kg IM/IV q 6 hr × 4 days	Decreased
Pancuronium				
Perlman et al.	24	<1,500 g	0.1 mg/kg IV prn 7 days	Decreased
Fresh frozen plasma				
Beverley et al.	73	<1,500 g or <32 wk	10 mL/kg qd 2 days	Decreased
Tranexamic acid				
Hensey et al.	100	<1,250 g or <1,500 g, ventilator	25 mg/kg IV 5 days	No change
Vitamin K_1 (antenatal)				
Pomerance et al.	53	24–34 wk	10 mg IM 4 hr before delivery	Decreased

*Adapted from Ment LR, Ehraenkranz RA, Duncan LM: Intraventricular hemorrhage of the preterm neonate: Prevention studies. *Semin Perinatol* 1988; 12:359–372.
ICH = intracranial hemorrhage.
[†]All received oral vitamin E 100 mg/kg.
[‡]No change in the severity.
[§]Blood levels were maintained at 3.0 to 3.5 μm/mL.
[‖]Reported increased severity.

ment of basement membrane, increase in platelet adhesiveness and capillary resistance, increasing local intrinsic thromboplastin release, and early closure of PDA.

Ethamsylate has been mainly used in Great Britain, and results of all clinical trials have been published (see Table 23–4). With the use of 12.5 mg/kg ethamsylate intramuscularly every 6 hours for about 4 days, Benson et al.[2] reported 11.3% reduction in IVH incidence: 18.5% (30/162) in the treated group vs. 29.8% (50/168) in the controls. In the treated infants who had previous bleeding, extension of hemorrhage seemed to be reduced, too. These data are impressive; however, additional trials are needed before routine clinical use of this drug can be recommended for IVH prophylaxis.

Pancuronium

Perlman et al.[9] (see Table 23–4) initially reported that "fluctuations" in anterior cerebral artery velocity waveforms were more frequent in those preterm infants who later developed IVH and that muscle paralysis with pancuronium abolished the fluctuations. In a subsequent prospective controlled trial[8] they showed a significant reduction in the incidence of IVH in infants paralyzed with pancuronium.

The findings of this study have not been replicated, and whether fluctuations in cerebral artery velocity indeed suggest a risk for hemorrhage is yet to be established. Because velocity fluctuations measured by hand-held Doppler equipment could reflect motion artifacts, Kuban et al.[4] strongly question this assumption. Although routine use of pancuronium has been suggested, we must consider its various side effects and complications. Until more definitive results become available, a *routine* use of pancuronium for prevention of IVH does not appear justified.

Other Approaches

Three isolated reports in which tranexamic acid, fresh-frozen plasma, and maternally administered vitamin K_1 were used before delivery are summarized in Table 23–4. Because of the limited number of trials using these agents, the findings from these studies must be considered tentative.

CONCLUSIONS

At present, none of the preventive regimens proposed appears to have a significant impact on the incidence of severe IVH in extremely premature infants, a group in whom major IVH is still a great concern. *Antenatal phenobarbital, postnatal (early) indomethacin, and ethamsylate* seem to have promise; however, until more studies evaluate the magnitude of treatment effect on *severe* grades of IVH and relate it to risk-benefit ratios, final conclusions must be deferred. Both short-term side effects and long-term complications due to therapy must be considered before these agents are used routinely for IVH prophylaxis. Until such time, use of any of the agents discussed for the specific purpose of preventing IVH must be considered experimental.

REFERENCES

1. Bada HS, Green RS, Pourcyrous M, et al: Indomethacin reduces relative risks of severe intraventricular hemorrhage (abstract). *Pediatr Res* 1989; 25:353A.
2. Benson JWT, Dayton MR, Hayward C, et al: Multicentre trial of ethamsylate for prevention of periventricular hemorrhage in very low birthweight infants. *Lancet* 1986; 2:1297–1300.
3. Donn SM, Roloff DW, Goldstein GW: Prevention of intraventricular hemorrhage in preterm infants by phenobarbitone: A controlled trial. *Lancet* 1981; 2:215–217.
4. Kuban KCK, Skouteli H, Cherer A, et al: Hemorrhage, phenobarbital and fluctuating cerebral blood flow velocity in the neonate. *Pediatrics* 1988; 82:548–553.
5. Kuban KK, Leviton A, Krishnamoorthy KS, et al: Neonatal intracranial hemorrhage and phenobarbital therapy. *Pediatrics* 1986; 77:443–450.
6. Leffler CW, Busija DW, Beasley DG, et al: Maintenance of cerebral circulation during hemorrhagic hypotension in newborn pigs: Role of prostanoids. *Circ Res* 1986; 59:562–567.
7. Ment LR, Ehraenkranz RA, Duncan LM: Intraventricular hemorrhage of the preterm neonate: Prevention studies. *Semin Perinatol* 1988; 12:359–372.
8. Perlman JM, Goodman S, Kreusser KL, et al: Reduction in intraventricular hemorrhage by elimination of fluctuating cerebral blood-flow velocity in preterm infants with respiratory distress syndrome. *N Engl J Med* 1985; 312:1353–1357.
9. Perlman JM, McMenamin JB, Volpe JJ: Fluctuating cerebral blood-flow velocity in respiratory-distress syndrome. *New Engl J Med* 1983; 309:204–209.
10. Phelps DL, Rosenbaum AL, Isenberg SJ, et al: Tocopherol efficacy and safety for preventing retinopathy of prematurity: A randomized, controlled, double-masked trial. *Pediatrics* 1987; 79:489–500.
11. Porter FL, Marshall RE, Moore J, et al: Effect of phenobarbital on motor activity and intraventricular hemorrhage in preterm infants with respiratory disease weighing less than 1500 grams. *Am J Perinatol* 1985; 2:63–66.
12. Shankaran S, Cepeda EE, Ilagan N, et al: Antenatal phenobarbital for the prevention of neonatal intracerebral hemorrhage. *Am J Obstet Gynecol* 1986; 154:53–57.
13. Volpe JJ: *Neurology of the Newborn,* ed 2. Philadelphia, WB Saunders Co, 1987, pp 311–361.

24

Parenteral Nutritional Therapy

William C. Heird, M.D.

Sudha Kashyap, M.D.

The first report of the long-term efficacy of parenterally administered nutrients in supporting growth and development in young animals and in regrowth in depleted adult patients appeared in the late 1960s.[8] The major
difference between the technique described in this report and those in the
many previous unsuccessful attempts reported sporadically since it was first
suspected[24, 47] that ingested nutrients could be absorbed from the intestine
into the bloodstream was that a hypertonic nutrient infusate was infused
continuously through a catheter inserted into the superior vena cava rather
than directly into a peripheral vein. The rationale for the successful technique
was that the rapid blood flow within the superior vena cava immediately
diluted the hypertonic infusate, thus preventing damage to the vessel and
permitting delivery of required amounts of protein, energy, electrolytes, minerals, and vitamins without delivery of excessive fluid.

This dramatic demonstration of normal growth and development in an
infant with multiple atresias of the small intestine who was nourished exclusively by this technique for several months[46] was the stimulus for the now
widespread use of parenteral nutrition in pediatric patients. The technique
has been used most frequently in infants requiring multiple operative procedures for correction of congenital or acquired lesions of the gastrointestinal
tract and in infants and children with intractable diarrhea. In such patients
the ability to maintain or improve nutritional status with only parenterally
administered nutrients no doubt has played a major role in reducing the
formerly dismally low survival rates to the high survival rates currently seen.[23]

Low-birth-weight (LBW) infants account for a large percentage of pediatric
patients who receive parenteral nutrients. Approximately 7% of all infants
born in the United States fall into this category, and many of these infants,
particularly those who weigh less than 1,500 g at birth (more than 1% of all

births), cannot tolerate adequate amounts of enterally delivered nutrients until they are several weeks of age. Since endogenous nutrient stores in these infants are limited[49] and their rate of ongoing energy expenditure is relatively high, they are at great risk for development of malnutrition or actual starvation during the early neonatal period. The total endogenous nutrient stores in the 1,000 g infant, for example, are sufficient to support survival without exogenous nutrients for only about 5 days.[24] For this reason, parenteral nutrition therapy is a firmly established aspect of neonatal care throughout the developed world. Virtually all infants who weigh less than 1,500 g at birth receive at least some, if not all, of their total nutrient intake for the first several days of life by the parenteral route.

Despite this widespread use of parenterally delivered nutrients in nutritional management in infants who cannot tolerate enteral nutrients, the therapy is associated with a variety of problems. In addition, a number of aspects of the technique remain poorly understood. The techniques of parenteral nutrition advocated in this chapter are those followed with reasonable success for the past 20 years at Babies Hospital in New York. Also, since it is likely that a more thorough understanding of all aspects of the technique will further enhance efficacy, unsolved problems related to the technique are discussed.

TECHNIQUES USED FOR PARENTERAL NUTRITION THERAPY

The basic concept of long-term parenteral nutrition therapy is continuous infusion of a hypertonic nutrient solution into a vessel with rapid blood flow. In infants, the nutrient solution is infused by way of an indwelling catheter, usually placed in the superior vena cava just above the right atrium through a surgical cutdown in either the internal or external jugular vein. The proximal portion of the catheter is usually tunneled subcutaneously to exit some distance from the site of insertion, usually the anterior chest. This maneuver helps protect the catheter from inadvertent dislodgement as well as contamination by microorganisms, and makes maintenance and care of the catheter exit site easier.

Catheters placed in the inferior vena cava just below the right atrium should be equally effective, but since introduction of a catheter through a cutdown in the groin area theoretically increases the risk of infection, inferior vena cava catheters have not been so popular as superior vena cava catheters. However, if such catheters are placed under strictly sterile conditions and tunneled subcutaneously to an exit site on the abdominal wall or the thigh, the risk of infection appears to be no greater than that associated with superior vena cava catheters.[41]

Because polyvinyl catheters have a tendency to become rigid after they have been in place for only a short time, Silastic catheters, which remain soft and flexible, are preferable. In recent years, Silastic catheters with a polyvinyl cuff on the portion that is tunneled subcutaneously have become popular. The cuff promotes fibroblast proliferation, which in turn helps secure the catheter in place and therefore increases the life of the single catheter. Such catheters are particularly useful for administering parenteral nutrient in the home setting, a practice that has increased dramatically over the past few years.

Radiographic confirmation of correct catheter position prior to its use for nutrient infusion is mandatory; otherwise, the hypertonic nutrient may be infused into an undesired site. Regular and meticulous care of the central venous catheter is also essential for prolonged, safe, complication-free use and seems to be the most important factor in preventing infection. It is recommended that the occlusive dressing placed at the catheter exit site at the time of insertion be changed at least three times a week. At each dressing change, which should be performed using sterile technique, the skin area should be cleaned thoroughly, first with a defatting agent and then with an antiseptic agent. An antiseptic ointment and a fresh occlusive dressing should then be applied. Use of the catheter for purposes other than delivery of the nutrient infusate, particularly for blood transfusions and blood sampling, should be discouraged, and preferably forbidden. With meticulous care, a single catheter, particularly one with a polyvinyl cuff, can be used safely for several months.

Because of the considerable effort, personnel, and expense required to reduce the complications of central vein delivery of concentrated nutrient mixtures to an acceptable level, many advocate use of parenteral nutrition regimens in which infusion occurs through a peripheral vein. Since the glucose concentration of such regimens cannot be much greater than 10%, this route of delivery limits the nutrient intake that can be provided without excessive fluid intake. For example, if fluid intake is limited to a total volume of 150 mL/kg/day, which may be somewhat excessive for small infants prone to development of patent ductus arteriosus, and the intake of intravenous lipid emulsion is limited to 2 g/kg/day, the maximum energy intake that can be delivered is approximately 75 kcal/kg/day.[24] The growth achievable with such a regimen is less than that achievable with a conventional central vein parenteral nutrition regimen, which permits delivery of at least a 50% greater energy intake. Despite this limitation, there are a number of patients for whom peripheral vein regimens may be preferable (discussed later).

The assumed simplicity of nutrient delivery by way of a peripheral vein vs. a central vein is deceiving. The supervision required for successful peripheral vein delivery is certainly equal to that required for successful central vein delivery. In addition, because a single infusion site rarely lasts for more than 24 hours, considerable time and effort are required to maintain peripheral vein infusions. Further, the complications per day of therapy associated with the two routes of delivery, although different in nature and seriousness, are similar.[29] Thus the choice of delivery route for parenteral nutrients should be based on the individual patient's clinical condition and nutritional needs rather than on the perceived ease or difficulty of a particular technique.

CHOICE OF PARENTERAL NUTRIENT REGIMEN

Any infant who is unable to tolerate enteral feedings for a significant period of time is likely to benefit from parenterally administered nutrients. However, the indications for central vs. peripheral vein delivery are less clear. One reasonable guideline is to gauge the extent to which an infant's endogenous nutrient stores are likely to be eroded by inadequate nutrient intake. For example, a large infant whose enteral feedings must be withheld for only a few days is unlikely to experience significant erosion of endogenous nutrient stores, whereas a small infant or a large infant with preexisting nutritional depletion is likely to experience significant erosion of already limited endogenous stores with even a short period of starvation.

Another guideline concerns the goal of parenteral nutrition therapy. A parenteral nutrition regimen that can be delivered by peripheral vein will maintain existing body composition and may support some growth, although not rapid growth; a central vein regimen, on the other hand, will support normal rates of growth and even some catch-up growth. Hence the peripheral route of delivery is a reasonable choice in a normally nourished infant who is likely to tolerate an adequate enteral regimen within 1 to 2 weeks, but central vein delivery is a more reasonable choice for an infant who is likely to be intolerant of enteral feedings for longer than 2 weeks. This distinction also takes into account the practical difficulties of maintaining peripheral vein infusions for much longer than 2 weeks.

Although most infants require parenteral nutrients as their major source of nutrition for 10 to 20 days (e.g., intolerance of enteral feedings, postoperative complications, necrotizing enterocolitis, many surgically correctable lesions, intractable diarrhea), it is often difficult or impossible to predict how long parenterally administered nutrients will be required. Hence the choice between peripheral and central vein nutrient delivery is usually made on the basis of factors such as nutritional status, duration of illness, and clinical course prior to beginning parenteral nutrition. The nutritional status of a larger infant who becomes intolerant of enteral feedings within the first few days of life (e.g., the term infant with a surgically correctable lesion of the intestine) is likely to be reasonable, and such an infant might reasonably be assigned a peripheral vein regimen. On the other hand, a central vein regimen is a more reasonable choice for a smaller neonate who requires parenteral nutrition for the same condition (e.g., a small-for-gestational-age infant with the same surgically correctable lesion) or an infant who requires parenteral nutrition after a complicated clinical course characterized by inadequate nutritional intake (e.g., one with intractable diarrhea or some infants with necrotizing enterocolitis).

INFUSATE COMPOSITION AND DELIVERY

The parenteral nutrition infusate intended either for central vein or pe-

TABLE 24–1.
Composition of Nutrient Infusate

Component	Central Vein (vol/kg/day)	Peripheral Vein (vol/kg/day)
Crystalline amino acids (g)	3–4	2.5–3.0
Glucose (g)	20–30	15
Lipid emulsion (g)	0.5–3.0	0.5–3.0
Sodium (mEq)	3–4	3–4
Potassium* (mEq)	2–4	2–4
Calcium (mg)	40–80	40–80
Magnesium (mEq)	0.25	0.25
Chloride (mEq)	3–4	3–4
Phosphorus* (mmol/L)	1–2	1–2
Zinc (μg)	200	200–400
Copper (μg)	20	—
Iron[†]	—	—
Other trace minerals[‡]	—	—
Vitamins[§]	—	—
Total volume	120–130	150

*Hyperphosphatemia develops frequently if daily phosphorus intake exceeds 1.4 mmol/kg, the amount given with daily potassium intake 2 mEq/kg as a mixture of KH_2PO_4 and K_2HPO_4. If potassium intake >2 mEq/kg/day is required, additional potassium should be given as KCl.

[†]Iron dextran (Imferon) can be added to infusate in patients requiring prolonged parenteral nutrition therapy. We arbitrarily limit the dose to 0.1 mg/kg/day. Alternatively, the indicated IM dose can be used intermittently as either the sole source of iron or an additional dose.

[‡]See text and Table 24–4.

[§]M.V.I.-Pediatric is a lyophilized product. When reconstituted as directed, 5 mL added to daily infusate provides 80 mg vitamin C, 700 μg vitamin A, 10 μg vitamin D, 1.3 mg thiamine, 1.4 mg riboflavin, 1.0 mg pyridoxine, 17 mg niacin, 5 mg pantothenic acid, 7 mg vitamin E, 20 μg biotin, 140 μg folic acid, 1 μg vitamin B_{12}, and 200 μg vitamin K_1.

ripheral vein delivery must include a source of both nitrogen and energy as well as adequate electrolytes, minerals, and vitamins. Infusates suitable for central and peripheral vein delivery are shown in Table 24–1.

One of several crystalline amino acid mixtures (Table 24–2) is usually used as the nitrogen source. Three of the mixtures (TrophAmine, Aminosyn-PF, and Neopham) are considered "pediatric" mixtures. On balance, the limited data available suggest that these mixtures result in a more normal plasma amino acid pattern[3, 25, 26] and also may be used more efficiently. In addition, the incidence of hepatic dysfunction in the first clinical trial of TrophAmine was lower than expected.[25] Whether this will be confirmed in more appropriate studies and, if so, the reason for the lower incidence is

TABLE 24–2.
Amino Acid Content (mg/2.5 g) of Commercially Available Amino Acid Mixtures

Amino Acid	Aminosyn	Aminosyn-PF	Travasol (B)	FreAmine III	TrophAmine	Neopham
Isoleucine	180	191	120	175	204	12
Leucine	235	297	155	228	350	269
Lysine	180	170	145	182	204	217
Methionine	100	45	145	132	83	50
Phenylalanine	110	107	155	140	121	104
Threonine	130	129	105	100	104	138
Tryptophan	40	45	45	38	50	54
Valine	200	161	115	165	196	137
Histidine	75	79	109	71	121	81
Cystine	0	0	0	<6	<8	98
Tyrosine	11	16	10	0	58*	20
Taurine	0	18	0	0	6	0
Alanine	320	175	518	178	133	242
Aspartate	0	132	0	0	79	157
Glutamate	0	206	0	0	125	272
Glycine	320	96	518	350	92	81
Proline	215	204	104	280	171	214
Serine	105	124	0	148	96	146
Arginine	245	308	258	238	304	159

*Mixture of L-tyrosine and N-acetyl-L-tyrosine.

not clear. Other special-purpose mixtures (e.g., mixtures of essential amino acids for patients with renal failure and a mixture designed for patients with liver failure) also are available.

The amount of amino acids provided usually ranges from 2 to 4 g/kg/day. An amino acid intake of about 2.5 g/kg/day results in nitrogen retention comparable to that observed in healthy, enterally fed, term infants, but an intake of 3.0 g/kg/day is required to achieve a rate of nitrogen retention equal to the intrauterine rate.[51]

Glucose is the predominant energy source of most parenteral nutrition regimens. An intake greater than 15 g/kg/day is rarely tolerated by any infant on the first day of therapy, and the amount tolerated by LBW infants is frequently less. Thereafter, glucose intake usually can be increased by 2 to 5 g/kg/day, until the desired intake is achieved. Some advocate the use of insulin to increase glucose tolerance. In our experience, the amount required is quite variable; thus it is used only in those infants who are particularly intolerant.

Any infant who receives a fat-free parenteral nutrition regimen will develop essential fatty acid deficiency within a relatively short time. Preterm and nutritionally depleted infants do so within days, particularly if their growth is rapid.[11] For this reason, sufficient amounts of a parenteral lipid emulsion to prevent essential fatty acid deficiency (i.e., 0.5 to 1.0 g/kg/day) are indicated. This amount, however, provides only 5 to 10 kcal/kg/day.

Two general types of parenteral lipid emulsions are available in the United States (Table 24–3). These include emulsions of soybean oil (Intralipid, Liposyn III) and an emulsion of soybean plus safflower oil (Liposyn II), all with a triglyceride concentration of either 10% or 20%. Egg yolk phospholipid is the emulsifying agent of all emulsions. Thus the major difference among available emulsions is related to the different fatty acid patterns of soybean vs. safflower oil.

Since tolerance of parenteral lipid emulsions is variable and intolerance is associated with adverse effects on both pulmonary gas exchange[15, 42] and reticuloendothelial cell function,[35] it is recommended that the dose of emulsion be limited to 2 g/kg/day in LBW infants and 3 g/kg/day in older infants.[7] A recent study suggests that a 20% soybean oil emulsion (Intralipid) is cleared more rapidly than the 10% emulsion, presumably because of the lower free liposome content of the 20% emulsion.[17] If this finding is confirmed, it may be possible to increase the maximum dose recommendations for both the LBW and older infant.

Convenient additive preparations of electrolytes, minerals, and vitamins have been available for many years. Since the requirements for these electrolytes vary from patient to patient, the amounts shown in Table 24–1 should not be considered absolute requirements. The amount of calcium suggested for either the peripheral or central vein regimen almost certainly is inadequate for optimal skeletal mineralization. However, provision of more calcium without decreasing the phosphate content will likely result in precipitation of calcium phosphate.

TABLE 24–3.
Suggested Parenteral Intake of Vitamins

Vitamin	Preterm Infants (amount/kg/day)*	Term Infants and Children (amount/day)†
Vitamin A (μg)	280	700
Vitamin E (mg)	2.8	7
Vitamin K (μg)	80	200
Vitamin D (μg)	4	10
(IU)	160	400
Ascorbic acid (mg)	25	80
Thiamin (mg)	0.48	1.2
Riboflavin (mg)	0.56	1.4
Pyridoxine (mg)	0.4	1.0
Niacin (mg)	6.8	17
Pantothenate (mg)	2.0	5
Biotin (μg)	8.0	20
Folate (μg)	56	140
Vitamin B_{12} (μg)	0.4	1.0

*Total daily dose should not exceed that recommended for term infants and children. A dose of 2 mL reconstituted M.V.I.-Pediatric provides the recommended amount/kg/day of all vitamins except ascorbic acid.
†These amounts are provided by 5 mL of reconstituted M.V.I.-Pediatric.

The amounts of vitamins listed in Table 24–1 are particularly tenuous, but can be provided conveniently using available products. Since both zinc and copper deficiency develop relatively frequently if these nutrients are not provided, these trace minerals should be components of the infusates in any patient likely to require parenteral nutrients for more than 1 to 2 weeks. Other essential trace minerals (e.g., chromium,[30] selenium,[33] molybdenum[1]) should be added to the infusates in patients who require parenteral nutrients exclusively for a longer time.

Recommendations for parenteral vitamin and trace mineral intake have been revised recently. The most recent recommendations[16] are summarized in Tables 24–4 and 24–5.

Whether delivered by central or peripheral vein, the nutrient infusate should be delivered at a constant rate by means of one of several available constant infusion pumps. Some consider use of a 0.22 μm membrane filter between the catheter and the administration tubing optional; we believe this precaution is advisable.

Many patients tolerate the same infusate for the total duration of parenteral nutrition; others require frequent adjustment of the intake of one or more nutrients. For this reason, ability to change the composition of the infusate in response to clinical and chemical monitoring or to increase the volume in response to diarrheal and other ongoing losses is important.

TABLE 24–4.
Recommended Parenteral Intake of
Trace Minerals*

Trace Mineral	Preterm Infants (μg/kg/day)	Term Infants (μg/kg/day)
Zinc	400	250[†]
Copper	20	20
Selenium	2.0	2.0
Chromium	0.20	0.20
Manganese	1.0	1.0
Molybdenum	0.25	0.25
Iodide	1.0	1.0

*If parenteral nutrients are used as a supplement for tolerated enteral feedings or as the sole source of nutrients for <4 weeks, only zinc is needed.
[†]100 mg/kg/day in infants >3 months of age.

COMPLICATIONS OF PARENTERAL NUTRITION

The complications associated with parenteral nutrition can be classified into 2 categories: those related to the technique, particularly the presence of an indwelling catheter (catheter-related complications), and those related to the infusate (metabolic complications).

The major catheter-related complication is infection. Many of the infusate components support growth of various microorganisms,[13, 38] but most infec-

TABLE 24–5.
Composition (Amount/Liter) of Currently Available Parenteral
Lipid Emulsions

Component	Soybean Oil Emulsion (Intralipid*)	Soybean-Safflower Oil Emulsion (Liposyn II)
Soybean oil (g)	100[†]	50[†]
Safflower oil (g)	—	50[†]
Egg yolk phospholipid (g)	12	up to 12
Glycerol (g)	22.5	25
Fatty acids (% of total)		
16:0	10	8.8
18:0	3.5	3.4
18:1	26	17.7
18:2	50	65.8
18:3	9	4.2
Particle size (μm)	0.5	0.4

*Liposyn III also is a soybean oil emulsion.
[†]A 20% emulsion is also available, containing twice as much of the oils but roughly the same amounts of all other ingredients.

TABLE 24–6.
Metabolic Complications of Parenteral Nutrition and Their Most Common Causes

Complication	Most Common Cause
Complications related to metabolic capacity	
Hyperglycemia	Excessive intake (either excessive concentration or excessive infusion rate relative to tolerance); change in metabolic state (e.g., infection; post-surgery)
Hypoglycemia	Sudden cessation of infusion; excessive insulin
Azotemia	Excessive nitrogen intake; inadequate fluid intake
Electrolyte, mineral (major and trace) and vitamin disorders	Excessive or inadequate intake
Hypertriglyceridemia	Excessive lipid intake relative to rate of hydrolysis
Complications related to infusate composition	
Abnormal plasma aminograms	Amino acid pattern of nitrogen source
Hypercholesterolemia/ phospholipidemia	Characteristics of lipid emulsion
Abnormal fatty acid pattern of serum and tissue lipids	Characteristics of lipid emulsion or its route of metabolism
Hepatic disorders	Unknown

tions appear to result from improper care of the catheter, particularly failure to follow meticulously the requirement for frequent changes of the catheter exit site dressing, rather than from a contaminated infusate. Other catheter-related complications of central vein parenteral nutrition include malposition, dislodgement, and thrombosis, including superior (or inferior) vena cava thrombosis. Malposition can be avoided by radiographic confirmation of the location of the catheter tip prior to infusion of the hypertonic nutrient infusate, and reconfirmation is indicated thereafter. It is unlikely that other catheter-related complications can be completely avoided. However, careful attention to all procedures involving the catheter and infusion of the nutrient mixture will maintain the incidence of these complications at an acceptable level.

The most common complication of peripheral vein infusion of nutrients is thrombophlebitis. Skin and subcutaneous sloughs secondary to infiltration of the hypertonic infusate also are relatively common. Infection is much less common with peripheral vein delivery than with central vein delivery, and is more likely to result from contaminated infusate.

The metabolic complications of parenteral nutrition and their probable cause are summarized in Table 24–6. These complications can be subdivided into two general categories: those related to the patient's limited metabolic capacity for the various components of the infusate and those related to the nature of available infusate components. Many of the metabolic complications related to the patient's tolerance of the infusate are likely to be decreased with the less concentrated peripheral vein regimens. However, since infusates delivered by central vein and peripheral vein are qualitatively similar, the latter group of complications should be similar regardless of the route of delivery.

Glucose intolerance generally is less frequent with peripheral vein delivery, which limits glucose intake to 15 g/kg/day. However, some LBW infants cannot tolerate even this limited amount of glucose. With both routes of delivery, electrolyte and mineral disorders usually result from provision of either too much or too little of the particular nutrient in relation to need. For example, the very LBW infant frequently experiences greater urinary sodium losses and therefore requires greater intake. Electrolyte disorders also can result from hyperglycemia and attendant osmotic diuresis.

Some earlier complications related to composition of the amino acid mixtures are no longer problems. Metabolic acidosis, which was common with early crystalline amino acid mixtures, was related to the fact that these mixtures contained hydrochloride salts of the cationic amino acids.[18] Currently available mixtures contain either free cationic amino acids or acetate salts and hence do not cause acidosis; some, in fact, appear to result in mild metabolic alkalosis.[21] Hyperammonemia, another early metabolic problem in patients who received protein hydrolysates[31] and one of the early crystalline amino acid mixtures,[19] also is no longer a serious problem. In patients receiving the crystalline amino acid mixture, and probably those receiving the hydrolysates, this complication resulted from inadequate arginine intake.[19] All currently available parenteral amino acid mixtures appear to contain adequate arginine to circumvent this problem (i.e., >0.5 mmol/kg/day; see Table 24–2). In our experience, any parenteral nutrition regimen causes an increase in blood ammonia concentration; however, symptomatic hyperammonemia does not occur with currently available amino acid mixtures.

None of the currently available amino acid mixtures results in a completely normal plasma amino acid pattern.[47] Based in part on the long-recognized coexistence of mental retardation and elevated plasma amino acid concentrations in patients with various inborn errors of metabolism (e.g., phenylketonuria) and in part on the known relationship between an inadequate intake of a specific amino acid and a low plasma concentration of that amino acid, these abnormal plasma amino acid patterns are of some concern. From animal studies, it is clear that the abnormal plasma amino acid pattern associated with administration of parenteral nutrition regimens is accompanied by an abnormal tissue amino acid pattern.[22] Although this relationship is not necessarily direct, the abnormal plasma and tissue amino acid patterns suggest the possibility of adverse effects on ongoing protein synthesis as well as the concentration of various neurotransmitters within the central nervous system. These questions have not been studied sufficiently to warrant major concern or to allay fears.

Some of the newer parenteral amino acid mixtures (e.g., Troph-Amine)[25, 26] circumvent the problem of elevated plasma amino acid concentrations. However, all available mixtures result in very low plasma concentrations of cyst(e)ine and tyrosine, presumably because these amino acids, both of which are considered indispensable in newborns, are either unstable or insoluble in aqueous solution and therefore are not included in appreciable amounts in any available parenteral amino acid mixture. One mixture (TrophAmine) contains a soluble tyrosine derivative (*N*-acetyl-L-tyrosine), and infants receiving parenteral nutrition regimens with this mixture as the nitrogen source have somewhat higher (nonetheless low) plasma tyrosine concentrations than infants receiving regimens with other mixtures as the nitrogen source.[25, 26, 37, 50] In addition, cysteine hydrochloride, added separately when the nutrient infusate is prepared, results in higher plasma cyst(e)ine concentrations.[25, 26] However, much further research is required to determine if these additives effectively provide the requirements, respectively, for tyrosine and cyst(e)ine.

Perhaps the most pressing metabolic problem related to the composition or metabolism of available parenteral lipid emulsions is the resulting fatty acid pattern of serum and tissue lipids associated with use of available parenteral lipid emulsions. All available emulsions contain adequate amounts of the essential fatty acids linoleic and linolenic acid, the parent fatty acids, respectively, of the *n*-6 and *n*-3 fatty acid families. However, none contains the longer chain, more unsaturated fatty acids of either family (see Table 24–3). Since the infant may be unable to elongate and desaturate the parent fatty acids,[6] this lack gives rise to two concerns.

First, arachidonic acid, an elongated and desaturated derivative of linoleic acid, is a precursor of many prostaglandin series. Thus, if the infant is unable to convert linoleic acid to arachidonic acid, infants receiving available lipid emulsions, theoretically, may develop arachidonic deficiency and in turn derangements in prostaglandin production. Indeed, Friedman and Frolich[12] found that the arachidonic content of serum lipids in infants receiving a currently available soybean oil emulsion (i.e., Intralipid) was low and that this was associated with low urinary excretion of a stable metabolite of prostaglandin E. Although not associated with known clinical abnormalities, this association is disturbing, but has received very little attention.

Second, appreciable amounts of the longer chain, more unsaturated members of both the *n*-3 and *n*-6 fatty acid families accumulate during development,[4, 5] particularly in the developing CNS. Thus the possibility that the infant cannot convert the parent fatty acid of either family to the longer chain, more unsaturated derivatives of each family gives rise to concern regarding the fatty acid pattern of tissue lipids. Currently this concern is primarily theoretical. No data are available to indicate that the fatty acid pattern of lipids deposited by infants receiving only parenteral nutrients is abnormal. Further, if this pattern is abnormal, the extent to which it may be associated with functional abnormalities is unknown.

ASSURING THE SAFETY AND EFFICACY OF PARENTERAL NUTRITION REGIMENS

Continuous monitoring to detect both metabolic and catheter-related complications as well as actual parenteral intake of various nutrients and the clinical results of this intake is necessary for successful parenteral nutrition. The nursing time required to prevent infiltration of the nutrition infusate delivered by peripheral vein and to assure long-term function of the central vein catheter is considerable and cannot be provided in the usual clinical setting. Moreover, adequate monitoring requires personnel who are familiar with the intricacies of the intravenous infusion apparatus, including the many varieties of constant-infusion pumps that are an absolute necessity both for central vein and peripheral vein delivery.

The monitoring schedule shown in Table 24–7 has been followed for a number of years at Babies Hospital. This schedule allows detection of metabolic complications in sufficient time to permit correction by altering the infusate, but is somewhat simpler than many suggested schedules. For example, checking the urine regularly for the presence of glucose (at least three times daily, perhaps even more frequently during the first few days of the

TABLE 24–7.
Suggested Monitoring Schedule for Infants Receiving
Parenteral Nutrition

Variables to Be Monitored	Suggested Frequency (per week)*	
	Initial Period	Later Period
Growth variables		
Weight	7	7
Length	1	1
Head circumference	1	1
Metabolic variables		
Blood or plasma		
Electrolytes	2–4	1
Ca, Mg, P	2	1
Acid base status	2	1
Urea nitrogen	2	1
Albumin	1	1
Liver function studies	1	1
Lipids†		
Hemoglobin	2	1
Urine glucose	2–6/day	2/day
Prevention and detection of infection		
Clinical observations (activity, temperature)	Daily	Daily
White blood cell count and differential	As indicated	As indicated
Cultures	As indicated	As indicated

*"Initial Period" refers to the time before full intake is achieved as well as any period of metabolic instability (i.e., postoperative period, presence of infection); "Later Period" refers to the time during which the patient is in a metabolic steady state.
†See text.

technique) and determining blood glucose concentrations only when glucosuria is present rather than frequent determinations of blood glucose concentration, as often suggested, appears to be adequate; if the urine is free of glucose, it is safe to assume that the blood glucose concentration is not sufficiently high to cause problems. Dextrostix determinations of blood glucose concentration are useful in monitoring for hypoglycemia (e.g., following either infiltration of a peripheral vein infusion or sudden cessation of a central vein infusion) but are not sufficiently accurate for detection of troublesome degrees of hyperglycemia.

The suggested chemical monitoring schedule also omits routine determinations of plasma osmolality, which can easily be predicted from the plasma sodium concentration; that is, in the absence of hyperglycemia, plasma osmolality can be estimated sufficiently accurately as twice the plasma sodium concentration.

Derangements of the plasma amino acid pattern incident to use of available parenteral amino acid mixtures are predictable from the pattern of the mixture of amino acids used.[47] Thus, unless an underlying abnormality of amino acid metabolism is suspected, this expensive and often difficult determination is superfluous.

The hepatic dysfunction that develops during the course of parenteral nutrition in many patients[39] usually resolves without sequelae, but may in a few patients progress to cirrhosis and death. Although the cause of this disorder is not known, careful assessment and monitoring of hepatic function are necessary. The indices listed in Table 23–7 are adequate for such monitoring. More specific indices may be helpful if dysfunction is detected.

Perhaps the most problematic aspect of chemical monitoring concerns that necessary to ensure safe and efficacious use of parenteral lipid emulsions. The usual practice, if any, is to inspect the plasma periodically for presence of lipemia. However, neither visual inspection nor nephelometry is effective for detecting elevated plasma triglyceride or free fatty acid concentrations[43]; rather, actual chemical determinations are required. However, microtechniques for these assays are not routinely available, and if available usually are not available daily; making the required monitoring impossible. A reasonable compromise is to restrict intake of these emulsions to the maximum dose recommended (i.e., 2 g/kg/day for the LBW infant and 3 g/kg/day for the older infant)[7] and to inspect the plasma periodically, either visually or by nephelometry. More frequent inspection is necessary during the initial period of parenteral nutrition and when the patient develops a clinical condition likely to interfere with triglyceride hydrolysis. Determinations of triglyceride and free fatty acid concentrations once or twice weekly may or may not be helpful. Other serum lipid abnormalities associated with use of parenteral lipid emulsions (hypercholesterolemia, hyperphospholipidemia, deranged free fatty acid patterns of serum and tissue lipids) are predictable and unavoidable with use of currently available emulsions. In addition, the clinical relevance of these abnormalities is unknown. Thus monitoring to detect these is less important.

EXPECTATIONS OF PARENTERAL NUTRITION

In infants, a parenteral nutrition regimen delivering 2.5 to 3.0 g/kg/day of amino acids and 100 to 120 kcal/kg/day reliably produces a weight gain of 10 to 15 g/kg/day and nitrogen retention of 200 to 300 mg/kg/day. Increases in length also occur in infants receiving these intakes. But the rate of increase in length usually lags behind the rate of increase in weight, frequently resulting in a weight for length exceeding the 50th percentile. Since it is possible to maintain weight for length at or near the 50th percentile, it is likely that the disproportionate growth is a result of excessive energy intake. The problem of disproportionate growth applies only to patients who are dependent on parenteral nutrients for months rather than weeks. In the usual patient, weight for length is frequently low when parenteral nutrition is started, and the disproportionate increase in weight relative to length is not necessarily undesirable. On the other hand, it is likely that rapid rates of increase in weight represent deposition of large amounts of fat. Hence there is no convincing reason to provide energy intakes that result in rapid rates of weight gain, particularly if weight for length is appropriate.

A parenteral nutrition regimen providing 2.5 g/kg/day of amino acids and only 60 kcal/kg/day delivered by peripheral vein reliably results in positive nitrogen retention and either maintains weight or decreases weight loss.[2] As discussed earlier, such regimens may be particularly useful in the LBW infant and the reasonably well-nourished older infant who must forego enteral feeding for only a brief period. Somewhat greater amino acid and energy intakes can be delivered by peripheral vein regimens, and these greater intakes will result in some, albeit perhaps not optimal, weight gain. According to Zlotkin et al.,[51] LBW infants receiving a regimen providing 3 g/kg/day of amino acids and 80 kcal/kg/day, which can be delivered by peripheral vein, results in rates of weight gain and nitrogen retention equivalent to intrauterine rates.

Since the one unquestioned clinical indication for use of parenteral nutrition is to maintain or restore nutritional status in patients with deranged gastrointestinal function, the consequences of this therapy with respect to gastrointestinal function are of considerable interest. In healthy animals, parenteral nutrition, like starvation, results in an appreciable decrease in enteric mucosal mass.[10, 20, 32, 34] However, parenteral nutrition following a period of starvation prevents further decrease in mucosal mass but does not support regrowth of the mucosa, as occurs in starved animals that are refed by the enteral route.[40] The effect of parenteral nutrition on enteric hydrolase activities is less clear. Some studies show that the specific activity of some hydrolases decreases relative to that of control animals[34]; others show no difference in hydrolase activity between control animals and animals given parenteral nutrition.[20] These discrepancies may be related to the nature of the diet consumed by the control animals of the various studies.

The few available clinical studies of the effects of parenteral nutrition on intestinal tract structure and function do not demonstrate morphologic involution.[14, 44] On the other hand, hydrolase activities, which usually are low when parenteral nutrition is instituted, are not fully restored until enteral intake is reinstituted.

Two recent studies in LBW infants suggest that infants who receive seemingly negligible amounts of enterally delivered nutrients during the period of parenteral nutrition are more easily weaned from parenteral to enteral nutrients.[9, 45] The mechanism of this apparent effect is not known, but may be related to the different pattern of release of enteric hormones between fed and unfed (i.e., parenterally fed) infants.[36]

REFERENCES

1. Abumrad NN, Schneider AJ, Steel D, et al: Amino acid intolerance during prolonged total parenteral nutrition reversed by molybdenate therapy. *Am J Clin Nutr* 1981; 34:2551–2559.
2. Anderson TL, Muttart C, Bieber MA, et al: A controlled trial of glucose vs glucose and amino acids in premature infants. *J Pediatr* 1979; 94:947–951.
3. Bell EF, Filer LJ Jr, Wong AP, et al: Effects of a parenteral nutrition regimen containing dicarboxylic amino acids on plasma, erythrocyte, and urinary amino acid concentrations of young infants. *Am J Clin Nutr* 1983; 37:99–107.
4. Clandinin MT, Chappell JE, Leong S, et al: Intrauterine fatty acid accretion rates in human brain: Implications for fatty acid requirements. *Early Hum Devel* 1980; 4:121–129.
5. Clandinin MT, Chappell JE, Leong S, et al: Extrauterine fatty acid accretion in infant brain: Implications for fatty acid requirements. *Early Hum Devel* 1980; 4:131–138.
6. Clandinin MT, Chappell JE, Heim PR, et al: Fatty acid utilization in perinatal de novo synthesis of tissues. *Early Hum Devel* 1981; 5:355–366.
7. Committee on Nutrition, American Academy of Pediatrics: Use of intravenous fat emulsions in pediatric patients. *Pediatrics* 1981; 68:738–743.
8. Dudrick SJ, Wilmore DW, Vars HM, et al: Long term parenteral nutrition with growth, development, and positive nitrogen balance. *Surgery* 1968; 64:134–142.
9. Dunn L, Hulman S, Weiner J, et al: Beneficial effects of early hypocaloric enteral feeding on neonatal gastrointestinal function: Preliminary report of a randomized trial. *J Pediatr* 1988; 112:622–629.
10. Feldman EJ, Dowling RH, McNaughton J, et al: Effects of oral versus intravenous nutrition on intestinal adaptation after small bowel resection in the dog. *Gastroenterology* 1976; 70:712–719.
11. Friedman Z, Danon A, Stahlman MT, et al: Rapid onset of essential acid deficiency in the newborn. *Pediatrics* 1976; 58:640–649.
12. Friedman Z, Frolich JC: Essential fatty acids and the major urinary metabolites of the E prostaglandins in thriving neonates and in infants receiving parenteral fat emulsions. *Pediatr Res* 1979; 13:926–932.
13. Goldman DA, Martin WT, Worthington JW: Growth of bacteria and fungi in total parenteral nutrition solutions. *Am J Surg* 1973; 126:314–318.
14. Greene HL, McCabe DR, Merenstein GB: Intractable diarrhea and malnutrition in infancy: Changes in intestinal morphology and disaccharidase activities during treatment with total intravenous nutrition or oral elemental diets. *J Pediatr* 1975; 87:695–704.

15. Greene HL, Hazlett D, Demaree R: Relationship between intralipid-induced hyperlipidemia and pulmonary function. *Am J Clin Nutr* 1976; 29:127–135.
16. Greene HL, Hambridge KM, Schanler R, et al: Guidelines for the use of vitamins, trace elements, calcium, magnesium, and phosphorus in infants and children receiving total parenteral nutrition: Report of the Subcommittee on Pediatric Parenteral Nutrient Requirements from the Committee on Clinical Practice Issues of the American Society for Clinical Nutrition. *Am J Clin Nutr* 1988; 48:1324–1342.
17. Haumont D, Deckelbaum RJ, Richelle M, et al: Plasma lipid and plasma lipoprotein concentrations in low birth weight infants given parenteral nutrition with 20% compared to 10% Intralipid. *J Pediatr* 1989; 115:787–793.
18. Heird WC, Dell RB, Driscoll JM Jr, et al: Metabolic acidosis resulting from intravenous alimentation mixtures containing synthetic amino acids. *N Engl J Med* 1972; 827:943–948.
19. Heird WC, Nicholson JF, Driscoll JM Jr, et al: Hyperammonemia resulting from intravenous alimentation using a mixture of synthetic L-amino acids: A preliminary report. *J Pediatr* 1972; 81:162–167.
20. Heird WC, Tsang HL, MacMillan R, et al: Effect of total parenteral alimentation on rat small intestine (abstract). *Pediatr Res* 1974; 8:107.
21. Heird WC: Studies of pediatric patients receiving Aminosyn as the nitrogen source of total parenteral nutrition, in *Current Approaches to Nutrition of the Hospitalized Patient.* Chicago, Abbott and Ross Laboratories, 1977, pp 45–49.
22. Heird WC, Malloy MH: Brain composition of beagle puppies receiving total parenteral nutrition, in Itka V (ed): *Nutrition and Metabolism of the Fetus and Infant.* The Hague, Nijhoff, 1979, pp 365–375.
23. Heird WC: Nutritional support of the pediatric patient, in Winters RW, Greene HL (eds): *Nutritional Support of the Seriously Ill Patient.* New York, Academic Press, 1983, pp 157–179.
24. Heird WC: Parenteral nutrition, in Grand RJ, Sutphen JL, Dietz WH Jr (eds): *Pediatric Nutrition: Theory and Practice.* Boston, Butterworth, 1987, pp 747–761.
25. Heird WC, Dell RB, Helms RA, et al: Amino acid mixture designed to maintain normal plasma amino acid patterns in infants and children requiring parenteral nutrition. *Pediatrics* 1987; 80:401–408.
26. Heird WC, Hay W, Helms RA, et al: Pediatric parenteral amino acid mixture in low birth weight infants. *Pediatrics* 1988; 81:41–50.
27. Helfrick FW, Abelson NM: Intravenous feeding of a complete diet in a child: A report of a case. *J Pediatr* 1944; 25:400–403.
28. Helms RA, Christensen ML, Mauer EC, et al: Comparison of a pediatric versus standard amino acid formulation in preterm neonates requiring parenteral nutrition. *J Pediatr* 1987; 110:466–472.
29. Jacobowski D, Ziegler MD, Perreira G: Complications of pediatric parenteral nutrition: Central versus peripheral administration (abstract). *J Parenteral Enteral Nutr* 1979; 3:29.
30. Jeejeebhoy KN, Chu RC, Marliss EB, et al: Chromium deficiency, glucose intolerance, and neuropathy reversed by chromium supplementation, in a patient receiving long-term total parenteral nutrition. *Am J Clin Nutr* 1977; 30:531–538.
31. Johnson JD, Albritton WL, Sunshine P: Hyperammonemia accompanying parenteral nutrition in newborn infants. *J Pediatr* 1972; 81:154–161.

32. Johnson LR, Copeland EM, Dudrick SJ, et al: Structural and hormonal alterations in the gastrointestinal tract of parenterally fed rats. *Gastroenterology* 1975; 68:1177–1183.

33. Kien CL, Ganther HE: Manifestations of chronic selenium deficiency in a child receiving total parenteral nutrition. *Am J Clin Nutr* 1983; 37:319–328.

34. Levine GM, Deren JJ, Steiger E, et al: Role of oral intake in maintenance of gut mass and disaccharidase activity. *Gastroenterology* 1974; 67:975–982.

35. Loo LS, Tang JP, Kohl S: The inhibition of leukocyte cellular cytotoxicity to herpes simplex virus in vitro and in vivo by intralipid. *J Infect Dis* 1982; 146:64–70.

36. Lucas A, Bloom SR, Aynsley-Green A: Metabolic and endocrine effects of depriving preterm infants of enteral nutrition. *Acta Paediatr Scand* 1983; 72:245–249.

37. Malloy MH, Rassin DK, Richardson CJ: Total parenteral nutrition in sick preterm infants: Effects of cysteine supplementation with nitrogen intakes of 240 and 400 mg/kg/d. *J Pediatr Gastroenterol Nutr* 1984; 3:239–244.

38. McKee KT, Melly MA, Greene HL, et al: Gram-negative bacillary sepsis associated with use of lipid emulsion in parenteral nutrition. *Am J Dis Child* 1979; 133:649–650.

39. Merritt RJ: Cholestasis associated with total parenteral nutrition. *J Pediatr Gastroenterol Nutr* 1980; 5:9–22.

40. Mones RL, Heird WC, Rosensweig SN: Unpublished data.

41. Mulvihill SJ, Fonkalsrud EW: Complications of superior versus inferior vena cava occlusion in infants receiving central total parenteral nutrition (abstract). *J Pediatr Surg* 1984; 19:752.

42. Perreira GR, Fox WW, Stanley CA, et al: Decreased oxygenation and hyperlipidemia during intravenous fat infusions in premature infants. *Pediatrics* 1980; 66:26–30.

43. Schreiner RL, Glick MR, Nordschow CD, et al: An evaluation of methods to monitor infants receiving intravenous lipids. *J Pediatr* 1979; 94:197–200.

44. Schwachman H, Lloyd-Still JD, Khaw KT, et al: Protracted diarrhea of infancy treated with intravenous alimentation: II: Studies of small intestinal biopsy results. *Am J Dis Child* 1973; 125:365–368.

45. Slagle TA, Gross SJ: Effect of early enteral substrate on subsequent feeding intolerance. *J Pediatr* 1988; 113:526–531.

46. Wilmore DM, Dudrick SJ: Growth and development of an infant receiving all nutrients by vein. *JAMA* 1968; 203:860–864.

47. Winters RW, Heird WC, Dell RB, et al: Plasma amino acids in infants receiving parenteral nutrition, in Greene HL, Holliday MA, Munro RH (eds): *Clinical Nutrition Update: Amino Acids.* Chicago, American Medical Association, 1977, pp 147–154.

48. Wretlind A: Total parenteral nutrition. *Surg Clin North Am* 1978; 58:1055–1070.

49. Ziegler EE, O'Donnell AM, Nelson SE, et al: Body composition of the reference fetus. *Growth* 1986; 40:329–341.

50. Zlotkin SH, Bryan MH, Anderson GH: Cysteine supplementation to cysteine-free intravenous feeding regimens in newborn infants. *Am J Clin Nutr* 1981; 34:914–923.

51. Zlotkin SH, Bryan MH, Anderson GH: Intravenous nitrogen and energy intakes required to duplicate in utero nitrogen accretion in prematurely born human infants. *J Pediatr* 1981; 99:115–120.

25

Jaundice

Kwang-sun Lee, M.D.
Albert D. Moscioni, Ph.D.
Jung-hwan Choi, M.D., Ph.D.

Unconjugated bilirubin is potentially toxic to the brain. Not all unconjugated hyperbilirubinemia in the newborn period requires treatment, however. Although a number of drugs have demonstrated effectiveness in lowering serum bilirubin concentration, most have failed to gain wide clinical use because of their potential toxicity and untoward complications. Phenobarbital and phototherapy have received approval, under certain clinical situations, for treatment of neonatal jaundice.

There are five approaches for management of neonatal jaundice: exchange transfusion, induction of hepatic conjugating enzyme by drug, interference of heme degradation by drug, interruption of enterohepatic circulation of bilirubin by oral administration of absorptive substances that sequester bilirubin and excrete it in stool, and phototherapy. In this chapter exchange transfusion is not discussed.

DRUGS THAT ACCELERATE HEPATIC BILIRUBIN CONJUGATION

More than 200 chemical compounds have been listed as inducers of drug-metabolizing enzymes, especially those of the liver.[5] A large number of these chemical agents are capable of inducing cellular endoplasmic reticular membrane enzymes, including those families involved in both phase 1 and phase 2 detoxification mechanisms of either xenobiotic or endogenous substances. Of those drugs that have been examined as possible therapeutic agents for neonatal jaundice, the majority involve induction of the enzyme that catalyzes hepatic conjugation of bilirubin, uridine diphosphate (UDP)–glucuronyl transferase.[38] These are phenobarbital, ethanol, nikethamide (Coramine), certain organochlorine insecticides (especially DDT), addictive drugs such as heroin, diazepam (Valium), antipyrine (phenazone), and clofibrate. Because of known and potential toxicity, only a few have been administered to human infants. Previous studies of these and other drugs are summarized in Table 25–1. Among these, the barbiturates have received the greatest interest and acceptance as therapeutic agents to control neonatal hyperbilirubinemia.[6, 38]

Phenobarbital

The reduction in serum bilirubin level by phenobarbital is attributed to an increased level of hepatic glucuronyl transferase activity. Phenobarbital also increases non–bile salt–dependent bile flow and elevates the concentration of the hepatic intracytoplasmic anion binding protein (Y protein) that preferentially transports bilirubin to smooth endoplasmic reticulum where the bilirubin glucuronyl transferase resides. The major rate-limiting step in bilirubin elimination in human newborns is at hepatic conjugation of bilirubin, however.

Treatment of pregnant women with phenobarbital lowers serum bilirubin concentrations in their newborn infants. Maurer et al.[22] noted markedly reduced serum bilirubin levels during the first 4 days of life in newborns of mothers who had received an average oral dose of phenobarbital of 60 mg/kg/day for 2 weeks or longer prior to delivery. Rh- and ABO-sensitized and premature babies were excluded from this study, however. In another study[36] phenobarbital was administered to pregnant women or their infants. It was effective when given to either mothers or newborns, but a most pronounced reduction in serum bilirubin level occurred when it was given both to mothers prior to delivery and to their newborn infants.

Phenobarbital administration to low-birth-weight (LBW) infants yields a less impressive decrease in serum bilirubin level than in full-term newborns.[36] Vasmain et al.[39, 40] observed that phenobarbital administration, 5 mg/kg intramuscularly for 3 days, lowered serum bilirubin levels in both full-term and LBW infants on the fourth and fifth days of life. Although the decrease in serum bilirubin level was significant in the LBW infants, its reduction was less remarkable than in full-term newborns. Similarly, Sinniah et al.[34] found little or no effect in LBW infants, but significantly lower serum bilirubin levels in infants with normal birth weight.

Higher doses of phenobarbital produce much greater decreases in serum bilirubin levels.[35] In a group of 21 premature newborns administered phenobarbital orally at 30 mg/kg/day, serum bilirubin levels of the treated group never exceeded 18 mg/dL; however, at this dose marked sedative effects were noted. Zwacka and Frenzel[42] reported a significant reduction in bilirubin concentrations in premature infants beginning on the third day of life when they were given phenobarbital 10 mg/kg intramuscularly twice daily during the first 2 days of life.

In premature infants a longer course of phenobarbital treatment was

TABLE 25–1.
Therapeutic Agents Used to Treat Neonatal Jaundice

Drug (Trade Name)	Subject	Dose	Route of Administration[†]	Neonate Status[‡]	Outcome (efficacy)[§]	Reference
Antipyrine	Pregnant woman	300 mg/day ≥8 days	PO	FTN	+	Lewis and Friedman, 1979[17]
Clofibrate	Neonate	50 mg/kg	PO	FTN	+	Lindenbaum et al., 1981[18]
Nonenzyme inducers						
Orotic acid	Neonate	200 mg/day 1st 4 days	PO	FTN	+	Matsuda and Shirahata, 1966[21]
	Neonate	125 mg/day bid 1st 6 days	PO	FTN	–	Gray and Mowat, 1971[9]
	Neonate	150 mg/day bid 1st 6 days	PO	LBW	+	Kintzel et al., 1971[13]
	Neonate	100 mg/day bid 1st 5 days	PO	FTN	–	Schwarze et al., 1971[39]
Aspartic acid	Neonate	200 mg/day 1st 4 days	PO	FTN	+	Matsuda and Shirahata, 1966[21]
	Neonate	100 mg/day bid 1st 6 days	PO	PMN	–	Gray and Mowat, 1971[9]
Uridine diphosphoglucose	Neonate	3 mg/kg/day 1st 7 days	IM	FTN	–	Salazar de Sousa et al., 1975[30]
D-Penicillamine	Neonate	300–400 mg/kg/day 2–5 days	PO, IV	HDN	+	Lakatos et al., 1976[15]
				FTN	+	
				PMN	+	
Vitamin E	Neonate	50 mg/kg/day 1st 3 days	IM	LBW	±	Gross, 1979[10]
				VLBW	+	
Substances That Interfere With Enteric Reabsorption of Bilirubin						
Activated charcoal	Neonate	0.75 g q4hr from 4 hr of age	PO	FTN	+	Ulstrom and Eisenklam, 1964[37]
Agar	Neonate	250 mg/feeding 1st 5 days	PO	FTN	+	Poland and Odell, 1971[28]
	Neonate	125 mg q3hr 1st 4 days	PO	LBW	–	Maurer et al., 1973[23]
	Neonate	250 mg q4hr, 6 meals/ day, 1st 3 days	PO	FTN	–	Moller, 1974[24]
Polyvinylpyrrolidone	Neonate	700 mg/kg/day 1st 7 days	PO	LBW	–	Romagnoli et al., 1975[29]
Cholestyramine	Neonate	2 g/kg/day 1st 3 days	PO	PMN	+	Ploussard et al., 1972[26]
	Neonate	250 mg q4hr days 2–8	PO	PMN	–	Schmid et al., 1963[31]

FTN = full-term newborn; HDN = newborn with hemolytic disease; LBW = low birth weight; PMN = premature newborn; VLBW = very low birth weight.

needed to demonstrate the effect. Cao et al.,[2] in a study of LBW infants, observed that a significant reduction in serum bilirubin level occurred after 4 to 6 days of treatment. Carswell et al.[3] observed similarly that in their group of preterm newborns with gestational ages of 36 weeks or less, significantly lower peak bilirubin levels were recorded after 5 days of treatment with phenobarbital.

Alterations in the side groups of the barbiturate ring structure may enhance the potency of phenobarbital for the treatment of neonatal jaundice (especially in the premature newborn) without enhancing its sedative effects. A barbiturate analog, the anti-inflammatory drug bucolome (1-cyclohexyl-5n-butyl-barbituric acid), has been demonstrated to lower serum bilirubin levels by a mechanism similar to that of phenobarbital but without hypnotic side effects. Recently Segni et al.[33] investigated its potential use for the treatment of neonatal hyperbilirubinemia in premature newborns. In a total of 50 newborns between 33 and 36 weeks gestational age who weighed less than 2.5 kg, half were randomly assigned to a treatment group and received oral bucolome at 30 mg/kg for 5 days. Serum bilirubin levels were found to be consistently lower in the treated infants from the fourth day of treatment. Twelve percent of the control infants had levels of serum bilirubin above 18 mg/dL, compared with none in the treated group; 52% of the controls reached levels above 12 mg/dL, compared with only 16% of the treated group. No sedative effects were recorded at the dosage used.

In conclusion, phenobarbital is effective for reducing serum bilirubin levels. Its effect is noted in infants with advanced gestational age, and little or no effect is observed in infants with gestational ages 32 weeks or less. At least 3 days of treatment is needed before its effect is noted. The drug is potentially addictive, may lead to excessive sedation in the newborn, and has other potent metabolic effects in addition to those on bilirubin metabolism. For these reasons the use of phenobarbital has not achieved wide application but has been reserved largely for very specific high-risk populations. For example, in the unexplained severe hyperbilirubinemia of the newborn seen in the Greek coastal islands, the frequency of kernicterus has been significantly reduced by general administration of phenobarbital to pregnant women during the last trimester. A dosage of 60 mg/day is sufficient for maternal administration, and 5 mg/kg/day in neonates. Phenobarbital also is useful in the differentiation of types 1 and 2 glucuronyl transferase deficiency.

Other Drugs

Orotic and aspartic acids are biochemical precursors of uridine, which then incorporate into uridine diphosphoglucose. The latter is the immediate precursor for uridine diphosphate glucuronic acid, which as the second substrate for glucuronyl transferase, donates the glucuronic acid group to bilirubin and to the other endogenous and exogenous substances that require glucuronide conjugation. Studies by Matsuda and Shirahata[21] in full-term newborns and by Kintzel et al.[13] in LBW newborns showed a small but significant reduction in serum bilirubin levels after 4 to 6 days of oral treatment[9]; others, however, were unable to reproduce these effects.

DRUGS THAT INTERFERE WITH HEME DEGRADATION

Recently, tin (Sn)–protoporphyrin (heme) has come under investigation for clinical use in neonatal unconjugated hyperbilirubinemia.[12] Tin-protoporphyrin is a synthetic heme analogue that potently inhibits the activity of heme oxygenase, the rate-limiting enzyme for the degradation of heme to bile pigment. Administration of this compound has been shown to decrease serum bilirubin concentrations in newborn rats, newborn rhesus monkeys, adult rats with hemolytic anemia, and human newborn infants. Tin-protoporphyrin is also a potent photosensitizer and forms a singlet oxygen that can accelerate photodegradation of bilirubin.[19] But this photodynamic action of tin-porphyrin may potentially injure cell membranes and lead to cytolysis.[27] In a clinical study,[12] a group of newborn infants received tin-protoporphyrin, 0.75 μmol/kg body weight, two or three times at 24-hour intervals. Compared with the control group, the treated infants had not dramatic but significantly lower serum bilirubin levels and also required less frequent phototherapy. Although the dose used was small, a few developed mild skin photosensitivity. In newborn rhesus monkeys, administration of tin-protoporphyrin produced ulceration of the skin.[7] Precise details on alterations in heme catabolism and its potential side effects are not fully known at this time and must await further animal and human trials.

DRUGS THAT INTERFERE WITH ENTERIC ABSORPTION OF BILIRUBIN

The bile pigment that reaches the duodenum is reabsorbed as unconjugated bilirubin and returned to the liver by way of the enterohepatic circulation. In the newborn, the enterohepatic reabsorption pathway may be exaggerated, and one of the factors contributing in physiologic jaundice. The theory of treatment is that oral administration of an inert nonabsorbable substance with a high affinity for bilirubin may prevent or reduce reabsorption of bilirubin from the intestine.

By administering activated charcoal to full-term infants within the first 12 hours of life, Ulstrom and Eisenklam[37] observed a significantly lower serum level of bilirubin than in untreated controls. Poland and Odell,[28] administering formula supplemented with agar to a group of full-term newborns from birth to the fifth day of life, observed no rise in serum bilirubin concentration after the thirteenth hour of life and found an increased amount of bilirubin in the feces within the first 5 days, as compared with the control group. Later studies, however, in premature and LBW newborns[23, 29] and in a group of full-term infants[24] showed less convincing results.

Ploussard et al.[26] were able to show a significant decrease in bilirubin levels on the second and third days of life in premature infants who received polyvinylpyrrolidone orally. Schmid et al.[31] were unable to measure a fall in serum bilirubin levels in premature infants as a result of cholestyramine oral treatment. The possible side effects of these agents need more investigations. Long-term administration of cholestyramine, for instance, has been reported to cause steatorrhea, deficiency of fat-soluble vitamins and folic acid, intestinal obstruction, and hyperchloremic acidosis.

Other Agents

The daily administration of vitamin E in newborns may reduce the rate of red blood cell hemolysis and decrease bilirubin production.[10] In infants with birth weight $\leq$ 1,500 g, vitamin E administration produced a significant decrease in the serum bilirubin level on the third day of life and a significant decrease in peak serum bilirubin levels during the first week of life.

D-Penicillamine has been investigated in a series of studies by Lakatos et al.[15] Its administration to premature and full-term newborn infants with hemolysis and hyperbilirubinemia resulted in a significant reduction in serum bilirubin levels and frequency of exchange transfusion. The apparent action of the drug in lowering bilirubin levels seems to derive from its capacity to chelate copper (Cu^{++}) ions; the complex thus formed becomes involved in the degradation of bilirubin by an unknown mechanism to a colorless, water-soluble, and readily excretable product.

PHOTOTHERAPY

Phototherapy has emerged as the most widely used form of therapy for the treatment and prophylaxis of neonatal unconjugated hyperbilirubinemia. In nearly all infants phototherapy reduces or blunts the rise in serum bilirubin concentrations regardless of maturity, presence or absence of hemolysis, or degree of skin pigmentation. The initial report from the Collaborative Study on the Effectiveness and Safety of Phototherapy, undertaken under the auspices of the National Institute of Child Health and Human Development, reveals that infants receiving phototherapy require significantly fewer exchange transfusions and, more important, have an incidence of gross kernicterus that is not different from those who did not receive phototherapy but had exchange transfusions alone to control hyperbilirubinemia.[1] Phototherapy has been used in Europe and Latin America for the past 15 to 20 years and in the United States since the early 1970s. No serious long-term side effects have been reported thus far.

Phototherapy is used either as therapy or as prophylaxis. A guide for phototherapy is shown in Table 25–2. Prophylactic phototherapy is indicated for very LBW (<1,500 g) infants, starting within the first day of life and for

TABLE 25–2.
Guidelines for Use of Phototherapy

Birth weight (g)	Indications for Phototherapy
<1,500	Start during first 24 hr of life regardless of serum bilirubin concentration
1,500–1,999	Without hemolysis at 10 mg/dL, with hemolysis at 8 mg/dL
2,000–2,499	Without hemolysis at 12 mg/dL, with hemolysis at 10 mg/dL
≥2,500	Not recommended unless a specific indication exists (see text)

at least 4 or 5 days. This recommendation reflects careful consideration of the risk-benefit ratio of exchange transfusion vs. phototherapy in this high-risk group of infants.

In our center phototherapy is not recommended as a primary mode of treatment in full-term infants with birth weight ≥2,500 g unless there is a specific indication for its use. In term infants, exchange transfusion carries very low risk of morbidity and mortality. Moreover, the great majority of term infants with serum bilirubin concentrations 10 to 15 mg/dL rarely reach the level for the exchange, 20 mg/dL, even without phototherapy. In this group of infants phototherapy may only prolong the unnecessary hospitalization and the separation of the infant from the family. Uncertainty remains regarding the potential long-term side effects of phototherapy. However, in any newborn infants (including full-term) with any of the following conditions or complications, phototherapy is recommended: (1) serious cardiovascular or other disease that may increase morbidity or mortality risk of the exchange; (2) a serious complication with previous exchange transfusion; (3) expectation of multiple exchange transfusions; (4) difficulty of using umbilical vessels for the exchange route (e.g., abdominal surgery, omphalocele); and (5) potential graft-vs.-host reaction from the exchange (e.g., in acquired or inherited immune deficiencies).

Three independent mechanisms have been proposed to explain the action of phototherapy in reducing serum bilirubin concentrations in newborn infants. The first and major pathway is geometric photoisomerization of unconjugated bilirubin IXa (Fig 25–1).[20] Unconjugated bilirubin IXa is usually in the 5Z, 15Z configuration. In this form the –COOH group of each carboxymethyl side chain interacts by means of three hydrogen bonds with the C=O and N–H group of the pyrrole rings in the opposite half-molecule. As a result, the ionization of the two –COOH groups is inhibited, and therefore the molecule is nonpolar and water-insoluble. When illuminated, unconjugated bilirubin undergoes Z to E isomerization. With tetrapyrrolic bilirubin IX, either one or both of the bridge double bonds can undergo isomerization, yielding potentially three isomers: 5E, 15Z; 5Z, 15E; and 5E, 15E. The E configuration spatially precludes hydrogen bonding of the molecule, which therefore becomes free to ionize, rendering the E isomer more polar than the Z isomer. At least two pairs of geometric photoisomers have been identified in vivo. The first pair, photoisomers IA and IB, is presumably the two possible E, Z isomers. The second pair, photobilirubins IIA and IIB, is most likely two rotamers of the 5E, 15E isomer. Both pairs presumably are formed rapidly in the skin, subcutaneous tissue, and capillaries. Being more polar, all of these isomers partition into the plasma, continuously shifting the equilibrium to promote more isomer formation. These isomers are rapidly taken up by the liver and transported into bile. These photoisomers are destabilized by bile acids, rapidly reverting to native unconjugated bilirubin IX ZZ. The rotameric isomers remain mostly intact and are the major polar photoproducts found in bile. This photoisomerization pathway may be responsible for more than 80% of the augmented bilirubin elimination during the phototherapy. Geometric photoisomerization is not the only isomerization pathway open to a photoexcited bilirubin, however. The proximity of the side chain double bond at C-3 to the adjacent pyrrole ring allows intramolecular cyclization, again rendering the bilirubin molecule more polar[25] (see Fig 25–1). This structural isomer of bilirubin, called "lumirubin," is also excreted into bile without hepatic conjugation. This second pathway is responsible for less than 10% of bilirubin elimination under phototherapy.

The third pathway of phototherapy involves a variety of oxidation reactions with bilirubin, resulting from an autosensitized reaction involving singlet oxygen. The products formed by these reactions are multiple but include biliverdin, dipyrroles, and monopyrroles. Many of these products are colorless, nonreactive in the van den Bergh test, and presumably excreted by the liver and kidney without need for conjugation. Compared with the photoisomerization pathway, the oxidation mechanism appears to play a very minor role in photocatabolism of unconjugated bilirubin in vivo.

In applying phototherapy, banks of eight to 10 fluorescent lamps are placed approximately 12 to 16 inches above an unclothed infant lying in an open radiant warmer or an incubator. A shield of the corrective type of Plexiglas should be placed between the lamps and the infant to absorb the

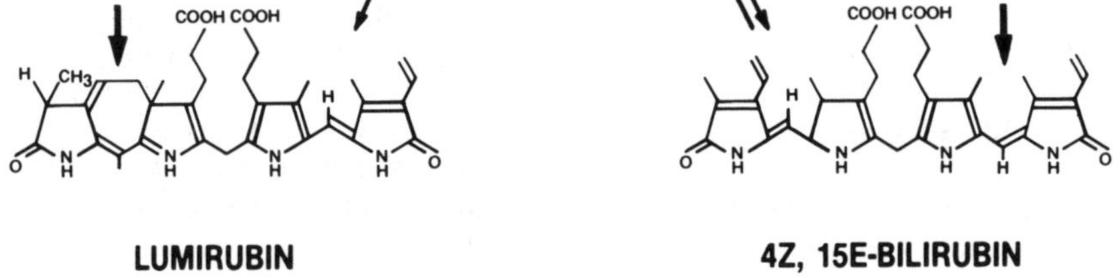

structural

geometric

LUMIRUBIN

4Z, 15E-BILIRUBIN

FIG 25–1.
Geometric (configurational) and structural photoisomerization products of bilirubin IXa.

small amount of ultraviolet light emitted by most fluorescent lamps and to guard against injury from lamp explosion. For phototherapy various kinds of fluorescent lamps have been used, including daylight, cool white, green, blue, and special blue types. Bilirubin absorbs light maximally in the blue range (from 420 to 500 nm), with peak absorption for albumin-bound bilirubin at 460 nm and for unbound bilirubin at 440 nm.[16] Daylight and cool white lamps have a spectral peak between 550 and 600 nm and thus are less effective than special blue lamps, which have a narrow spectral range and peak between 420 and 480 nm.[11] It has been suggested that phototherapy with green light (peak at 525 nm) is as effective as that with blue light and better than white light in reducing serum bilirubin concentrations.[41] Green light lacks the untoward side effects of dizziness and nausea often noted in those working under blue light. However, further careful study is needed to determine the effectiveness of green light, a precise comparison with the blue by determining net reduction in serum bilirubin concentrations at each same increment of irradiance, and also the long-term side effects.

A standard phototherapy unit with eight new daylight lamps operating under optimal conditions will provide clinically significant minimally effective levels of phototherapy (approximately 5 μW/cm^2/nm). According to current knowledge, a saturation point for bilirubin degradation appears to correspond to the energy output provided by a standard phototherapy unit with four daylight and four special blue lamps (approximately 11 μW/cm^2/nm).[11] Increasing the distance from the lamp to the skin surface of the infant results in diminution of light energy by a factor equal to the square of the increase in distance. Skin pigmentation does not reduce the effectiveness of phototherapy. With time in use, fluorescent lamps reduce the energy output to a degree that varies from one type of lamp to another. A meter for monitoring lamp energy output should be used routinely during treatment.

Home phototherapy[8] may be an effective and safe alternative to prolonged hospitalization for the healthy full-term neonate with jaundice. However, complications of home phototherapy that might result from inadequate nursing care include corneal abrasion, eye patch misuse, excessive weight loss, and temperature derangements. Application of home phototherapy without initial evaluation of more significant causes for jaundice is another great risk. The Committee on Fetus and Newborn of the American Academy of Pediatrics[4] has not endorsed this treatment, but has issued guidelines for its use.

The effect of high-intensity light exposure on the eyes of newborn human infants is uncertain, but studies in animals indicate that retinal degeneration may occur after several days of continuous exposure. The eyes of all newborns exposed to phototherapy should be covered with sufficient layers of opaque material to ensure against the potential injury. There is increased insensible and intestinal water loss during phototherapy. In addition, stools are slightly looser and more frequent.

A well-recognized side effect of phototherapy is the "bronze baby" syndrome.[14] In this disorder the serum, urine, and skin become brown-black (bronze) several hours or more after an infant is placed under the phototherapy lamp. All infants with this syndrome have recovered without apparent sequelae. In nearly all patients conjugated hyperbilirubinemia and retention of bile acids have been noted either before light exposure or after the syndrome has developed. This syndrome is reproduced in Gunn rats when their smaller bile ducts were obstructed by precipitated bile pigment during phototherapy. Photobilirubin II is degraded to brown pigment in vitro and converted to brown pigment when administered to Gunn rats in vivo. It seems likely, then, that the bronze color of the plasma and urine in bronze baby syndrome results from retention of bile pigment photoproducts when their biliary excretion is impaired by concomitant cholestasis.

Congenital erythropoietic porphyria is another syndrome in which phototherapy is contraindicated. Exposure to visible light of moderate to high intensity will produce severe bullous lesions on the exposed skin and may produce hemolysis. Other possible dangers of phototherapy include overheating of the infant, unproved potential long-term effects on endocrine and sexual maturation, and on DNA repairing mechanism of skin epithelial cells, with the remote possibility of skin cancer later in life.

REFERENCES

1. Brown AK, Kim MH, Wu PYK, et al: Efficacy of phototherapy in prevention and management of neonatal hyperbilirubinemia. *Pediatrics* 1985; 75(suppl):393–400.
2. Cao A, et al: Phenobarbital effect on serum bilirubin levels in underweight infants. *Helv Paediatr Acta* 1973; 28:231–238.
3. Carswell F, Kerr MM, Dunsmore IR: Sequential trial of effect of phenobarbital on serum bilirubin or preterm infants. *Arch Dis Child* 1972; 47:621–625.
4. Committee on fetus and newborn. Home phototherapy. *Pediatrics* 1985; 76:136.
5. Conney AH: Pharmacological implications of microsomal enzyme induction. *Pharmacol Rev* 1967; 19:317–366.
6. Conney AH, Jacobson MM, Levin W: Effects of drugs on the metabolism of bilirubin and other normal body constituents. *Birth Defects* 1976; 12:275–292.
7. Cornelius CE, Rodgers PA: Prevention of neonatal hyperbilirubinemia in rhesus monkeys by tin-protoporphyrin. *Pediatr Res* 1984; 18:728–730.
8. Grabert BE, Wardwell C, Harburg SK: Home phototherapy: An alternative to prolonged hospitalization of the full-term, well newborn. *Clin Pediatr* 1986; 25:291–294.
9. Gray DW, Mowat AP: Effects of aspartic acid, orotic acid and glucose on serum bilirubin concentrations in infants born before term. *Arch Dis Child* 1971; 46:123–124.
10. Gross SJ: Vitamin E and neonatal bilirubinemia. *Pediatrics* 1979; 64:321–323.
11. Hammerman C, Eidelman AI, Lee KS, et al: Comparative measurement of phototherapy: A practical guide. *Pediatrics* 1981; 67:368–372.
12. Kappas A, Drummond GS, Simionatto CS, et al: Control of heme oxygenase and plasma levels of bilirubin by a synthetic heme analogue, tin-protoporphyrin. *Hepatology* 1984; 4:336–341.
13. Kintzel HW, Hinkel GK, Schwarze R: The decrease in the serum bilirubin level in premature infants by orotic acid. *Acta Paediatr Scand* 1971; 60:1–5.

14. Kopelman AE, Brown RS, Odell GB: The "bronze" baby syndrome: A complication of phototherapy. *J Pediatr* 1972; 81:466–472.
15. Lakatos L, et al: D-Penicillamine therapy of neonatal jaundice: Comparison with phototherapy. *Acta Paediatr Acad Sci Hung* 1976; 17:93–102.
16. Lee KS, Gartner LM: Spectrophotometric characteristics of bilirubin. *Pediatr Res* 1976; 10:782–788.
17. Lewis PJ, Friedman LA: Prophylaxis of neonatal jaundice with maternal antipyrine treatment. *Lancet* 1979; 1:300–301.
18. Lindenbaum A, et al: Traitement curatif de l'ictere du nouveau-né a terme par le clofibrate. Essai thérapeutique contrôlé en double avengle. *Arch Fr Pediatr* 1981; 1 (suppl):867–873.
19. McDonagh AF: Purple versus yellow: Preventing neonatal jaundice with tin-porphyrins. *J Pediatr* 1988; 113:777–781.
20. McDonagh AF, Lightner DA: "Like a shrivelled blood orange": Bilirubin, jaundice, and phototherapy. *Pediatrics* 1985; 75:443–455.
21. Matsuda I, Shirahata T: Effects of aspartic acid and orotic acid upon serum bilirubin level in newborn infants. *Tohoku J Exp Med* 1966; 90:133–136.
22. Maurer HM, et al: Reduction in concentration of total serum-bilirubin in offspring of women treated with phenobarbitone during pregnancy. *Lancet* 1968; 2:122–124.
23. Maurer HM, et al: Controlled trial comparing agar, intermittent phototherapy, and continuous phototherapy for reducing neonatal hyperbilirubinemia. *J Pediatr* 1973; 82:73–76.
24. Moller J: Agar ingestion and serum bilirubin values in newborn infants. *Acta Obstet Gynecol Scand* 1974; 29(suppl):61–63.
25. Onishi SK, Itoh S, Isobe K: Wavelength-dependence of the relative rate constants for the main geometric and structural photoisomerization of bilirubin IXa bound to human serum albumin. *Biochem J* 1986; 236:23–29.
26. Ploussard JP, et al: Ineret et limite de l'utilisation d'un capteur intestinal de la bilirubine non conjuguee (polyvinyl-pyrrolidone) dans l'ictere du premature. *Arch Fr Pediatr* 1972; 29:373–390.
27. Poh-Fitzpatrick MG: Molecular and cellular mechanisms of porphyrin photosensitization. *Photodermatol* 1986; 3:148–157.
28. Poland RL, Odell GB: Physiologic jaundice: The enterohepatic circulation of bilirubin. *N Engl J Med* 1971; 284:1–6.
29. Romagnoli C, et al: Agar in the management of hyperbilirubinaemia in the premature baby. *Arch Dis Child* 1975; 50:202–204.
30. Salazar de Sousa J, Sanches N, Paes MVR: Esperimento terapeutico con l'uridindifosfosglucosio (UDPG) nella iperbilirubinemia fisiologica del neonato. *Minerva Pediatr* 1975; 27:1162–1165.
31. Schmid R, et al: Lack of effect of cholestyramine resin on hyperbilirubinemia of premature infants. *Lancet* 1963; 2:938–939.
32. Schwarze R, Kintzel HW, Hinkel GK: The influence of orotic acid on the serum bilirubin level of mature newborn. *Acta Paediatr Scand* 1971; 60:705–708.
33. Segni G, Polidori G, Romagnoli C: Bucolone in prevention of hyperbilirubinemia in preterm infants. *Arch Dis Child* 1977; 52:549–550.
34. Sinniah D, Tay LK, Dugdale AE: Phenobarbitone in neonatal jaundice. *Arch Dis Child* 1971: 46:712–715.
35. Theile H, Reich J: Die Wirkung von Phenobarbital auf den Bilirubinspiegel bei Fruhgeborenen. *Helv Paediatr Acta* 1970; 25:77–82.

36. Trolle D: Decrease of total serum-bilirubin concentration in newborn infants after phenobarbitone treatment. *Lancet* 1968; 2:705–708.
37. Ulstrom RA, Eisenklam E: The enterohepatic shunting of bilirubin in the newborn infant: I. Use of oral activated charcoal to reduce normal serum bilirubin values. *J Pediatr* 1964; 65:27–37.
38. Vaisman SL, Gartner LM: Pharmacologic treatment of neonatal hyperbilirubinemia. *Clin Perinatol* 1975; 2:37–58.
39. Vaisman S, Ebenssperger I, Hering E: Hyperbilirubinemia del recien nacido y fenobarbital: II. Recien nacido de bajo peso. *Rev Child Pediatr* 1971; 42:315–319.
40. Vaisman S, et al: Hyperbilirubinemia del recien nacido y fenobarbital: I. Recien nacido de termino. *Rev Child Pediatr* 1971; 42:245–250.
41. Vecchi C, Donzell GP, Migliorini MG, et al: Phototherapy for neonatal jaundice: Clinical equivalence of fluorescent green and special blue lamps. *J Pediatr* 1986; 108:452–456.
42. Zwacka G, Frenzel J: Untersuchungen zur Beeinflüssung der Hyperbilirubinemia unreifer Neugeborener durch Kurzzeit-induktion mit Phenobarbital. *Padiatr Padol* 1971; 6:102–107.

26

Use of Blood Products in Neonates and Small Infants

Ruth Andrea Seeler, M.D.

RED BLOOD CELL TRANSFUSION

In neonates receiving assisted ventilation it is a common practice to maintain a hemoglobin level of 13 g/dL or hematocrit 40% or greater and to transfuse whenever 5% to 10% of the blood volume has been sampled. When using packed blood cells the change in hematocrit is equal to the number of cubic centimeters (milliliters) infused per kilogram body weight of the child.

Special Blood Bank Considerations

Because neonates do not respond to polysaccharide antigens, the American Association of Blood Banks (AABB) standards allow for repeated booster erythrocyte (RBC) transfusion in infants younger than 4 months old without compatibility testing, provided the initial test revealed no alloantibodies. Neonates do not seem to form white blood cell antibodies either.[11] If the infant has undergone an exchange transfusion, a new blood sample is required before further transfusion to assure compatibility of the exchanged blood with erythrocytes for subsequent transfusions.

The neonate's poor immune response makes it possible for the blood banks to use 1 unit per day of type O Rh-specific washed RBCs for all infants needing transfusions on that day. Another advantage of using type O RBCs is the avoidance of transfusion reactions resulting from unrecognized ABO hemolytic disease of the newborn. Because of the relative weakness of A and B antigens on fetal erythrocytes, the direct Coombs' test can be negative in presence of transplacental anti-A and anti-B antigens. However, when adult RBCs are infused, with their strong A and B antigens, a hemolytic transfusion reaction may result.[10a]

Complications

Non-A, Non-B Hepatitis

An estimated 5% to 10% of patients who have received multiple transfusions will develop non-A, non-B hepatitis, and in approximately two thirds of these patients, whether icteric or not, the hepatitis will become chronic. In an attempt to decrease this risk, the AABB now requires donor screening for hepatitis B core (HBc) antibody. There is active research on methods to sterilize both the fluid and cellular blood components, not only for non-A, non-B hepatitis but also for other viral agents [human immunodeficiency virus (HIV), hepatitis B virus, cytomegalovirus (CMV)]. It is hoped that the promising results using the light-active psoralins[1] will become clinically useful.

Human Immunodeficiency Virus

Current donor screening and testing have reduced the risk of HIV transmission drastically to about one case in 10,000 to 100,000 transfusions. Because of these risks, however, transfusions should be viewed as a lifesaving therapy, not a routine therapy.

Cytomegalovirus

Cytomegalovirus infection can be spread by RBC transfusion.[27, 28] Low-birth-weight infants lose their maternal antibody quickly and then become susceptible to infection by way of transfusion. Such transfusion infection can be confirmed by restriction endonuclease techniques.[27]

Providing the infant with blood products solely from CMV-negative donors is not simple because of the high prevalence (50% to 70%) of CMV antibodies in the general population. There is mounting evidence that frozen deglycerolized erythrocytes do not transmit CMV[3, 26]; however, such techniques are cumbersome and expensive and are not available in all blood banks. After deglycerolization, erythrocytes have only a 24-hour half-life; thus, the use of frozen RBCs may be a practical approach in large neonatal intensive care units where such a packed cell unit is used to supply all of the babies needing RBCs on a given day.

Because the CMV virus is attached to the leukocytes, there have been attempts to render CMV antibody-positive blood noninfectious by leuko-depletion.[10, 14] Luban et al.[14] concluded that this procedure was effective in reducing transfusion CMV infections in babies who received no other cellular blood products.

Radiation will not reduce CMV infectiousness, and it is technically difficult for a blood bank to provide leukodepleted platelet or granulocyte concentrates. Therefore, when premature infants born to CMV-negative mothers require either platelet or granulocyte concentrates, the donor should be CMV negative. If the infant is born to a CMV-positive mother, one needs to be sure the baby still has a protective titer before using CMV-positive donor blood.[27]

To date, fresh-frozen plasma and cryoprecipitate have not been implicated in transmitting CMV infections. This is probably due to the freeze-thaw cycle, with consequent destruction of white blood cells.

Phototherapy Heat Injury

For infants receiving phototherapy, care must be taken to prevent heat-induced hemolysis of the RBCs while in the intravenous tubing.[17] Such iatrogenic hemolysis has led to the need for exchange transfusion as well as to hemoglobinuria.

Graft-vs.-Host Disease

Immunodeficient or immunocompromised persons may develop graft-vs.-host disease (GVHD) following transfusion, due to engraftment of histoincompatible T cells. Although rare, GVHD is almost uniformly fatal, and the lack of any effective therapy mandates prevention. At high risk for transfusion GVHD are infants with congenital immunodeficiencies (particularly severe combined immunodeficiency, Wiskott-Aldrich syndrome, and DiGeorge syndrome) and infants who received in utero transfusion(s).[18, 19]

All cellular blood products have been incriminated in transfusion-related GVHD. Platelet concentrates and granulocyte concentrations are heavily contaminated with lymphocytes. Fresh-frozen plasma and cryoprecipitate have yet to be reported to cause GVHD.[19]

There is consensus that only washed irradiated packed erythrocytes should be used for intrauterine transfusion. Infants who have received an intrauterine transfusion and require exchange transfusions after birth should be given only irradiated erythrocytes.[19] In those cases where GVHD has been reported, the lymphocytes were from the donor of the blood used at the exchange transfusion. The usual irradiation of 1,500 to 2,500 rad (cGy) will render the lymphocytes nonviable and has no negative effect on erythrocyte survival. Should the infants require platelet transfusion because of associated severe thrombocytopenia, the platelets should be irradiated.

Whole Blood

All of the requirements for packed RBCs apply equally to whole-blood transfusion. Many neonatologists are using reconstituted whole blood (1 unit packed RBCs and 1 unit ABO-compatible plasma) for exchange transfusion. Acute hemorrhagic blood loss is likewise treated with packed cells and a volume expander, such as saline solution or albumin. If there is a coagulation disturbance, fresh-frozen plasma may be used to reconstitute the RBCs. All of this takes precious time, and it is better to use packed cells than to leave the baby in shock while the blood bank either reconstitutes a unit or searches for a unit of blood.

Designated Donors

Often parents want to donate blood for their child or to designate a relative as a donor. This may be considered for nonemergency transfusions, because the AABB standards mandate that a designated donor be as safe as an autologous donor. Thus all of the routine screening tests [HIV, HBc, hepatitis B surface antigen (HBSag), ALT (alanine transaminase), serology, CMV] cannot be waived and usually take $1^1/_2$ to 2 days to complete. All of these tests must be completed before the blood can be transfused.

POLYCYTHEMIA-HYPERVISCOSITY

Definition

In contrast to most disease entities, the definition of polycythemia-hyperviscosity syndrome in the newborn is anything but precise.[21, 22] A consensus is emerging in which peripheral venous hematocrit 65% or greater is required for the diagnosis of polycythemia.[21] Management of this condition is likewise not standardized. The incidence of hyperviscosity-polycythemia syndrome varies from 1.8% at sea level to approximately 5% in mile-high Denver. All workers agree that the incidence of polycythemia-hyperviscosity is much more common than the number of infants who have the potential to become impaired by central nervous system damage. There is consensus that for symptomatic infants a partial exchange transfusion is recommended.

Partial Exchange Transfusion

Considering the gastrointestinal complications[2, 13] and infectious risks, there is a compelling case against using fresh-frozen plasma for partial exchange transfusion. Many neonatal centers are using crystalloid (either 0.9% sodium chloride or Ringer's lactate) rather than either albumin or pasteurized protein solution. The goal after the partial exchange transfusion is to have final hematocrit 50% to 55%.[23]

The conventional formula for calculating the volume is:

$$\frac{\text{Blood volume} \times (\text{Baby's Hct} - \text{Desired Hct})}{\text{Baby's Hct}}$$

A partial exchange should be done in 10 mL increments.

HEMOTHERAPY IN INFANTS WITH SEPSIS

Granulocyte Transfusion

Both qualitative and quantitative granulocyte defects have been among the numerous documented immune defects in neonates. In an attempt to overcome this, granulocyte transfusions have been used in a limited number of studies.[6, 9] There has been no demonstrable benefit of granulocyte transfusion when the infant's bone marrow granulocyte reserve was adequate.

Improved survival has been demonstrated in a limited number of infants with neutropenia and marrow granulocyte precursor depletion. The granulocyte transfusions were given repeatedly, usually every 12 hours, for either five transfusions or until such time as the infant's own granulocyte reserve recovered. The effectiveness of the repeated granulocyte transfusion was measured by clearing of bacteremia and by survival. The effectiveness of granulocyte transfusions cannot be measured by a white blood cell count after transfusion, because the granulocytes circulate for only minutes to hours.

Research in this area has been hampered by the logistic difficulties of quickly providing an adequate granulocyte concentrate for neutropenic infants with bone marrow depletion. The granulocytes per se have not had any recognized systemic effects in the relatively few infants studied. Because granulocyte concentrates are very heavily contaminated with lymphocytes, most researchers routinely irradiate the granulocytes. To date there have been no cases of GVHD, but fewer than 50 infants have been studied. It is prudent to have the granulocyte concentrates irradiated because with wider experience GVHD is almost to be anticipated. If the infants were born to CMV-negative mothers, the donors should be CMV negative; or if the infant is older than 1 month of age, it is probably wise to use a CMV-negative donor, because the infant's transplacental maternal antibody may be at a nonprotective level.

Neutrophil Replacement by Exchange Transfusion

The difficulty in repeatedly providing granulocyte concentrates has stimulated interest in exchange transfusion for septic neutropenic infants because of the additional theoretical benefit of removing endotoxin.[22] Granulocyte function is impaired with refrigeration. The logistics therefore require that the blood bank be able to immediately do all of the screening tests (HIV, hepatitis B antigen, HBc antibody, liver enzymes, CMV, sickle test) on the donor in the hours before the blood is actually drawn.

Intravenous Immunoglobulin (See also Chapter 16)

In a group of mothers who received 24 g/day immunoglobulin for 5 days and whose infants were greater than 32 weeks gestation, there was a significant reduction in the incidence of septicemia in infants born to mothers with ruptured membranes or chorioamnionitis.[24] In other studies, intravenous IgG (IV IgG) was administered on a weekly basis to the premature infants. Infants less than 1,500 g receiving IV IgG (0.5 g/kg/wk) prophylaxis had fewer infections, less septicemia, and fewer deaths than neonates of similar weight in the same nursery.[7] Even better results were reported with a European gammaglobulin enriched with IgM.[12]

Recombinant Colony-Stimulating Factors

There are currently adult trials of recombinant granulocyte-monocyte colony-stimulating factors (Rh-GM-CSF) and granulocyte stimulating factor (Rh-G-CSF) that hold potential value for treating septic neutropenia in neonates. These glycoproteins have the ability to drive the pleuripotential stem cell or the granulocyte-committed cell to faster granulocyte production. Recombinant CSFs are proving to be clinically useful in adults, shortening the neutropenic period following bone marrow transplantation and restoring normal granulopoiesis in some patients with aplastic anemia. This is an exciting area of research with wide clinical potential.[6]

THROMBOCYTOPENIA

Unlike almost all other laboratory values, the platelet number in healthy newborns and premature infants is not gestationally related, normal values being in excess of 150,000/mm³. As with older children, clinical bleeding is not a problem so long as the platelet count exceeds 50,000/mm³.

The differential diagnosis of thrombocytopenia in the newborn is extensive, and I have found it clinically useful to approach the problem as outlined in Table 26–1. When the thrombocytopenia is a secondary phenomenon, treatment of the underlying condition will correct the low platelet count.

For symptomatic bleeding, except in immune-mediated severe thrombocytopenia, platelet concentrates should be administered. The platelet concentrates are heavily contaminated with leukocytes and probably should be irradiated (definitely for any infant who received an in utero transfusion). The platelets from 1 unit of blood will increase the full-term infant's platelet count to approximately 50,000 to 75,000/mm³. In cases where there is ongoing platelet destruction, such high platelet counts will not be achieved. Random donor platelet concentrates will be of little or no value in immune thrombocytopenia (see next section).

Immune Thrombocytopenia(s)

Neonatal immune thrombocytopenia occurs in well-defined clinical situations: mothers with idiopathic thrombocytopenic purpura (ITP) or systemic lupus erythematosus and neonatal alloimmune thrombocytopenia (NAT). It is beyond the scope of this chapter to discuss management of subsequent pregnancies in detail, and only highlights are covered. Readers are referred to Bussell et al.[5] for in depth analysis of this rapidly changing field.

Maternal ITP
Approximately 8.3% of healthy women were found to have laboratory-confirmed thrombocytopenia during the third trimester of pregnancy. These

TABLE 26–1.
Differential Diagnosis of Neonatal Thrombocytopenia

Immune-mediated
    Maternal idiopathic thrombocytopenia purpura (with or without splenectomy)
    Maternal systemic lupus erythematosus
    Neonatal alloimmune platelet antibodies
    Severe Rh hemolytic disease of the newborn
Infectious
    Group B streptococcus bacteremia
    Gram-negative bacteremia, especially *Escherichia coli*
    Toxoplasmosis
    Syphilis
    Herpes simplex
    Cytomegalic inclusion disease (CMV)
    Rubella
Increased peripheral destruction
    Kasabach-Merritt syndrome (giant hemangioma)
    Maternal preeclampsia
    Abruptio placentae
    Renal vein thrombosis
    Large artery thrombosis
    Necrotizing enterocolitis
    Indwelling vascular catheter
Megakaryocytic hypoplasia syndromes
    Thrombocytopenia and absent radius syndrome
    Wiskott-Aldrich syndrome
    Congenital amegakaryocytic thrombocytopenia
    Trisomy 13 and 18
Tumors and leukemia
    Congenital leukemia
    Placental chorangioma
    Disseminated neuroblastoma
Metabolic disorders
    Ketogenic hyperglycemia
    Methylmalonic aciduria
    Isovaleric acidemia
    Propionic acidemia
Unusual factors
    Intralipid infusion
    Hyperviscosity (polycythemia)
    Phototherapy
    Exchange transfusion
    Congenital thyrotoxicosis
    Mechanical ventilation

women were without a history of ITP before pregnancy, had platelet counts in excess of 80,000/mm³, and all had healthy infants.[4] This has been labeled "pseudo ITP pregnancy." It is critically important that this phenomenon be recognized so that a mother not be treated for ITP[4] and subjected to medical therapy and cesarean section delivery.

The major problem with true ITP is the difficulty in predicting the clinical severity in the infant. Approximately 50% of infants are unaffected. It should be noted that women who have had ITP in childhood and are now in remission and receiving no therapy are totally cured and are not at risk of having an affected child. The predictive problem pertains to women who developed ITP as adults, are receiving steroids, or have had a splenectomy.

Infants born to mothers with ITP or a history of adult ITP should have daily platelet counts, because the platelets may decline from the initial values at birth.[25] If the platelet count goes below 50,000/mm³, the baby should receive IV IgG therapy. Originally the dose given was 0.4 g/kg/day for 5 days; but more recently 1 g/kg, repeated if needed, has been used. The baby should be examined weekly, and if platelet count declines to less than 50,000/mm³ during the second or third week, a booster dose of IV IgG given. Because of the normal decay of transplacental IgG, it is unlikely that further therapy will be needed.[8, 16] With 0.4 g/kg IV IgG, approximately 20,000/mm³ rise per day is expected, and approximately 40,000 to 50,000/mm³ rise in platelet with 1 g/kg dose. The expected platelet increase is measured 18 to 24 hours after conclusion of the infusion.

Neonatal Alloimmune Thrombocytopenia

Neonatal alloimmune thrombocytopenia is caused by fetomaternal incompatibility, usually for platelet antigen (PL^{a1}), although others have been involved, for example, Pen and Bak[2] antigens. The accepted incidence of one or two cases per 10,000 live births may be much too low; prospective studies are identifying many more mildly affected infants.[15] Approximately 50% of symptomatic children have been born to primigravidas, and subsequent infants are more severely affected. Clinical manifestations range from asymptomatic mild thrombocytopenia to severe thrombocytopenia with hemorrhage, including in utero intracranial hemorrhage and porencephalic cyst formation prior to the onset of labor.[29] Mothers who have had a child with NAT should be referred to centers with particular expertise in this area.

The thrombocytopenia seen in NAT is the most severe that has been documented in the neonatal period, and platelet counts under 10,000/mm³ are not unusual. Therapy should be the prompt administration of IV IgG at a dose of 0.4 g/kg/day for 5 days or 1 g/kg. In ongoing hemorrhage, the mother should undergo platelet pheresis, in which the platelets are washed to eliminate the offending antibody and then resuspended in appropriate ABO-compatible plasma. Because of the rarity of these antigen-negative individuals, it is almost fruitless to search for platelet concentrates in random donors negative for the offending antigen. Because there is not sufficient time to identify the antigen, washed pheresed maternal platelets are recommended for these infants. Platelets from random donors will be destroyed, and steroids are ineffective.

SELECTED PLASMA COAGULATION DISORDERS

Hemophilia A

Hemophilia A is a sex-linked disease with an estimated 25% to 30% spontaneous mutation rate. Factor VIII is a large molecule and does not cross the placenta; thus the diagnosis can be established by factor assay in the newborn period. Values in newborns are similar to those in adults, 50% to 150%. In hemophilia the partial thromboplastin time (PTT) is greatly prolonged and the prothrombin time (PT) in the usual range for a neonate. Newly diagnosed factor VIII hemophilia should be treated only with 20 to 30 U/kg monoclonal purified or solvent detergent–purified factor VIII preparations, which are devoid of HIV and hepatitis viruses. The need for further doses should be determined in consultation with a pediatric hematologist.

Hemophilia B

Hemophilia B is also inherited in a sex-linked manner. The diagnosis in the newborn period is slightly more complicated because factor IX is vitamin K dependent. However, in vitamin K deficiency low levels of the other vitamin K–deficient factors (see below) and factor IX are usually found. If the factor IX level is below 15% and the infant has been given vitamin K, this is very suggestive for hemophilia B. Therapy for hemorrhage depends on its location. If there is a threat to the CNS or limb, the child should be given heat-treated concentrate, approximately 25 U/kg. Fresh-frozen plasma, 12 to 15 mL/kg, may also be given for less serious bleeding. The need for further doses should be determined in consultation with a pediatric hematologist.

Hemorrhagic Diseases of the Newborn

All newborn infants should receive 1 mg vitamin K intramuscularly as prophylaxis against vitamin K deficiency. Vitamin K is needed only for hepatic synthesis of the calcium binding site to precursors for factors II, VII, IX, and X. Because human milk contains very little vitamin K, the breast-fed infant may develop hemorrhagic symptoms after days to weeks. All commercial formulas have adequate amounts of vitamin K and thus protect the infant against hemorrhagic disease of the newborn. Because vitamin K is needed only for the attachment of the calcium binding site, the shortening of PT can be seen as soon as 1 hour after administration of vitamin K. If the hemorrhage is ongoing, fresh-frozen plasma, 12 to 15 mL/kg, can be given. Usually only single treatment is needed.[20]

Disseminated Intravascular Coagulation

The potential for disseminated intravascular coagulation (DIC) is great.[20] Infants have sepsis, and frequently also endotoxemia, tissue damage from indwelling catheters, hypoxemia, and shock. All are predisposed to DIC with its consumption of the labile clotting factors, thrombocytopenia, and increased fibrinolysis, yielding fibrin split products. Therapy for the cause of the DIC will usually arrest the process; however, the fibrin clots accumulating in the microcirculation are themselves detrimental, and replacement therapy may be needed until the primary process is controlled.

Exchange transfusion with fresh blood not only replaces the consumed clotting factors but also removes the fibrin degradation products, which are also anticoagulants, as well as removing endotoxin.[23] Another approach to DIC treatment is infusion of fresh-frozen plasma, 10 to 15 mL/kg every 10 to 12 hours, and monitoring of PT and PTT. Platelet concentrates will need to be given, because the platelets in whole blood that has been refrigerated are rendered relatively nonfunctional. One unit of platelets increases the platelet count to 50,000 to 75,000/mm^3. Most workers agree that there is no benefit from heparin treatment in neonatal DIC.[20, 23]

REFERENCES

1. Alter HJ, Morel PA, Dorman BP, et al: Photochemical decontamination of blood components containing hepatitis B and non-A, non-B virus. *Lancet* 1988; 2:1446–1450.
2. Black VD, Rumack CM, Lubchenco LO, et al: Gastrointestinal injury in polycythemia term infants. *Pediatrics* 1985; 76:225–231.
3. Brady MT, Milam JD, Anderson DC, et al: Use of deglycerolized red blood cells to prevent posttransfusion infection with cytomegalovirus in neonates. *Pediatr Infec Dis* 1984; 150:334–339.
4. Burrows RF, Kelton JG: Incidentally detected thrombocytopenia in healthy mothers and their infants. *N Engl J Med* 1988; 319:142–145.
5. Bussell JB, Berkowitz RL, McFarland JG, et al: Antenatal treatment of neonatal alloimmune thrombocytopenia. *N Engl J Med* 1988; 319:142–145.
6. Cairo MS: Neonatal neutrophil host defense. *Am J Dis Child* 1989; 143:40–45.
7. Chirico G, Duse M, Ugazio, et al: High-dose intravenous gammaglobulin therapy for passive immune thrombocytopenia in the neonate. *J Pediatr* 1983; 103:654–655.
8. Chirico G, Rondini G, Plebani A, et al: Intravenous gammaglobulin therapy for prophylaxis of infection in high-risk neonates. *J Pediatr* 1987; 110:437–443.
9. Christensen RD, Rothstein G, Anstall HB, et al: Granulocyte transfusion in neonates with bacterial infection, neutropenia and depletion of mature marrow neutrophils. *Pediatrics* 1982; 70:1–6.
10. Demmler GJ, Brady MT, Bijou H, et al: Posttransfusion cytomegalovirus infection in neonates: Role of saline-washed red blood cells. *J Pediatr* 1986; 108:762–765.
10a. Falterman CG, Richardson CJ: Transfusion reaction due to unrecognized ABO hemolytic disease of the newborn. *J Pediatr* 1980; 97:812–814.

11. Floss AM, Strauss, Goeken N, et al: Multiple transfusions fail to provoke antibodies against blood cell antigens in human infants. *Transfusion* 1986; 26:419–422.
12. Haque KN, Zaidi MH, Bahakim H: IgM-enriched intravenous immunoglobulin therapy in neonatal sepsis. *Am J Dis Child* 1988; 142 1293–1296.
13. Hein HA, Lathrop SS: Partial exchange transfusion in term, polycythemic neonates: Absence of association with severe gastrointestinal injury. *Pediatrics* 1987; 80:75–78.
14. Luban NLC, Williams AE, MacDonald MG, et al: Low incidence of acquired cytomegalovirus infection in neonates transfused with washed red blood cells. *Am J Dis Child* 1987; 141:416–419.
15. Mueller-Eckhardt C, Grubert A, Weisheit M, et al: 348 cases of suspected neonatal alloimmune thrombocytopenia. *Lancet* 1989; 1:363–366.
16. Newland AC, Boots MA, Patterson KG: Intravenous IgG for autoimmune thrombocytopenia in pregnancy. *N Engl J Med* 1984; 310:261–262.
17. Opitz JC, Baldauf MC, Kessler DL, et al: Hemolysis of blood in intravenous tubing caused by heat. *J Pediatr* 1988; 112:111–113.
18. Parkman P, Mosier D, Umansky I, et al: Graft-versus-host disease after intrauterine and exchange transfusions for hemolytic disease of the newborn. *N Engl J Med* 1974; 290:359–363.
19. Pisciotto P: Irradiated blood, in Kasprisin DO, Luban NLC (eds): *Pediatric Transfusion Medicine,* vol II. Boca Raton, Fla, CRC Press, 1987, pp 1–18.
20. Plunket DC: Bleeding syndromes of the newborn, in Kasprisin DO, Luban NLC (eds): *Pediatric Transfusion Medicine,* vol I. Boca Raton, Fla, CRC Press, 1987, pp 53–67.
21. Ramamurthy RS, Berlanga M: Postnatal alteration in hematocrit and viscosity in normal and polycythemic infants. *J Pediatr* 1987; 110:929–934.
22. Ramamurthy RS, Brans YW: Neonatal polycythemia: 1. Criteria for diagnosis and treatment. *Pediatrics* 1981; 68:168–174.
23. Seibel M, Gross S: Exchange transfusion in the neonate, in Kasprisin DO, Luban NLC (eds): *Pediatric Transfusion Medicine,* vol I. Boca Raton, Fla, CRC Press, 1987, pp 43–52.
24. Sidiropoulos D, Herrmann U Jr, Morell A, et al: Transplacental passage of intravenous immunoglobulin in the last trimester of pregnancy. *J Pediatr* 1986; 109:505–508.
25. Suarez CR, Anderson C: High-dose intravenous gammaglobulin (IVG) in neonatal immune thrombocytopenia. *Am J Hematol* 1987; 26:247–253.
26. Taylor BJ, Jacobs RF, Baker RJ, et al: Frozen deglycerolyzed blood prevents transfusion-acquired cytomegalovirus infections in neonates. *Pediatr Infect Dis* 1986; 5:188–191.
27. Tolpin MD, Stewart JA, Warren D, et al: Transfusion transmission of cytomegalovirus confirmed by restriction endonuclease analysis. *J Pediatr* 1985; 107:953–956.
28. Yeager AS, Grumet FC, Hafleigh EB, et al: Prevention of transfusion-acquired cytomegalovirus infections in newborn infants. *J Pediatr* 1981; 98:281–287.
29. Zalneraitis EL, Young RSK, Krishnamoorthy KS: Intracranial hemorrhage in utero as a complication of isoimmune thrombocytopenia. *J Pediatr* 1979; 95:611–614.

27

Drug Use in Medical, Surgical, and Radiologic Procedures

Shirley Reitz, Pharm.D.

Vivian Harris, M.D.

Tsu F. Yeh, M.D.

Drugs used during diagnosis or treatment must be effective in obtaining the desired end point without causing significant undesired toxicity. Special concerns in the neonate include increased drug absorption through skin, bilirubin displacement by highly protein-bound drugs, altered pharmacokinetics resulting from immature liver and kidney function, and increased sensitivity of the neonate to the depressive effects of many sedatives and anesthetics. Lack of verbal communication of pain has often left the neonate without adequate pharmacologic coverage. This chapter focuses on drugs that are commonly used for medical, surgical, and radiologic procedures.

TOPICAL ANTISEPTICS

General Principles

An antiseptic is a substance that kills or prevents the growth of microorganisms when applied to living tissue. It is desirable that an antiseptic be germicidal rather than germistatic, that it have a broad spectrum of germicidal activity, and that it have rapid onset and sustained activity. It should not produce local cellular damage or impair wound healing. Antiseptics that retain these characteristics and are commonly used include alcohol, chlorhexidine, iodophors, silver compounds, and dyes.

Alcohol

Ethanol 70% (rubbing alcohol) is bactericidal to most common pathogens but has poor efficacy against viruses and spores. It works by denaturation of soluble protein, and can be used for skin disinfection before minor procedures.

Isopropyl alcohol, used in concentrations of 70% to 100%, is slightly more germicidal than ethanol; however, it is also more irritating. As a vehicle for other germicidal agents, it increases their effectiveness.

Alcohol generally evaporates from the skin before significant absorption occurs; however, if the area is occluded, serious local damage may occur, especially in the preterm infant. Gluteal skin necrosis and high blood levels of methyl and ethyl alcohol have been described in a 27-week gestational age infant who underwent prolonged, difficult umbilical catheterization during which the sheet the infant was lying on became soaked with alcohol.[12] Similar skin lesions resulting from isopropyl alcohol have been reported in two infants.[29] Alcohol should be used only as impregnated swabs for local procedures (i.e., heelstick) in neonates.

Chlorhexidine

Hexachlorophene came under investigation and (finally) restricted use in the early 1970s after central nervous system toxicity in neonates was reported. Chlorhexidine gluconate has largely replaced hexachlorophene and is bactericidal to both gram-positive and gram-negative bacteria. It has a rapid onset of action, and up to 26% of the emulsion remains active on the skin as long as 29 hours. In addition to its use in prophylactic bathing of the infant, the 4% emulsion (Hibiclens) is also used as a surgical scrub, as a handwash for health care personnel, and as a skin wound cleanser and antiseptic. Although absorption through the skin of premature infants has been shown, no known toxic effects have been attributed to chlorhexidine.

Iodine and Iodophors

Iodine has been widely used because of its efficacy, low cost, and low toxicity to the tissues. It is effective against bacteria, spores, fungi, protozoa, and viruses, and is probably superior to any other agent as a skin disinfectant. Iodine solution USP (2% iodine, 2.5% sodium iodide) is used as an antiseptic in treating superficial wounds. Iodine tincture USP (2% iodine, 2% sodium iodide, and 50% alcohol) is more irritating to tissues and therefore less preferred.

Iodophors are organic complexes that serve as a sustained release reservoir for iodine. The active antiseptic in these products is iodine, which produces this effect by oxidizing microbial protoplasm. The percentage of active ingredient ranges from 1% in ointments to 0.75% in shampoos and skin antiseptics.

Iodophors, although less effective than iodine solution, are also less irritating, are nonstaining, and are less sensitizing. Povidone-iodine is a complex of I_2 with the pyrrolidone nitrogen of polyvinyl-pyrrolidone. Dilution of the 10% solution allows for dissociation of the I_2 carrier complex and higher concentrations of "free" iodine. Thus bactericidal activity is higher at 0.1% than at 10% concentration. Standard surgical scrub with 10% povidone-iodine (containing 1% "available" iodine) decreases cutaneous bacterial count by about 85%; effective antibacterial control is lost within about 1 hour, with normal bacterial counts returning in 6 to 8 hours. Pyati et al.[25] and others have shown that topical use of povidone-iodine solutions in neonates results in a significant increase in total serum iodine, decrease in serum thyroxin, and increase in urinary excretion of iodine. Transient hypothyroidism generally abates within 10 to 14 days. There have been no reports of permanent hypothyroidism in infants or children following the use of iodine-containing antiseptics.

Silver Compounds

The silver ion exerts its antimicrobial effect by denaturation of the microbial cell protein, disrupting the cell membrane and causing death of the organism. In general, the only two commonly used silver compounds are silver nitrate and silver sulfadiazine.

Silver nitrate has caustic, antiseptic, and astringent activities; the degree of action depends on the concentration being used and the amount of time it is allowed to act. The silver ion is precipitated by chloride and by proteins; therefore silver nitrate does not readily penetrate tissue, and the resultant silver precipitate may stain the tissue black. Silver nitrate is germicidal for gonococci and *Pseudomonas,* and is commonly used as 1% ophthalmic solution for the prevention of ophthalmia neonatorum. Following application of 1% silver nitrate ophthalmic solution, up to 90% of neonates experience mild chemical conjunctivitis, which rarely persists beyond 24 hours.

The antibacterial action of silver sulfadiazine 1% (Silvadene) is not entirely known; it may result both because sulfadiazine competitively inhibits *p*-aminobenzoic acid and the silver ion binds with deoxyribonucleic acid, preventing replication. Silver sulfadiazine is bactericidal against both gram-negative and gram-positive organisms. It is used primarily as an adjunct in the prevention and treatment of infection in burn patients. Unlike silver nitrate, silver sulfadiazine does not cause staining of the tissue. In addition, it does not bind with chloride ions, thereby eliminating potential electrolyte and acid-base disturbances. Transient leukopenia, occurring after 2 to 3 days of treatment, has been seen in many patients treated with silver sulfadiazine. Despite continued use, the leukopenia generally resolves in a few days.

Triple Dye

A single application of triple dye (gentian violet, brilliant green, and proflavine hemisulfate in 2:2:1 ratio) to the umbilical stump shortly after birth was shown by Pildes et al.[23] to be effective in significantly reducing staphylococcal colonization rates. Triple dye has been shown to be less effective than silver sulfadiazine in reducing colonization of group B streptococci and gram-negative organisms.[3]

ANALGESICS, ANESTHETICS

Neonates respond to painful procedures with a number of physiologic and behavioral alterations. Some have suggested that neonatal nerve pathways are insufficiently myelinated to transmit painful messages. Yet even during simple brief procedures, physiologic markers (heart rate, blood pressure, transcutaneous oxygen pressure [$tcPO_2$], respiratory rate) fluctuate widely. It has become incumbent on clinicians to recognize and treat neonatal pain.

Local Anesthetics

Local anesthetics block nerve conduction by preventing the large transient increase in permeability of the membrane to sodium ions, increasing the threshold for electrical excitability. They are nonirritating to tissue, and recovery from the nerve blockade is complete. The action of local anesthetics may be prolonged by the addition of a local vasoconstrictor (epinephrine) to the solution, keeping the anesthetic at the nerve site longer.

Lidocaine (xylocaine) produces a prompt, intense local anesthetic effect. It is available as an ointment (2.5%, 5.0%), solution and jelly for mucous membranes (2%, 4%, 10%), and solution for parenteral administration (0.5% to 20%). Lidocaine 1.0% (0.4 mL) has been advocated for regional anesthesia by dorsal penile nerve block during newborn circumcision.[17]

Procaine (Novacaine) is a shorter acting local anesthetic than lidocaine. In the body, it is hydrolyzed to p-aminobenzoic acid, which inhibits the action of sulfonamides. Procaine is available as a 1%, 2%, and 10% solution for injection.

Systemic toxicity may occur if local anesthetics are administered as a very large dose or as a rapid intravenous push. Central nervous system stimulation and convulsions are followed by depression and death secondary to respiratory failure. Decrease in the electrical excitability, conduction rate, and force of myocardial contractility lead to cardiovascular collapse. Rarely, hypersensitivity reactions can occur with local anesthetics, primarily with the ester type (procaine).

Systemic Anesthetics and Analgesics

Morphine
Morphine, a purified alkaloid found in opium, produces analgesia, drow-

siness, respiratory depression, decreased gastrointestinal motility, and alterations in the endocrine and autonomic nervous systems. Pharmacokinetic studies of morphine show decreased clearance and increased half-life in newborns in comparison with infants and older children, which may explain the prolonged duration of action in young infants.[19, 20] In addition, morphine-induced hypotension, decreased gut motility, and the potential for physiologic dependence with prolonged use make its use in neonates less attractive. Morphine doses range from 20 to 100 µg/kg/hr as continuous intravenous infusion to 100 to 200 µg/kg given intermittently every 3 to 4 hours.

Fentanyl

Fentanyl has become widely used for analgesia or anesthesia during surgery in neonates since its use was first described in 1981 by Robinson and Gregory.[26] Fentanyl is a synthetic, rapid-acting opioid with a potency approximately 150 times greater than that of morphine. It is metabolized in the liver and excreted mainly in the urine, with reported elimination half-life ranging from 6 to 32 hours.[5] Newborns appear to be more sensitive to the respiratory depressant effects of fentanyl; it is unknown whether this effect is due to altered CNS penetration of the drug, higher cerebral blood flow, altered protein binding, or differences in respiratory control mechanisms in the premature newborn. Fentanyl in a dose of 10 to 50 µg/kg blunts stress responses (heart rate, blood pressure, tcpo$_2$) in infants undergoing thoracic, abdominal, or genitourinary surgery. Duration of anesthesia was dose dependent; doses of 10 and 12.5 µg/kg produced reliable anesthesia for 75 and 90 minutes, respectively.[18]

Hypotension may rarely occur after administration of fentanyl; decreasing the rate of infusion of the dose will correct it. For this reason it is preferred to many other anesthetic agents in the hemodynamically unstable infant. With high doses and rapid administration, muscle rigidity has occurred. It is recommended that patients given fentanyl be administered pancuronium for muscle relaxation to facilitate ventilation.

Sufentanil, another synthetic narcotic closely related to fentanyl, has been used in infants. It is similar to fentanyl in terms of hemodynamic stability; however, it has the advantage of greater potency and shorter duration of action. Doses used in infants range from 5 to 15 µg/kg.[10, 14]

SEDATIVES

Chloral Hydrate

Chloral hydrate is a safe sedative hypnotic often used in children for mild sedation prior to special examinations or procedures. It is rapidly metabolized in the liver to trichloroethanol, an active metabolite. In general, sedation after a 25 to 50 mg/kg dose lasts 1 to 2 hours. Chloral hydrate is irritating to all mucous membranes. Acute toxicity includes hypotension, respiratory depression, and cardiac arrhythmias.

Diazepam

Diazepam has been used as both sedative and anticonvulsant in neonates. N-Desmethyldiazepam, the active metabolite of diazepam, has a very long half-life, and may accumulate in neonates with repeated dosing. Although this group of medications has a wide margin of safety, overdosage may require respiratory and cardiovascular support. The usual dose of diazepam is 0.1 to 1 mg/kg. Care must be taken during intravenous administration to prevent extravasation.

A better alternative to diazepam for sedation in neonates may be lorazepam; it is not metabolized to an active agent and has a shorter half-life, lowering the risk for accumulation. Doses range from 0.1 to 0.4 mg/kg.[7]

SKELETAL MUSCLE RELAXANTS

Pancuronium

Pancuronium (Pavulon) is a nondepolarizing (competitive) neuromuscular blocking agent that is approximately five times as potent as d-tubocurarine and has minimal cardiovascular and little histamine releasing or hormonal actions. It is frequently used as an adjunct to anesthetics prior to surgery to induce muscle relaxation, and in neonates is often used to reduce fighting the ventilator. It has been shown that the muscle paralysis induced by pancuronium may be potentiated by both aminoglycoside antibiotics and increased magnesium.

Studies have demonstrated that pancuronium can decrease the incidence of pulmonary barotrauma in infants with bronchopulmonary dysplasia,[24] prevent the development of pneumothoraces,[11] decrease fluctuations of intracranial pressure seen during noxious stimulation,[16] and eliminate fluctuating cerebral blood-flow velocity in preterm infants, thus potentially reducing the incidence and severity of intraventricular hemorrhage.[22] Pancuronium is not without toxic effects, including acute increase in blood pressure and heart rate,[27] decreased pulmonary compliance and increased total pulmonary resistance,[4] skeletal muscle disuse atrophy following prolonged use,[28] and joint contractures.[30] In addition to its toxic effects, pancuronium may mask seizure activity. Pancuronium does not have any sedative or analgesic properties; adjunctive therapy may be indicated.

The usual dose of pancuronium is 0.01 to 0.03 mg/kg given every 2 to 4 hours as needed. It is cleared from the body by the kidneys and thus may have a prolonged duration of action in renal failure.

Newer competitive skeletal muscle relaxants (e.g., atracurium) have been used in infants and children.[15] However, lack of studies in neonatal intensive care limit their use at this time.

OPHTHALMIC DRUGS

The primary ophthalmic drugs needed in neonates during examination are mydriatics. The compounding of cyclopentolate 0.5%, tropicamide 0.5%, and phenylephrine 2.5% into one solution (Caputo drops) yields an effective agent that combines the mydriatic effect of phenylephrine and tropicamide with the cycloplegic effect of cyclopentolate. One drop is placed in each eye every 5 minutes two to four times. Peak effect occurs within 1 hour; duration is 3 to 4 hours. Significant side effects to this combination have not been reported.

CONTRAST AGENTS USED IN RADIOLOGIC PROCEDURES

Contrast media available for radiologic procedures vary according to the type of study performed. For gastrointestinal studies there is air, barium, water-soluble agents, and radionuclides. For intravascular studies of either the genitourinary tract or heart and vessels there are water-soluble hyperosmolar ionic compounds or low osmolar nonionic compounds, and nuclear radiopharmaceuticals. There are also water-soluble contrast agents for computed tomographic scans.

Gastrointestinal Tract

Before a contrast study of the neonatal gastrointestinal tract is performed:

1. A plain abdominal film must be obtained because it gives useful, and often sufficient, information.
2. The infant must not be fed for at least 4 hours prior to contrast study.
3. A variety of feeding devices and contrast media should be readily available, as should restraining devices, heating devices for neonates, and suction apparatus in case of emergency.

Contrast media used in infants are air, barium, and water-soluble contrast agents.

Air

In many cases only air is needed as a contrast medium (e.g., duodenal atresia, pyloric stenosis). The distribution of the intestinal gas pattern is helpful for the diagnosis of certain abnormalities of the gastrointestinal tract (e.g., malrotation). Occasionally air contrast may identify the size of the colon and the location of the cecum. However, a gas-free abdomen does not always indicate intestinal obstruction, as a very sick infant on a ventilator may show a similar picture.

Barium

Barium is the contrast medium of choice because it is nontoxic, insoluble, and has a lower osmolarity than water-soluble contrast media. It also can be used in a dehydrated patient, and may be given in most conditions except suspected perforation. Barium sulfate comes in liquid, paste, and capsule form. Flavored liquids (fruit or chocolate) are available. In small infants, nonflavored barium should be used because, if aspirated, flavoring substances cause severe aspiration pneumonia.

Barium administration from a nursing bottle is preferred over administration through a nasogastric tube because the infant's ability to suck and swallow can be studied. Sterile barium should be used in neonates. The amount used should be as small as possible to avoid aspiration. Barium is used in gastrointestinal series to locate suspected obstruction; it is the agent of choice in distal intestinal obstruction in neonates.

Water Soluble Contrast Media

A water-soluble contrast medium is used when perforation of gut is suspected. It also is used for the first study postoperatively to detect any leaks. It is of greater advantage than barium for showing fistulas and sinuses. Water-soluble contrast medium is available as preparations of diatrizoate meglumine (Gastrografin) and diatrizoate sodium (Hypaque).

Water-soluble contrast media are readily absorbed from peritoneum and excreted by the kidneys; therefore they can be used when perforation is suspected. They give good opacification and coating of the esophagus, and are used in meconium ileus for therapeutic as well as diagnostic purposes. The disadvantages of water-soluble contrast are (1) unpleasant bitter taste; (2) severe pulmonary edema if aspirated; (3) hyperosmolarity, which causes loss of fluid into the bowel lumen, leading to aggravation of hypovolemia, dehydration, shock, and even death; and (4) poor visualization in the small intestine (the contrast materials become diluted very quickly by water entering the gut due to the high osmolarity).

Low osmolar water-soluble agents have been on the market since 1972. These include metrizamide, iopamidol, ioxaglate, and iohexol. All are triiodinated derivatives of benzoic acid and do not dissociate in solution. They can be diluted to an isotonic solution and still provide excellent images of the bowel. They cause no harmful shifts of fluid from the body into the bowel lumen. Absorption is low, and they offer excellent prolonged visualization. There is less irritation to the peritoneum or lung when aspiration occurs in infants. These agents are recommended for studies in patients with swallowing disorders, esophageal obstruction, or fistula and those with high risk for perforation.

Genitourinary Tract

Two radiologic procedures are commonly done in neonates: excretory urography and voiding cystourethrography.

Excretory Urography

Contrast media used in excretory urography are diatrizoate sodium (Hypaque 50%), diatrizoate meglumine (Renografin 60%), and iothalamate meglumine (Conray 60%). Meglumine compounds are preferred in neonates because of their low sodium content. The recommended dosage in newborns is 3 to 4.4 mL/kg^2 (in infants older than 1 month the dosage is 1.5 to 2.0 mL/kg[21]) injected intravenously over a maximum of 1 to 2 minutes. Injection into the femoral vein should be avoided because local extravasation causes severe tissue necrosis.

The contrast agents are hyperosmolar and can lead to hypertonic dehydration. Local extravasation of contrast agent can lead to tissue necrosis and sloughing of skin. Overdose can lead to pulmonary edema and even death. There is a risk of renal damage in a dehydrated infant.

The newer nonionic compounds metrizamide, iohexol, and iopromide are advantageous in the first weeks of life, when glomerular filtration rates are low and when high osmolality may depress renal function of the immature kidney.[13]

When some form of kidney disease has been suspected, renal nuclear imaging using technetium 99m diethylenetriaminepentaacetic acid (Tc-99m DTPA) can delineate the degree of obstruction and physiology. A diuretic scan using Tc^{99m} DTPA can be achieved by administering 0.3 to 0.4 mg/kg furosemide intravenously. When urinary tract infection is suspected, renal cortical imaging with Tc^{99m} dimercaptosuccinic acid (DMSA) or Tc^{99m} glucoheptonate is useful for showing pyelonephritis or bacterial nephritis.[8]

Voiding Cystourethrogram

The purpose of the voiding cystourethrogram is to evaluate the bladder and urethra and to detect vesicoureteral reflux. Media used in the procedure are diatrizoate sodium (Hypaque sodium 25%), diatrizoate meglumine (Cystografin 30%), iothalamate meglumine (Cysto-Conray), and acetotrizoate sodium (Cystokon). The dosage varies depending on the capacity of the bladder. It can be given by catheter; the main purpose of this method is to evaluate the reflux. The procedure also can be done as a part of excretory urography, which causes less vesical irritation and has a decreased risk of infection. The contrast agent should not be injected forcefully by syringe; it should be hung in a bottle approximately 2 feet above the table so that it can flow in by gravity. The height of the bottle should be less than 1 m to avoid rupture of bladder caused by increased pressure. Filling of the bladder should be checked intermittently. In a patient with urinary tract infection, the test should be done at least 2 weeks after the infection has subsided, because infection by itself can give rise to reflux.

Complications of the procedure include infection if catheterization is not done under aseptic conditions and if unsterile contrast agent is used, damage to the urethra, and renal pain secondary to massive reflux. A high concentration of contrast agent can cause cystitis (irritation of bladder mucosa). Radionuclide examination using Tc-99m decreases radiation exposure, and by permitting constant visualization is a sensitive indicator of reflux.[1]

Nuclear Radiopharmaceuticals

Computed tomography is useful in evaluating renal mass due to tumor, hydronephrosis, cystic disease, or infection. Contrast material for kidney and bladder CT studies is a water-soluble high-osmolality compound (e.g., Hypaque 60%, 2 to 3 mL/kg up to 120 mL). This is injected as a rapid intravenous bolus after scout radiographs are obtained. Oral contrast material is given to outline the bowel. Because any part of the stomach or upper small bowel may simulate a mass lesion on CT, oral contrast material is necessary to avoid these confusing pseudomasses. Oral contrast, 5 mL diatrizoate meglumine (Gastrografin) diluted in 180 mL fluid, is given 30 to 45 minutes prior to scanning. Fruit-flavored drinks may be used to mask the taste. Neonates require 50 mL of diluted contrast material to outline the stomach and small bowel; 100 mL for the entire small bowel.[6]

Peripheral angiography is infrequently performed in children. The new low osmolar agents are valuable for use with digital subtraction angiography and may be considered in patients with cardiac dysfunction or a history of allergy or previous reaction to contrast media.[9] The new media reduce osmolality to 25% that of conventional contrast media, which reduces vasodilation during arteriography. Injection into the carotid and vertebral arteries may produce systemic effects of bradycardia and drop in aortic pressure with high osmolar agents. Alteration in myocardial contractility is less affected by the nonionic media.

REFERENCES

1. American Academy of Pediatrics. Committee on Radiology: Report on water soluble contrast material. *Pediatrics* 1978; 62:429–432.
2. Ansell G: Fatal overdose of contrast medium in infants. *Br J Radiol* 1970; 46:333–334.
3. Barrett FF, Mason EO, Fleming D: The effect of three cord-care regimens on bacterial colonization of normal newborn infants. *J Pediatr* 1979; 94:796–800.
4. Bhutani VK, Abbasi S, Sivieri EM: Continuous skeletal muscle paralysis: Effect on neonatal pulmonary mechanics. *Pediatrics* 1988; 81:419–422.
5. Collins C, Koren G, Crean P, et al: Fentanyl pharmacokinetics and hemodynamic effects in preterm infants during ligation of patent ductus arteriosus. *Anesth Analg* 1985; 64:1078–1080.
6. Daneman A: *Pediatric Body CT*. New York, Springer-Verlag, 1987.

7. Deshmukh A, Wittert W, Schnitzler E, et al: Lorazepam in the treatment of refractory neonatal seizures. *Am J Dis Child* 1986; 140:1042–1044.

8. Firlit C, Shkolnik A, Weiss S: The localization of urinary tract infection with 99m Tc glucoheptonate scintigraphy. *Pediatr Radiol* 1986; 16:403–406.

9. Fletcher BD, Jacobstein MD, Morrison SC: Intravenous digital subtraction angiography (IVDSA) in children. *Pediatr Radiol* 1984; 14:425–430.

10. Greeley WJ, de Bruijn NP, Davis DP: Sufentanil pharmacokinetics in pediatric cardiovascular patients. *Anesth Analg* 1987; 66:1067–1072.

11. Greenough A, Wood S, Morley CJ, et al: Pancuronium prevents pneumothoraces in ventilated premature babies who actively expire against positive pressure inflation. *Lancet* 1984; 1:1–3.

12. Harpin V, Rutter N: Percutaneous alcohol absorption and skin necrosis in a preterm infant. *Arch Dis Child* 1982; 517:477–479.

13. Harvey LA, Caldicott WJH, Kurue A: The effect of contrast media on immature renal function. *Radiology* 1983; 148:429–432.

14. Hickey PR, Hansen DD: Fentanyl- and sufentanil-oxygen-pancuronium anesthesia for cardiac surgery in infants. *Anesth Analg* 1984; 63:117–124.

15. Kalli I, Meretoja OA: Infusion of atracurium in neonates, infants and children. *Br J Anaesth* 1988; 60:651–654.

16. Kelly MA, Finer NN: Nasotracheal intubation in the neonate: Physiologic responses and effects of atropine and pancuronium. *J Pediatr* 1984; 105:303–309.

17. Kirya C, Werthmann MW: Neonatal circumcision and penile dorsal nerve block—a painless procedure. *J Pediatr* 1978; 92:998–1000.

18. Koehntop DE, Rodman JH, Brundage DM, et al: Pharmacokinetics of fentanyl in neonates. *Anesth Analg* 1986; 65:227–232.

19. Koren G, Butt W, Chinyanga H, et al: Postoperative morphine infusion in newborn infants: Assessment of disposition characteristics and safety. *J Pediatr* 1985; 107:963–967.

20. Lynn AM, Slattery JT: Morphine pharmacokinetics in early infancy. *Anesthesiology* 1987; 66:136–139.

21. Nogardy MB, Dunbar JS: The technique of roentgen investigation of urinary tract in infants and children, in Kaufmann HJ (ed): *Progress in Pediatric Radiology*, vol 3, *Genitourinary Tract*. Chicago, Year Book Medical Publishers, 1970, pp 3–50.

22. Perlman JM, Goodman S, Kreusser KL, et al: Reduction in intraventricular hemorrhage by elimination of fluctuating cerebral blood-flow velocity in preterm infants with respiratory distress syndrome. *N Engl J Med* 1985; 312:1353–1357.

23. Pildes RS, Ramamurthy RS, Vidyasagar D: Effect of triple dye on staphylococcal colonization in the newborn infant. *J Pediatr* 1973; 82:987–990.

24. Pollitzer MJ, Reynolds EOR, Shaw DG, et al: Pancuronium during mechanical ventilation speeds recovery of lungs of infants with hyaline membrane disease. *Lancet* 1981; 1:346–348.

25. Pyati SP, Ramamurthy RS, Krauss MT, et al: Absorption of iodine in the neonate following topical use of povidone-iodine. *J Pediatr* 1977; 91:825–828.

26. Robinson S, Gregory GA: Fentanyl-air-oxygen anesthesia for ligation of patent ductus arteriosus in preterm infants. *Anesth Analg* 1981; 60:331–334.

27. Runkle B, Bancalari E: Acute cardiopulmonary effects of pancuronium bromide in mechanically ventilated newborn infants. *J Pediatr* 1984; 104:614–617.

28. Rutledge ML, Hawkins EP, Langston C: Skeletal muscle growth failure induced in premature newborn infants by prolonged pancuronium treatment. *J Pediatr* 1986; 109:338–342.
29. Schick JB, Milstein JM: Burn hazard of isopropyl alcohol in the neonate. *Pediatrics* 1981; 68:587–588.
30. Sinha SK, Levene MI: Pancuronium bromide induced joint contractures in the newborn. *Arch Dis Child* 1984; 59:73–79.
31. Yaster M: The dose response of fentanyl in neonatal anesthesia. *Anesthesiology* 1987; 66:433–435.

INDEX

A

Absorption, 6–8
  alimentary tract and, 8–10
  epidermis and, 10
  after intramuscular or subcutaneous administration, 10
  oral, factors affecting, 9
  percutaneous, 10
Acenocoumarol: in breast milk, 25
Acetotrizoate sodium: in voiding cystourethrography, 383
Acetylsalicylic acid (see Aspirin)
Acidosis
  correction during resuscitation, 94–95
  in renal failure, treatment, 281
Acyclovir: in herpes simplex virus infection, 215
Afferent input increase: in apnea, 44
Agar: in jaundice, 356
Age
  -related causes of heart failure, 148
  -specific percentiles for systolic blood pressure in boys, 113
Air: as contrast medium in gastrointestinal tract procedures, 381–382
Airway
  management during resuscitation, 92

pressure, continuous positive, in apnea, 44
resistance
  effects of diuretics on, 56
  effects of isoproterenol, metaproterenol and atropine on, 61
Alcohol
  as antiseptic, 376
  in breast milk, 28
Aldactone: in bronchopulmonary dysplasia, 59
Alimentary tract: and absorption, 8–10
Alloimmune thrombocytopenia: blood products in, 371–372
Alpha-methyldopa: in breast milk, 27
Alprostadil in congenital heart disease, 140–144
  complications, 144
  contraindications, 140–141
  dilution instructions for, 142
  dosage, 141–142
  indications, 140–141
  pharmacology, 140
  route of administration, 141–142
  side effects, 144
Alveolus: mammary gland, milk-blood barrier of, 23
Amines: sympathomimetic, during resuscitation, 96

387